IMPROVING CARE IN THE NURSING HOME

IMPROVING CARE IN THE NURSING HOME

Comprehensive Reviews of Clinical Research

Laurence Z. Rubenstein
Darryl Wieland

editors

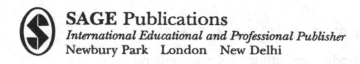

SAGE Publications
International Educational and Professional Publisher
Newbury Park   London   New Delhi

For information address:

SAGE Publications, Inc.
2455 Teller Road
Newbury Park, California 91320

SAGE Publications Ltd.
6 Bonhill Street
London EC2A 4PU
United Kingdom

SAGE Publications India Pvt. Ltd.
M-32 Market
Greater Kailash I
New Delhi 110 048 India

Printed in the United States of America

Library of Congress Cataloging-in-Publication Data

Main entry under title:

Improving care in the nursing home : comprehensive reviews of clinical
  research / [edited by] Laurence Z. Rubenstein, Darryl Wieland.
      p.   cm.
  Includes bibliographical references and index.
  ISBN: 978-0-8039-4307-0
  1. Nursing home care.   I. Rubenstein, Laurence Z.   II. Wieland,
Darryl.
  [DNLM: 1. Nursing Homes—organization & administration—United
States.   2. Homes for the Aged—organization & administration
—United States.   3. Health Services for the Aged—United States.
WT 27 AA1 I3 1993]
RC954.3.I45   1993
362.1′6—dc20
DNLM/DLC   93-14334
for Library of Congress   CIP

93 94 95 96 10 9 8 7 6 5 4 3 2 1

Sage Production Editor: Rebecca Holland

Contents

Acknowledgments

We, the editors, are grateful for the small grant from the Health Services Research and Development Service of the Department of Veterans Affairs (HSR&D #87098) that allowed us to pursue this project. James W. Davis, M.D., Elizabeth Clark, Ph.D., and Karen R. Josephson, M.P.H., were all part of the original study group leading to the planning of the book. We thank Christine Smedley of Sage for her valuable editorial assistance and Wendy Barnett, Beverley Philbrook, and Mae Homestead, who assisted with manuscript preparation. Thanks also to Adina Katz, GRECC Administrative Officer, for helping us keep our oars in the water. Finally, we thank our uncomplaining families for supporting us through this and a multitude of other labors.

Introduction:
Clinical Research in the Nursing Home

LAURENCE Z. RUBENSTEIN
DARRYL WIELAND

The size and scope of nursing home (NH) care has increased dramatically in the past 40 years. Since 1950, the number of persons living
in U.S. NHs at any one time has grown more than fivefold—from
under 300,000 in 1950 to over 15,000,000 in 1990 (1,2). Currently, over
20% of health care expenditures for persons age 65 years and over
goes for NH care, about half coming from government sources,
primarily Medicaid (2).

This growth has been spurred by increasing numbers and longer
survival of elderly disabled people, changing demographics and
family structures that have left more of these disabled elders to fend
for themselves outside traditional family care environments, and
financial incentives from governmental programs that have encouraged the growth of the NH industry.

Not uncharacteristically for health services, this growth has preceded the existence of clinical research to guide its structures, function, and direction. Much of how NH care is structured and delivered
is determined by tradition or has been developed empirically rather
than based upon a logical progression of what has been shown to be
scientifically effective. As in many areas of health care, research into
the effectiveness of an intervention generally comes after general
deployment of the services.

There has also been a tremendous growth in areas of clinical
research in the NH over the past two decades. Research has been of
diverse types (e.g., medical, psychosocial, epidemiologic, health services), from many disciplines (e.g., medicine, nursing, social work,
psychology, anthropology, pharmacy), covering a multitude of topics (e.g., drug use, infections, rehabilitation, quality of life). The

present volume is a concerted effort to bring together and synthesize the major parts of this expanding body of clinical research, particularly research examining the effectiveness of clinical interventions. It is hoped that this will be both a useful chronicle of research progress as well as a clinically helpful compendium of current knowledge.

The volume is organized by chapters into the major topic areas of NH research. In most cases, the chapters are intended to include the vast majority of published clinical research studies pertaining to the topic. We have tried to include chapters representing each of the major active areas of clinical NH research. However, we acknowledge that some areas of research relevant to NH care have been left out— mostly because the published body of knowledge in those areas was relatively small.

Although much of NH care has evolved without the benefit of research, substantial progress has been made in NH care in a number of major areas directly as a result of and proportional to the intensity of the research devoted there. The chapters in this volume reflect this progress in practice as well as the progress in research productivity per se. For example, much has improved in the past two decades in the care of persons with common problems such as behavior disorders, incontinence, depression, and deconditioning. As well, we have learned much about what causes falls and how to assess and control the quality of care. Although we still have much to learn, we have learned a great deal about the epidemiology of pain, infections, and pressure sores in NHs, and research in these areas is extremely active.

The chapters are heterogeneous and have been organized in a rather arbitrary sequence, beginning with research on rehabilitation and proceeding with research on medication use, medical syndromes (infections, pressure sores, incontinence, bowel problems, nutritional problems, falls, pain), psychologic issues (depression, behavior problems), and ending with research on quality of care. The format of the review chapters, building around detailed tables of the research literature, was designed to make maximum use of space. The accompanying text is intended to provide summary narrative of the specific data in the tables and put the information into context, rather than repeat the tables.

Some chapters are more extensive than others, reflecting the variability in size of the research bodies themselves. Similarly, the depth and quality of the research data are quite variable—some areas are still fairly primitive and limited to descriptive studies and case series, whereas others are fairly well matured and include large randomized trials.

All these areas are still very much in progress, and this volume can do little more than review the state of the art as of this point in time. Our anticipation is that in a short time, all of these chapters will need to be extensively revised and new chapters written to account for the continuing substantial progress in NH research. We hope that this effort to compile and synthesize clinical research in NHs will be a positive step in accelerating this research effort toward further clinical progress.

References

1. Scanlon, W. J., & Feder, J. (1985). The long term care marketplace: An overview. In Healthcare Financial Management Association (HFMA) (Ed.), *Long-term care: Challenges and opportunities*. Oak Brook, IL: Author.
2. U.S. Senate Special Committee on Aging. (1987). *Aging America: Trends and projections* (LR 3377-188-D12198). Washington, DC: U.S. Department of Health and Human Services.

1

Rehabilitation in the Nursing Facility

CATHERINE GILL, M.S., M.H.A., P.T.
JANET A. HOWELLS, M.S., P.T.
ELIZABETH H. HOFFMAN, O.T.R.

INTRODUCTION

The need for rehabilitation in nursing homes (NHs) appears to be tremendous, judging from the high prevalence of functional dependency and disability. Of persons admitted to NHs from short-stay hospitals, 95% require assistance or are dependent in bathing, 84% in dressing, 74% in transfers, 74% in toileting, and 46% in eating; of all NH residents, 71% require assistance or are unable to ambulate, and 85% require assistance with instrumental activities of daily living (IADLs) (84). Yet, according to data collected in 1985, physical therapy, occupational therapy, and speech/language pathology services were available in only 56%, 54%, and 44% of Medicare- and/or Medicaid-certified facilities (84). Availability of rehabilitation services in NHs should increase, as the Omnibus Budget Reconciliation Act of 1987 (OBRA) specifies: "If specialized rehabilitation services are required in the resident's comprehensive plan of care, the facility must provide [or obtain] the required services." The regulatory goal is to "provide the highest practicable physical, mental, and psychosocial well-being" to NH residents. The assumption underpinning these reforms is that rehabilitation programs can be effective for NH residents.

The goal of rehabilitation is "to restore an individual to his/her former functional and environmental status, or alternately, to maintain or maximize remaining function" (117). Rehabilitation services in NHs are provided primarily by occupational and physical therapists

1

and speech/language pathologists, in coordination with nursing, dietary, social services, and activity departments' plans of care. Although all rehabilitation services are prescribed by physicians, physicians often have minimal involvement in rehabilitation programs, due largely to the low reimbursement rates by Medicare and Medicaid for physicians' NH visits.

S. J. Brody (1985) points out that although rehabilitation services seem to be available for the short-stay resident, NH care is notable for a "virtual absence of rehabilitation services for needy long-term residents," again due to funding limitations. As will be outlined below, long-term residents, comprising 78% of the total of NH residents at a given time (84), have as much need for services as those with more typical "rehabilitation diagnoses." For them, rehabilitation is necessary to minimize the disability from chronic or degenerative conditions. In these cases, the therapist typically develops programs to maintain residents' current functioning, teaches compensatory techniques to both residents and staff, and provides equipment to compensate for lost function.

In the present chapter, we describe a number of rehabilitation approaches intended to improve function, together with study data indicating their effectiveness in various older populations, including NH populations where available.

REHABILITATION APPROACHES TO IMPROVE FUNCTION

Reconditioning

Age-related declines in aerobic capacity and strength are well documented. However, due to the heterogeneous nature of the aged population, it is unclear how much of the noted decline can be attributed to "normal aging," to sedentary life-style, or to concomitant disease processes. What is clear is that these declines often bring older persons very near their functional "threshold," such that further decrements due to illness or injury may render an older person unable to perform everyday activities. This deconditioning below the threshold is a common sequela of hospitalization in older adults (55,54) and is often treated by physical and occupational therapists in skilled nursing facilities. In these cases, the focus of the rehabilitation process is on strengthening weakened muscles and improving aerobic capacity so that a person's prior level of function can be regained.

A number of studies have described improvements resulting from aerobic training programs in older persons (Table 1.1). Hagberg et al. (1989) reported an increase in VO_2max of 22% after a 26-week endurance treadmill program. Heart rates at submaximal work loads were significantly decreased. Benestad (1965) also reported a lower heart rate at submaximal work load after endurance training, but did not find a change in VO_2max. However, his intervention was limited to 6 weeks, which may be of insufficient duration for an older population. In women 52-79 years of age, Adams and deVries (1973) reported a significant increase in physical work capacity and VO_2max, along with a significant decrease in heart rate at each of 4 submaximal work loads as compared to controls. Similar results were also found in a study of older men (36). Barry and associates (1966) reported a 38% improvement in both aerobic and anaerobic capacity after 3 months of training in subjects with an average age of 70 years. Stamford (1972) also found a significant decrease in heart rate response at submaximal work loads after 12 weeks of a daily walking program. These studies give important positive evidence concerning the aerobic trainability of older adults. Unfortunately, the subjects of these studies are unrepresentative of the majority of persons residing in NHs. All but Stamford's study utilized community-dwelling subjects, and persons with cardiac or pulmonary disease were excluded.

Nevertheless, the literature has begun to document that individuals with even a very low level of aerobic conditioning—more characteristic of NH residents—can achieve significant improvements with a much lower intensity of training than previously reported. A walking program modified to keep exercise heart rates below 120 bpm was sufficient to challenge the cardiovascular systems of a subgroup of subjects with cardiac ischemia and/or arrhythmias (36). After 6 weeks of training, work capacity in these subjects increased 34.5%. Persons who had been institutionalized long term for psychiatric problems showed an improved heart rate response to submaximal work loads after an endurance training program at only 50% of their predicted maximal heart rates (109). In another study (10), subjects who underwent a training program at 30%-45% or 60%-75% of maximal heart rate showed significant declines in absolute and relative oxygen uptake and heart rates with exercise, with no significant differences in training responses between the groups. Sidney and Shephard (1978) reported that although the optimal regimen for cardiorespiratory response to endurance training is a high-frequency, high-intensity program, exercise at 120-130 bpm was sufficient to induce a training response.

No study has attempted actual aerobic training with older adults in NHs, and resident characteristics such as cardiac or pulmonary disease, neurological impairments, and extreme old age will make performing these studies all the more difficult as standard testing of aerobic capacity may be impossible in persons with arthritis, balance instability, or significant lower extremity weakness (99). Many medications used in this population can affect the assessment of both training intensity and training response, and the type of exercise used for training will need to accommodate the resident's multiple medical and/or functional problems. However, in light of the profound deconditioning that occurs with bed rest and lack of regular physical exercise for most residents, the literature suggests that regular exercise programs of lesser intensity could have significant impact on the NH population by improving muscle strength, joint flexibility, and submaximal exercise tolerance and translate to improved abilities. Although a progressive walking program is one way to induce a training response, arm ergometers or resistive cycling in a seated position can be used for those persons who because of imbalance or severely impaired endurance are not functionally ambulatory.

NH rehabilitation more often focuses on strengthening, rather than improving aerobic capacity. Medicare, which will not reimburse for treatments that lead to residents' "walking repetitiously or merely improving distance or endurance," will pay for strengthening. Several studies document that significantly increased strength can be obtained in older persons through a program of resistance training. Aniansson et al. (1980) and Frontera et al. (1988), both utilizing men in their 60s and 70s, found significant strength gains following a 12-week exercise program. Moritani and deVries (1980) reported a 23% increase in elbow flexion strength measured isometrically in similarly aged men following an 8-week resistive dumbbell training program. Hagberg and associates (1989) found a 9% increase in lower extremity strength and an 18% increase in upper extremity strength following a 26-week training program. (These latter results are significantly lower than the gains reported in other studies, but during the first 13 weeks participants used only light to moderate weights.) Frontera et al. (1988) had their subjects exercise at 80% of one repetition maximum for 12 weeks and reported 227% increase in dynamic strength in knee flexion and 107% and 117% increased in left and right knee extension. These studies, although important, are all of limited applicability to our population, as the researchers utilized only community-dwelling elders.

Two published studies have looked at resistance training specifically for older adults in NHs. Fiatarone et al. (1990) found that in nine subjects who completed a high-intensity resistance training program, quadriceps strength improved an average of 174%. This improvement allowed two subjects to abandon canes for ambulation; of three residents who had initially been unable, one could now rise from a chair without using his arms. This study was limited to subjects who were ambulatory, representing only 29.3% of the NH population (84). Fisher et al. (1991) used an institutionalized population more representative of that found in NHs. Their subjects had a variety of chronic diseases and only had to be able to walk five steps and transfer to the exercise bench. Of the 14 subjects who completed the study, overall muscle endurance improved 35% and strength 15%. Anecdotal improvements in activity levels and independence of the subjects were also reported. However, subject responses varied widely. If those who made no improvements were removed from the analysis, endurance improved 80% to 300%, strength 30% to 150%. The training program was limited to 6 weeks and the resistance never exceeded 50% of maximal; the Fiatarone study lasted 12 weeks and had subjects training at up to 80% of one repetition maximum.

Both these studies demonstrate that both strength and functional gains could be made in as little as 8 weeks in an older, institutionalized population, but this work needs repeating with larger numbers of subjects. Replication is currently under way, but it will still be a few years before results are available. Research is also needed to determine why some long-term residents, for example, the more frail residents in Fisher's study, do not show any improvements following therapy programs. The ability to predict which residents would benefit from rehabilitation is needed in order to best utilize limited health care resources.

Activities of Daily Living (ADL) Training

Training in ADLs is often a major component of the rehabilitation program for patients in NHs. It includes not only instruction in techniques to compensate for any residual deficits, but also prescription of and instruction in the use of assistive or adaptive equipment. Despite its importance in promoting independence in older persons, long-term benefits of ADL-specific training have not been studied. Several papers report improvements in global scores on various measures of ADL following rehabilitation programs (8,21,2,27,48).

Only one study assessed the functional outcome of an ADL-specific training activity. Shillam et al. (1983) reported that all subjects seen for a bathing training program showed statistically significant improvement in their bathing ability. Because withholding a treatment accepted as the standard of care is not ethical, this study was limited by lacking a control group. Although the subjects were being seen specifically for a bathing program, one may assume they were also receiving other rehabilitation services as they were referred from an inpatient rehabilitation ward. Thus, one cannot conclude that the bathing program was alone responsible for the increased independence in bathing. More studies of this type, albeit better designed, are very much needed to identify which ADL tasks require specific retraining programs, and what program components (e.g., strengthening, increasing range of motion, equipment training) are most beneficial.

Dysphagia

Eating and swallowing disorders are not a part of the normal aging process and appear to increase the risk of death. Aspiration pneumonia has been reported to cause 65% of deaths from terminal illness and 6% of deaths acutely following stroke (39). Siebens et al. (1986) reported a fourfold increase in mortality for dependent versus independent NH feeders. Normal swallow mechanisms decline with age (32,75,94), but these losses have not been associated with dysphagia. Although clinically there seems to be an increased prevalence of swallowing disorders in persons in NHs, the true prevalence is not known. In the only study of NH residents, Siebens et al. (1986) found that of 240 residents, 26% demonstrated abnormal pharyngeal function and 30% abnormal oral motor function on bedside evaluation. However, this may underestimate the problem, as bedside evaluations have been shown to be inadequate to detect aspiration in patients without external signs of swallowing dysfunction (107).

The high prevalence of dysphagia in NH residents may be secondary to other common conditions. These include stroke, Parkinson's disease, multiple sclerosis, cancer, and cervical spondylosis (83,57,70). In assessing 38 patients with a new onset of stroke suspected of having a swallowing disorder, Veis and Logemann (1985) found that 82% had a delayed swallowing reflex, 58% had reduced pharyngeal peristalsis, and 50% had reduced lingual control. Seventy-six percent had more than one swallowing disorder. Forty-five percent of patients with new strokes unscreened for swallowing problems clinically demonstrated dysphagia in a second study (47).

Due to its complexity, detection and treatment of dysphagia require an interdisciplinary approach. Swallowing dysfunction is often noticed by nursing staff or may be identified by speech or occupational therapists as part of their routine screenings of patients. A medical workup is then indicated to determine if the cause of the dysphagia is amenable to medical intervention. In a hospital setting this workup may include evaluations by a neurologist, ENT surgeon, or gastroenterologist as well as tests such as videofluoroscopic study, fiberoptic endoscopic evaluation of swallowing (FEES), or ultrasound. The major indicated assessment is the attainment of a videofluoroscopic study, when possible, to determine the phase(s) of the swallowing malfunction and the presence or absence of aspiration. This diagnostic process, as well as the treatment program, is coordinated in the NH by the speech/language pathologist. To be truly effective, the occupational therapist, physical therapist, and nursing and dietary staffs must also be involved. The rehabilitation process and roles of each discipline in the process are described elsewhere (83,49,81).

The efficacy of rehabilitation for this condition (consisting primarily of thermal stimulation; oral-motor exercises; and instruction in compensatory strategies such as turning or tilting the head, positioning of the food bolus, or supraglottic swallow) has not been systematically studied. Logemann (1989) discusses the possibility of investigating the effect of treatment on those persons whose swallows are expected to decline due to degenerative diseases, but this has yet to be done. Some have examined the effect of thermal stimulation to trigger the swallow reflex (71), but other investigators report responses to this treatment are ephemeral (49). In the meantime, we lack repeat-videofluoroscopic studies of long-term changes in swallowing mechanisms resulting from exercises or other treatment.

Adaptive Seating Programs

The literature available on adaptive seating strategies for the geriatric population is sparse. The prevalence of NH wheelchair use and the reason for such use was studied by Pawlson et al. (1986). In this study, 68% of residents used a wheelchair, including 25% of those who were able to ambulate. Wheelchair use began after moving to the NH for 52% of the residents, with the most frequent reason being physical impairment. With this high prevalence of wheelchair use, appropriate selection and modification of seating need to be addressed by therapists and nursing staff. In addition, the appropriateness of wheelchairs for mobility purposes for NH residents requires study, as well as the energy requirements of this type of mobility, patient autonomy, and staff attitudes toward residents in wheelchairs.

Hartigan (1982) addresses the many problems associated with using the standard collapsible wheelchair for long periods of sitting for the elderly. Most commonly cited problems include gluteal and sacral pressure ulcers, flexion deformities, and radial nerve paralysis. Settle (1987) also cited improper seating as a cause of pressure sores. Specifically identified were chairs that were too narrow or too wide, slack or incorrectly deep seat canvases, footrests incorrectly adjusted, improper backrest angle and height, and lack of an adequate cushion. Proper positioning in seating is a prerequisite to the use of many of the adaptive aids now on the market to promote function (111).

The goals for adaptive seating include to "minimize effects of abnormal tone and reflexes; accommodate, delay or prevent the development or progression of orthopedic deformities; increase functional skills; accommodate for impaired sensation; and provide comfort" (111). Proper positioning begins at the pelvis, as it acts as a base of support for the rest of the body. Lower extremities should be positioned in neutral rotation, and 90 degrees of hip, knee, and ankle flexion is ideal. Trunk support and accommodation for deformities such as scoliosis is critical. Upper extremity and head control should be provided if needed.

The adult head trauma patient is frequently seen in the NH setting. Roush and Emory (1990) addressed the needs of the coma-emerging patient for adequate seating by recommending that a basic wheelchair system be adjustable, allow for reclining, secure the client from falling, and allow for ease of transfers. Other institutions treating head trauma patients (67) have recommended the use of temporary, reusable adaptive seat inserts that can be modified for the individual undergoing rehabilitation prior to determining the long-term wheelchair prescription.

Hemiplegic patients were studied in a quasi-experimental design at a rehabilitation hospital (18). The use of seat boards and the combination of seat and backboards were studied in relation to the modification of sitting posture. The postural improvements noted would promote symmetry of trunk musculature and weight bearing, key principles in the neurodevelopmental treatment of hemiplegics. Limitations of this study included reliability of measurement and the use of a convenience sample.

Clinical observations indicate that changes in seating position can create dramatic improvements in function, but this has not been systematically studied. Changes in function occurring with changes in seating posture have been described in pediatric populations (59,60,61), but no such studies of older persons exist. The focus on the pediatric and younger adult populations in the literature may be tied to the vocational implications of improved function. In addition, reimbursement for interventions for seating and positioning is often limited, which may discourage the therapist from intervening. Studies demonstrating the functional impact of seating programs would go a long way toward increasing Medicare and Medicaid willingness to pay for such programs and thus improve the availability of such programs for nursing facility residents.

Positioning Strategies

Positioning strategies are utilized as a means of preventing pressure ulcers and contractures. Contractures are due to prolonged positions (due to immobility and/or pain) and central nervous system (CNS) damage causing spasticity and prolonged fixed postures (33,16). Eighty-four percent of a head trauma population had contractures upon admission to a rehabilitation facility (119); 80% of a NH population had moderate or severe limitations in at least one lower extremity joint (91). In spite of these statistics, clinical studies related to therapeutic positioning strategies in a NH setting could not be found.

Recommendations for positioning patients with CNS deficits include the use of custom-made bolsters manufactured by the therapist from blocks of foam cut with an electric knife and covered with fabric, and straps for positioning (15). Another case study with possible application to the adult population was the use of moldable vacuum packs made rigid through the use of suction to create customized positioning devices (96). Precautions cited included perspiration and skin integrity problems.

Techniques for the reduction of contractures include positioning, range of motion, serial casting, splinting, pharmacologic agents, and neurological blocks used in reducing spasticity (42,88). The use of prolonged stretching, as in dynamic splinting, was shown to be effective even in the case of long-standing contracture (77). The use of slow, prolonged stretching with moderate constant tension is supported by Kottke et al. (1966) in describing the plastic properties of connective tissue.

Another form of prolonged stretching is serial casting. Often used with head trauma patients, reduction of contractures in elbows, knees, and ankles have been reported (73,17,68). Knees were found to be the most resistant to treatment. Altered consciousness, contractures of long duration, and skin integrity compromise are precautions or contraindications to serial casting. In the NH, therapists' options are often limited to range of motion exercises, positioning, and splinting due to limited ongoing medical intervention.

As can been appreciated, the effectiveness of strategies to prevent and rehabilitate contractures in NH residents has been subject to little study. Because of the frequency of coexisting cognitive and skin integrity problems, many of the more aggressive contracture reduction techniques are contraindicated. The best strategy for dealing with contractures in any population is to prevent their occurrence. Longitudinal studies are needed to better identify NH patients at risk for contractures, including those residents who are not neurologically impaired.

Cognitive Retraining

Approximately 5% of the population over 65 and nearly 20% of that over 75 have some degree of clinically significant impairment of cognitive function (63). As these persons are likely to reside in NHs, physical therapists, occupational therapists, and speech/language pathologists serving these facilities are in position to participate in research and clinical management of these disorders. Yet rehabilitation approaches to cognitive dysfunction are not well documented in the geriatric rehabilitation literature. Comprehensive rehabilitation theory lacks a framework for understanding cognitive dysfunction, and evaluation and treatment approaches are only in an early state of development (5,26,37,90,118). Studies have been conducted to identify the functional changes that occur with the normal aging process (112,40,3), but questions as to when, why, and how these changes occur and how they relate to a physical illness or injury and the rehabilitative process are only now being asked (3).

Current information about the evaluation and treatment of cognitive dysfunction and its impact on the rehabilitation of daily living skills has been amply reviewed (37,118,92,9,7,38,41,95). The functional capabilities of the cognitively as well as physically impaired geriatric population are quite diverse. No single rehabilitation approach addresses the varied functional impairments seen clinically. The rehabilitation literature points to a gap between actual and potential levels of cognitive functioning (23). Assessment tools do not consistently differentiate between impairment due to physical factors versus psychological and/or social factors (28, 118). The literature discusses a variety of treatment approaches such as activity stimulation, milieu therapy, reality orientation programs, and behavioral approaches that can be incorporated into a patient's rehabilitation program. Minimal research has been conducted incorporating cognitive therapy programs into the rehabilitation process of cognitively impaired patients suffering from hip fracture, for example, in order to maximize the patient's functional outcome. Leer (1984) and Carter et al. (1983, 1988) describe studies demonstrating improvement in functional performance in subjects who received cognitive rehabilitation in addition to a standard rehabilitation program. For the most part, however, "Research efforts on memory and learning in the elderly have been focused primarily on differentiating the types and degrees of memory deficit that occur with increasing age, determining the effects of neurological changes on information processing, and ascertaining the effects of practice and/or the use of mediators (mnemonics)" (3). These areas of cognition are primarily evaluated by assessing recognition or recall. Research findings on cognition and aging are complex and inconclusive as they relate to ADL skills (19,20,34,104,93).

What is known suggests certain clinical approaches may help compensate for normal cognitive functional change in some individuals. With patients learning new information or skills, rehabilitation personnel must develop comprehensive evaluation tools and treatment approaches that incorporate cognitive function and therefore better predict outcome levels of functioning. There are a number of cognitive assessment tools available to therapists for identifying baseline abilities. These include the Mini-Mental State Examination (45), Test for Severe Impairment (4), Cognitive Level Evaluation (5), and the Bay Area Functional Performance Evaluation (58). These need to be more widely used in studies to evaluate the effectiveness of cognitive rehabilitation in improving functional skills and identifying those persons who benefit.

Aphasia

Related to rehabilitation of cognitive deficits is the rehabilitation for aphasia. Aphasia is one of the most common language disorders seen among the aged (25), affecting speech, auditory comprehension, reading, writing, gestures, and mathematics. It is "impairment, due to brain damage, of the capacity to interpret and formulate language symbols" (114). In the aging population its most common cause is stroke (25). Because of its often global impact on communication, in the absence of significant recovery and/or significant family support, persons with aphasia often remain in the NH following their rehabilitation process. They are then often mistakenly characterized by NH staff as demented, due to their difficulty in understanding or expressing responses using verbal communication (35).

Burns and Halper (1986) list the three goals of aphasia rehabilitation: (a) maximizing intact skills for compensation of deficits, (b) improving deficits areas through structured stimulation, and (c) inhibiting maladaptive behaviors. Wertz (1981) and others also recommend that treatment for aphasia include education of both patient and family so they can better cope with and manage the residual disability, as it is clear from the literature and clinical observation that not all patients improve and many patients do not regain their previous communication skills. Yet treatment for aphasia has been shown to be effective in important ways. Several studies demonstrated clinically and statistically significant improvements in subjects who received speech therapy as compared to nontreated controls in several aspects of speech and communication (51,116,100,13). These are summarized in Table 1.1. One study (74) did not find significant differences in impairments between treatment and nontreatment controls, but this result is questionable, because 55% of the treatment group received less than half of the treatment sessions, and treatment consisted of only 2 hours per week, which may be insufficient to obtain a response. Because the consensus from the literature is that treatment makes a difference in recovery, the focus of research in aphasia needs to move toward investigating the specifics of the treatment program. Nicholas and Helm-Estabrooks (1990) pose three questions other authors have also identified as needing study: (a) for what type of aphasia is a specific treatment effective, (b) at what point should a specific treatment begin—and end—for a particular type of aphasia, and (c) which (specific) language deficits are amenable to treatment and which are not?

Some studies have demonstrated similar improvement in older subjects (13), whereas others did not (79,56). A clear relationship between age and aphasia recovery is difficult because of probable interactions with severity of aphasia (105), etiology (35), and type of aphasia (86,52), all of which may affect aphasia prognosis (114,115).

None of the aphasia treatment efficacy research was conducted with subjects from NHs, although most utilized some subjects who are at least by age somewhat representative of this population. Residents might be expected to be further from their acute stroke events and therefore less likely to improve. Yet many patients may not have received an adequate trial of speech therapy in the acute setting and still possess rehabilitation potential. NH-based studies are clearly warranted. One additional issue regarding treatment for aphasia entails the use of personnel other than speech pathologists for treatment. Subjects in two studies (116,100) were randomly assigned to treatment groups with therapy provided either by a speech pathologist or trained volunteer. Those subjects who were in the group conducted by the volunteers showed improvements intermediate between those who received their therapy from a speech pathologist and those who received no treatment. Although sessions with a volunteer in no way substitute for skilled interventions by a speech/language pathologist, some benefits may be gained utilizing trained volunteers as an adjunct to skilled therapy or where skilled therapy is not available. This issue needs closer scrutiny, as the shortage of speech/language pathologists in NHs, especially in rural areas, leaves many residents little or no treatment. Even minimal changes made with nonlicensed personnel could significantly impact the quality of life for the long-term resident.

OUTCOMES OF GERIATRIC REHABILITATION

Numerous studies have investigated the outcomes from hospital rehabilitation in terms of both function and discharge placement. Hip fractures and strokes have been the two conditions most frequently investigated, and both these conditions are commonly treated in NHs. Unfortunately, very few studies report outcomes of patients who receive their rehabilitation in the NH. Moreover, because of the Medicare 3-hour rule, older persons or those with multiple medical problems are increasingly referred to NHs for their primary rehabilitation, which makes the need for NH rehabilitation research even more pressing. This section will summarize outcomes research studies for rehabilitation programs that could potentially apply in the NH, although only four were not actually performed there.

Functional Outcomes

Barnes (1984) investigated the frequency with which subjects returned to their previous level of ambulation in a NH rehabilitation program following a hip fracture. He found that whereas 96% became ambulatory, only 40% achieved their prefracture level of ambulation by the time of discharge from physical therapy. His definition of prefracture level of ambulation excluded persons functionally independent in ambulation but using a new assistive device. In another study, 62.5% of persons over the age of 90 who also received their rehabilitation in a NH regained independence in ambulation, although some needed an assistive device (66). Only 24% of persons who received their rehabilitation in "a hospital for patients with prolonged illness" had returned to prefracture level of ambulation by 6 months (65). Again, if independence in ambulation is used as the more functionally based outcome, 63% were independent at 6 months. The results compare favorably with outcomes from acute settings (62).

No study could be found that described the outcomes of persons who receive their primary rehabilitation in a NH following a stroke. Two studies looked specifically at the effect of age on functional progress following rehabilitation from a stroke. With subjects divided into four age groups (less than 55, 55-65, 66-75, or greater than 75 years), Adler et al. (1980) found no significant difference in functional gains as measured by the Gaylord Index. In the one subgroup in which a difference was noted—persons over age 75 with moderate impairment upon admission—the authors were unable to determine if it was due to less potential or simply a need for more time by older persons. Steinberg and Freedland (1990) found no significant outcome difference in persons over age 75 versus those under age 75 in five of seven ADLs. There was no discussion of why there were significant differences in the other two skills, eating and bowel management, yet not in other more difficult tasks such as bladder management and bathing. In persons over age 85 seen for rehabilitation for a variety of conditions, Parry (1983) found that 47% showed significant improvement and 32% had limited improvement. This issue of age differences in rehabilitation outcomes following stroke, as well as other conditions, clearly needs further study. Research also needs to identify what other factors may contribute to differences in functional outcomes following rehabilitation in NHs as compared to other settings.

Placement Outcomes

A large number of studies have looked at the factors affecting return to the community after rehabilitation. Age is a frequently cited factor (78,2,110), yet in Sweden, where there is a very aggressive approach to rehabilitation after hip fracture, 81% of persons over 80 years of age without significant additional diseases or impairments returned home (31). In the presence of these complications, the percent that went home dropped to 36%. Kaplan and Ford (1975) found that after rehabilitation in a skilled nursing facility (SNF), 61% were discharged from the SNF, and 61% of those (37% of the entire study population) returned to independent living. Thirty-six percent of persons judged to have poor rehabilitation potential seen in a "slow stream rehabilitation" program were discharged to home (87). Variables in addition to age and functional status determine discharge placement. McClatchie (1980) discusses the discrepancy between the amount of assistance needed by his subjects and the amount of support available in the home environment. This discrepancy is resolved by discharge to an institution. Although in McClatchie's study there was no relationship between age and availability of support in the home, E. M. Brody (1986) discusses the numbers of older persons who are widowed, divorced, or never married or who are childless or due to geography or long-standing alienation rarely see their children. Yet the role social support and other psychosocial factors play in determining discharge placement has not been adequately studied or ever addressed in a NH population. A study currently being conducted by the authors is investigating this issue, assessing the relative impact of physical and psychosocial factors on discharge outcomes from NH rehabilitation programs.

Rehabilitation After Rehabilitation

Snaedal et al. (1984) investigated outcomes of persons with hip fractures discharged to a chronic care hospital. These hospitals admitted "the very old, those in poor medical condition, fracture complications, or those living in unfavorable social conditions"—persons very much like those admitted to NH—for permanent placement. Yet, with rehabilitation, 12% of those surviving were able to go back to the community; at one year, 32% of those surviving returned to the community. O'Neil and associates (1987) also demonstrated positive outcomes for those persons who are thought not to have sufficient potential to enter traditional rehabilitation. Unfortunately, we do not know how to identify persons with "poor potential" who are likely to respond to therapeutic interventions. Nor is there any research documenting outcomes of those persons discharged to NHs who had supposedly "plateaued" during acute rehabilitation, yet continued to receive therapy at the NH. Although not a focus of the study, Granger and associates (1988) found that 13% of those discharged to

NHs after an acute rehabilitation program following a stroke were discharged back to the community. The studies concerning hip fracture also reported a similar population that was later discharged from a NH back to the community. This may be indicative of persons who were unable to tolerate a very aggressive program and needed the slower paced rehabilitation program a NH could provide. It may also include persons who simply needed a longer period of rehabilitation to achieve their goals. Home health therapy can be provided after discharge from an acute program; for those with no support in the home, services provided at the NH may allow some persons who would have been permanently institutionalized to return to the community. Research identifying those persons who need a slower pace or additional time to achieve equally positive outcomes will be difficult, but is required.

CONCLUSIONS

The refrain of this chapter is that rehabilitation in NHs has been largely ignored by researchers. Because of NH residents' age and medical complexity, one cannot blindly apply research findings from studies done in other settings to the NH population. What little research we do have indicates that rehabilitation can be effective for older persons, and clinically we see the benefits of it in our NH residents. In all areas, we need to develop, through well-designed research studies, realistic expectations of who would benefit from such services and ensure through reimbursement and regulatory policies that those services are provided.

REFERENCES

1. Adams, G. M., & deVries, H. A. (1973). Physiological effects of an exercise training regimen upon women aged 52-79. *Journal of Gerontology, 28*(1), 50-55.
2. Adler, M. K., Brown, C. C., & Acton, P. (1980). Stroke rehabilitation—Is age a determinant? *Journal of the American Geriatrics Society, 28*, 499-503.
3. Ager, C. L. (1988). Cognitive developmental changes. In L. J. Davis & M. Kirkland (Eds.), *The role of occupational therapy with the elderly* (pp. 69-78). Rockville, MD: American Occupational Therapy Association.
4. Albert, M., & Cohen, C. (1992). The test for severe impairment: An instrument for the assessment of patients with severe cognitive dysfunction. *Journal of the American Geriatrics Society, 40*, 449-453.
5. Allen, C. (1985). *Occupational therapy for psychiatric diseases: Measurement and management of cognitive disability.* Boston: Little, Brown.

6. Aniansson, A., Grimby G., Rundgren A., et al. (1980). Physical training in old men. *Age and Ageing, 9*, 186-187.
7. Applegate, W. B. (1987). Use of assessment instruments in clinical settings. *Journal of the American Geriatrics Society 35*, 45-50.
8. Applegate, W. B., Akins, D., VanderZwaag, R., et al. (1983). A geriatric rehabilitation and assessment unit in a community hospital. *Journal of the American Geriatrics Society, 31*(4), 206-210.
9. Arenberg, D. (1974). A longitudinal study of problem solving in adults. *Journal of Gerontology, 29*(6), 650-658.
10. Badenhop, D. T., Cleary, P. A., Schaal, S. F., et al. (1983). Physiological adjustments to higher or lower intensity exercise in elders. *Medicine and Science in Sports and Exercise, 15*(6), 496-502.
11. Barnes, B. (1984). Ambulation outcomes after hip fracture. *Physical Therapy, 64*(3), 317-323.
12. Barry, A. J., Daly, J. W., Pruett, E.D.R., et al. (1966). The effects of physical conditioning on older individuals: I. Work capacity, circulatory-respiratory function and work electrocardiogram. *Journal of Gerontology, 21*, 182-191.
13. Basso, A., Capitani, E., & Vignolo, L. A. (1979). Influence of rehabilitation on language skills in aphasic patients: A controlled study. *Archives of Neurology, 36*, 190-196.
14. Benestad, A. M. (1965). Trainability of old men. *Acta Medica Scandinavica, 178*, 321-327.
15. Bergen, A., Presperine, J., & Tallman, T. (1990). *Positioning for function*. Valhalla, NY: Valhalla Rehabilitation.
16. Boies, A. H. (1987). Management of contractures. *Home Healthcare Nurse, 5*(5), 40-41.
17. Booth, B. J., Doyle, M., & Montgomery, J. (1983). Serial casting for the management of spasticity in the head-injured adult. *Physical Therapy, 63*(12), 1960-1966.
18. Borello-France, D. F., Burdett, F. G., & Gee, Z. L. (1988). Modification of sitting posture of patients with hemiplegia using seat boards and backboards. *Physical Therapy, 68*(1), 67-71.
19. Botwinick, J. (1973). *Aging and behavior*. New York: Springer.
20. Botwinick, J. (1977). Intellectual abilities. In J. E. Birren & K. W. Schaie (Eds.), *Handbook of the psychology of aging* (pp. 580-605). New York: Van Nostrand Reinhold.
21. Breines, E. (1988). The functional assessment scale as an instrument for measuring changes in levels of function of nursing home residents following occupational therapy. *Canadian Journal of Occupational Therapy, 55*(3), 135-140.
22. Brody, E. M. (1986). Informal support systems in the rehabilitation of the disabled elderly. In S. J. Brody & G. E. Ruff (Eds.), *Aging and rehabilitation: Advances in the state of the art* (pp 87-104). New York: Springer.
23. Brody, E. M., Kleban, M. H., Lawton, M. P., et al. (1974). A longitudinal look at excess disabilities in the mentally impaired aged. *Journal of Gerontology, 29*, 79-84.
24. Brody, S. J. (1985). Rehabilitation and nursing homes. In E. L. Schneider (Ed.), *The teaching nursing home*. New York: Raven.
25. Burns, M. S., & Halper, A. S. (1986). Language disorders associated with aging. *Topics in Geriatric Rehabilitation, 1*(4), 15-27.
26. Burton, M., & Spall, R. (1981). The behavioral approach to nursing the elderly. *Nursing Times, 77*, 247-248.
27. Carey, R. G., Seibert, J. H., & Posavac, E. J. (1988). Who makes the most progress in inpatient rehabilitation? An analysis of functional gain. *Archives of Physical Medicine and Rehabilitation, 69*, 337-343.

28. Carroll, B. J., Feinberg, M., Smouse, P. E., et al. (1981). The Carroll rating scale for depression: I. Development, reliability and validation. *British Journal of Psychiatry, 138,* 194-200.

29. Carter, L. T., Howard, B. E., & O'Neil, W. A. (1983). Effectiveness of cognitive skill remediation in acute stroke patients. *American Journal of Occupational Therapy, 37*(5), 320-326.

30. Carter, L. T., Oliveira, D. O., Duponte, J., et al. (1988). The relationship of cognitive skills performance to activities of daily living. *American Journal of Occupational Therapy, 42*(7), 449-445.

31. Ceder, L., Thorngren, K., & Wallden, B. (1980). Prognostic indicators and early home rehabilitation in elderly patients with hip fractures. *Clinical Orthopaedics and Related Research, 152,* 173-184.

32. Cherney, L. R., & O'Neil, P. (1986). Swallowing disorders and the aged. *Topics in Geriatric Rehabilitation, 1*(4), 45-59.

33. Cherry, D. B. (1980). Review of the physical therapy alternatives for reducing muscle contracture. *Physical Therapy, 60*(7), 877-881.

34. Craik, F.I.M.L. (1977). Age differences in human memory. In J. E. Birren & K. W. Schaie (Eds.), *Handbook of the psychology of aging* (pp. 384-420). New York: Van Nostrand Reinhold.

35. Davis, G. A., & Holland, A. L. (1981). Age in understanding and treating aphasia. In D. S. Beasley & G. A. Davis (Eds.), *Aging: Communication processes and disorders* (pp. 207-228). New York: Grune & Stratton.

36. deVries, H. A. (1970). Physiological effects of an exercise training regimen upon men aged 52-88. *Journal of Gerontology, 25*(4), 325-336.

37. Diesfeldt, H. F. A., & Diesfeldt-Groenendijk, H. (1977). Improving cognitive performance in psychogeriatric patients: The influence of physical exercise. *Age and Ageing, 6,* 58-64.

38. Dietz, J. C., Tovar, V. S., Thorn, D. W., et al. (1990). The test of orientation for rehabilitation patients: Interrater reliability. *American Journal of Occupational Therapy, 44*(9), 784-790.

39. Elliott, J. L. (1988). Swallowing disorders in the elderly: A guide to diagnosis and treatment. *Geriatrics, 43*(1), 95-113.

40. Ernst, P., Badash, D., Beran, B., et al. (1977). Incidence of mental illness in the aged: Unmasking the effects of a diagnosis of chronic brain syndrome. *Journal of the American Geriatrics Society, 25,* 371-375.

41. Farver, P. F., & Farver, T. B. (1982). Performance of normal older adults on tests designed to measure parietal lobe functions. *American Journal of Occupational Therapy, 36,* 444-449.

42. Ferido, T., & Habel, M. (1988). Spasticity in head trauma and CVA patients: Etiology and management. *Journal of Neuroscience Nursing, 20*(1), 17-22.

43. Fiatarone, M. A., Marks, E. C., Ryan, N. D., et al. (1990). High-intensity strength training in nonagenarians. *Journal of the American Medical Association, 263*(22), 3029-3034.

44. Fisher, N. M., Pendergast, D. R., & Calkins, E. (1991). Muscle rehabilitation in impaired elderly nursing home residents. *Archives of Physical Medicine and Rehabilitation, 72,* 181-185.

45. Folstein, M. F., Folstein, S. E., & McHugh, P. R. (1975). Mini-Mental State—A practical method for grading the cognitive state of patients for the clinician. *Journal of Psychiatric Research, 12,* 189-198.

46. Frontera, W. R., Meredith, C. N., O'Reilly, K. P., et al. (1988). Strength conditioning in older men: Skeletal muscle hypertrophy and improved function. *Journal of Applied Physiology, 64*(3), 1038-1044.
47. Gordon, C., Hewer, R. L., & Wade, D. T. (1987). Dysphagia in acute stroke. *British Medical Journal, 295,* 411-414.
48. Granger, C. V., Hamilton, B. B., & Gresham, G. E. (1988). The stroke rehabilitation outcome study—Part I: General description. *Archives of Physical Medicine and Rehabilitation, 69,* 506-509.
49. Gray, R. P., Stefans, V., & Sowell, T. W. (1990). Rehabilitation of dysphagia. *Physical Medicine and Rehabilitation: State of the Art Reviews, 4*(1), 105-112.
50. Hagberg, J. M., Graves, J. E., Jimacher, M., et al. (1989). Cardiovascular responses of 70-79 year old men and women to exercise training. *Journal of Applied Physiology, 66*(6), 2589-2594.
51. Hagen, C. (1973). Communication abilities in hemiplegia: Effect of speech therapy. *Archives of Physical Medicine and Rehabilitation, 54,* 454-463.
52. Harasymiw, S. J., & Halper, A. (1981). Sex, age, and aphasia type. *Brain and Language, 12,* 190-198.
53. Hartigan, J. D. (1982). The dangerous wheelchair. *Journal of the American Geriatrics Society, 30*(9), 572-573.
54. Hirsch, C. H., Sommers, L., Olsen, A., et al. (1990). The natural history of functional morbidity in hospitalized older patients. *Journal of the American Geriatrics Society, 38,* 1296-1303.
55. Hoenig, H. M., & Rubenstein, L. Z. (1991). Hospital-associated deconditioning and dysfunction. *Journal of the American Geriatrics Society, 39,* 220-222.
56. Holland, A. L., Greenhouse, J. B., Fromm, D., et al. (1989). Predictors of language restitution following stroke: A multivariate analysis. *Journal of Speech and Hearing Research, 32,* 232-238.
57. Horner, J., & Massey, E. W. (1991). Managing dysphagia: Special problems in patients with neurologic disease. *Postgraduate Medicine, 89*(5), 203-213.
58. Houston, D., Williams, S. L., Blooner, J., et al. (1989). The Bay Area Functional Performance Evaluation: Development and standardization. *American Journal of Occupational Therapy, 43*(3), 170-183.
59. Hulme, J. B., Gallacher, K., Walsh, J., et al. (1987a). Behavioral and postural changes observed with use of adaptive seating by clients with multiple handicaps. *Physical Therapy, 67*(7), 1060-1067.
60. Hulme, J. B., Poor, R., Schulein, M., et al. (1983). Perceived behavioral changes observed with adaptive seating devices and training programs for multihandicapped, developmentally disabled individuals. *Physical Therapy, 63*(2), 204-208.
61. Hulme, J. B., Shaver, J., Acher, S., et al. (1987b). Effects of adaptive seating devices on the eating and drinking of children with multiple handicaps. *American Journal of Occupational Therapy, 41*(2), 81-89.
62. Jette, A. M., Harris, B. A., Cleary, P. D., et al. (1987). Functional recovery after hip fracture. *Archives of Physical Medicine and Rehabilitation, 68,* 735-740.
63. Kane, R. L., Ouslander, J. G., & Abrass, I. B. (1989). *Essentials of clinical geriatrics.* New York: McGraw-Hill.
64. Kaplan, J., & Ford, C. S. (1975). Rehabilitation for the elderly: An eleven year assessment. *Gerontologist, 15,* 393-397.
65. Katz, S., Ford, A. B., Heiple, K. G., et al. (1964). Studies of illness in the aged: Recovery after fracture of the hip. *Journal of Gerontology, 19,* 285-293.

66. Kauffman, T. L., Albright, L., & Wagner, C. (1987). Rehabilitation outcomes after hip fracture in persons 90 years old and older. *Archives of Physical Medicine and Rehabilitation, 68*, 369-371.
67. Keener, S. M., & Swigart, J. E. (1984). Early use of adaptable seating for patients with head trauma. *Physical Therapy, 64*(2), 206-207.
68. King, T. I. (1982). Plaster splinting as a means of reducing elbow flexor spasticity: A case study. *American Journal of Occupational Therapy, 36*(10), 671-673.
69. Kottke, F. J., Pauley, D. L., & Ptak, R. A. (1966). The rationale for prolonged stretching for correction of shortening of connective tissue. *Archives of Physical Medicine and Rehabilitation, 47*, 345-352.
70. Lambert, J. R., Tepperman, P. S., Jimenez, J., et al. (1981). Cervical spine disease and dysphagia. *American Journal of Gastroenterology, 76*, 35-40.
71. Lazzara, G., Lazaras, C., & Logemann, J. A. (1986). Impact of thermal stimulation on the triggering of the swallowing reflex. *Dysphagia, 1*, 73-77.
72. Leer, W. B. (1984). Block design training with stroke patients: A study on the effects of cognitive retraining on improving certain activities of daily living skills. *Dissertation Abstracts International, 45*(4-B), 1290-1291.
73. Lehmkuhl, L. D., Thoi, L. L., Baize, C., et al. (1990). Multimodality treatment of joint contractures in patients with severe brain injury: Cost, effectiveness, and integration of therapies in the application of serial/inhibitive casts. *Journal of Head Trauma Rehabilitation, 5*(4), 23-42.
74. Lincoln, N. B., McGuirk, E., Mulley, G. P., et al. (1984). Effectiveness of speech therapy for aphasic stroke patients: A randomized controlled study. *Lancet, 1*, 1197-1200.
75. Logemann, J. A. (1983). *Evaluation and treatment of swallowing disorders*. San Diego: College-Hill.
76. Logemann, J. A. (1989, Spring). Challenges for the speech-language pathologist working in dysphagia. *Hearsay*, pp. 6-10.
77. MacKay-Lyons, F. (1989). Low-load, prolonged stretch in treatment of elbow flexion contractures secondary to head trauma: A case report. *Physical Therapy, 69*(4), 292-296.
78. Magaziner, J., Simonsick, E. M., Kashner, T. M., et al. (1990). Predictors of functional recovery one year following hospital discharge for hip fracture: A prospective study. *Journal of Gerontology, 45*(3), M101-107.
79. Marshall, R. C., & Phillips, D. S. (1983). Prognosis for improved verbal communication in aphasic stroke patients. *Archives of Physical Medicine and Rehabilitation, 64*, 597-600.
80. McClatchie, G. (1980). Survey of the rehabilitation outcome of strokes. *Medical Journal of Australia, 1*, 649-651.
81. Milazzo, L. S., Bouchard, J., & Lund, D. A. (1989). The swallowing process: Effects of aging and stroke. *Physical Medicine and Rehabilitation: State of the Art Reviews, 3*(3), 489-499.
82. Moritani, T., & deVries, H. A. (1980). Potential for gross muscle hypertrophy in older men. *Journal of Gerontology, 35*(5), 672-682.
83. National Center for Health Services Research and Health Care Technology Assessment. (1989). *The role of speech-language pathologists in the management of dysphagia*. Rockville, MD: U.S. Department of Health and Human Services, Public Health Services.
84. National Center for Health Statistics. (1989). *Vital and health statistics* (DHHS Publication No. PHS 89-1758). Washington, DC: U.S. Government Printing Office.

85. Nicholas, M., & Helm-Estabrooks, N. (1990). Aphasia. *Seminars in Speech and Language, 11*(3), 135-144.
86. Obler, L. K., Albert, M. L., Goodglass, H., et al. (1978). Aphasia type and aging. *Brain and Language, 6,* 318-322.
87. O'Neil, T. J., McCarthy, K., & Newton, B. M. (1987). Slow-stream rehabilitation: Is it effective? *Medical Journal of Australia, 147,* 172-175.
88. Palmer, M., & Wyness, M. A. (1988). Positioning and handling: Important considerations in the care of the severely head-injured patient. *Journal of Neuroscience Nursing, 20*(1), 42-49.
89. Parry, F. (1983). Physical rehabilitation of the old, old patient. *Journal of the American Geriatrics Society, 31*(8), 482-484.
90. Paureel, R. (1974). Psychological effects of exercise therapy upon institutionalized geriatric mental patients. *Gerontologist, 14,* 157-161.
91. Pawlson, L. G., Goodwin, M., & Keith, K. (1986). Wheelchair use by ambulatory nursing home residents. *Journal of the American Geriatrics Society, 34,* 860-864.
92. Pearson, J. L., Teri, L., Reifler, B. V., et al. (1989). Functional status and cognitive impairment in Alzheimer's patients with and without depression. *Journal of the American Geriatrics Society, 37*(12), 1117-1121.
93. Perlmutter, M. (1978). What is memory aging the aging of? *Developmental Psychology, 14,* 330-345.
94. Pontoppidan, H., & Beecher, H. K. (1960). Progressive loss of protective reflexes in the airway with the advance of age. *Journal of the American Medical Association, 174*(18), 2209-2213.
95. Reisberg, B. L. (1985). Assessment tool for Alzheimer's type dementia. *Hospital and Community Psychiatry, 6,* 593-595.
96. Roberts, D. W. (1982). Positioning device for individuals with neuromuscular disabilities. *Physical Therapy, 62*(1), 33-34.
97. Roush, J. S., & Emory, N. (1990). Orthotics and seating systems. *Physical Medicine and Rehabilitation: State of the Art Reviews, 4*(3), 479-495.
98. Settle, C. (1987). Seating and pressure sores. *Physiotherapy, 73*(9), 455-457.
99. Shephard, R. J. (1987). *Physical activity and aging.* Rockville, MD: Aspen.
100. Shewan, C. M., & Kertesz, A. (1984). Effects of speech and language treatment on recovery from aphasia. *Brain and Language, 23,* 272-299.
101. Shillam, L. L., Beeman, C., & Loshin, P. M. (1983). Effect of occupational therapy intervention on bathing independence of disabled persons. *American Journal of Occupational Therapy, 3*(11), 744-748.
102. Sidney, K. H., & Shephard, R. J. (1978). Frequency and intensity of exercise training for elderly subjects. *Medicine and Science in Sports, 10*(2), 125-131.
103. Siebens, H., Trupe, E., Siebens, A., et al. (1986). Correlates and consequences of eating dependency in institutionalized elderly. *Journal of the American Geriatrics Society, 34,* 192-198.
104. Siegler, I. C. (1980). The psychology of adult development and aging. In E. W. Busse & D. G. Blazer (Eds.), *Handbook of geriatric psychiatry* (pp. 169-221). New York: Van Nostrand Reinhold.
105. Smith, A. (1971). Objective indices of severity of chronic aphasia in stroke patients. *Journal of Speech and Hearing Disorders, 36,* 167-207.
106. Snaedal, J., Thorngren, M., Ceder, L., et al. (1984). Outcomes of patients with a nailed hip fracture requiring rehabilitation in a hospital for chronic care. *Scandinavian Journal of Rehabilitative Medicine, 16,* 171-176.

107. Splaingard, M. L., Hutchins, B., Sulton, L. D., et al. (1988). Aspiration in rehabilitation patients: Videofluoroscopy versus bedside clinical assessment. *Archives of Physical Medicine and Rehabilitation, 69*, 637-640.
108. Stamford, B. A. (1972). Physiological effects of training upon institutionalized geriatric men. *Journal of Gerontology, 21*(4), 451-455.
109. Stamford, B. A. (1973). Effects of chronic institutionalization on the physical working capacity and trainability of geriatric men. *Journal of Gerontology, 28*(4), 441-446.
110. Steinberg, F. U., & Freedland, K. E. (1990, May). *Stroke rehabilitation in patients over the age of 75.* Paper presented at the 47th Annual Scientific Meeting of the American Geriatrics Society, Atlanta, GA.
111. Taylor, S. J. (1987). Evaluating the client with physical disabilities for wheelchair seating. *American Journal of Occupational Therapy, 41*(11), 711-716.
112. Tomlinson, B., Blessed, G., & Roth, M. (1970). Observations of the brain of demented old people. *Journal of Neurological Science, 11*, 205-243.
113. Veis, S. L., & Logemann, J. A. (1985). Swallowing disorders in persons with cerebrovascular accident. *Archives of Physical Medicine and Rehabilitation, 66*, 372-375.
114. Wertz, R. T. (1981). Aphasia management: The speech pathologist's role. *Seminars in Speech, Language and Hearing, 2*(4), 315-331.
115. Wertz, R. T. (1987). Language treatment for aphasia is efficacious, but for whom? *Topics in Language Disorders, 8*(1), 1-10.
116. Wertz, R. T., Weiss, D. G., Aten, J. L., et al. (1986). Comparison of clinic, home and deferred language treatment for aphasia. *Archives of Neurology, 43*, 653-658.
117. Williams, T. F. (1984). *Rehabilitation in the aging.* New York: Raven.
118. Wilson, L. A., Grant, K., Witney, P. M., et al. (1973). Mental status of elderly hospital patients related to occupational therapist's assessment of activities of daily living. *Gerontologica Clinica, 15*, 197-202.
119. Yarkony, G. M., & Sahgal, V. (1987). Contractures: A major complication of craniocerebral trauma. *Clinical Orthopaedics and Related Research, 219*, 93-96.

Table 1.1 Findings From Geriatric Rehabilitation Research

Author	Subjects	Setting	Intervention	Scale	Outcome
Conditioning					
Hagberg et al., 1989	16 in endurance grp 19 in resistance grp 12 in control grp 70-79 yrs	Community	Endurance—3x/wk x 26 wks @ up to 60-70% VO_2 max walking or jogging Resistance—3x/wk x 26 wks @ variable resistance on Nautilus machines	Naughton protocol	Endurance grp—22% inc in VO_2max Resistance grp—9% inc in lower body, 18% in upper body
Benestad, 1965	13 men, physically active Mean age 75.5 yrs	Community	3x/wk x 5-6 wks Treadmill up to 80% VO_2max	Bicycle ergometer	Dec HR at submaximal work loads No change in VO_2max
Adams & deVries, 1973	Exp—17 men, mean age 65.9 yrs Control—6 men, mean age 66.7 yrs	Senior village	3x/wk x 6 wks Exercise class of calisthenics, jog-walk, stretching	Bicycle ergometer	Physical work capacity inc 37%; VO_2max inc 20.8% Dec RHR and HR at submaximal work loads versus controls
deVries, 1970	Exp—66 men Modified exp—7 men Control—32 men Mean age 69.5 yrs	Senior village	3x/wk x 3 mos (mod exp grp x 6 wks) exercise class as above Exp grp—ex HR 145 Mod exp grp—ex HR 120	Bicycle ergometer	Exp grp—inc 29.4% VO_2max, 19.6% VC, 15.8% work capacity; signif. inc in strength mod exp grp—work capacity inc 34.5%
Barry et al., 1966	Exp—5 men, 3 women Mean age 70 yrs Control—2 men, 3 women Mean age 72 yrs	Community and RH	3x/wk x 3 mos Interval training on bicycle ergometer x 40'; 10-15 min conditioning ex	Bicycle ergometer	Dec submaximal ex HR; 38% inc VO_2max Inc work capacity

continued

Table 1.1 Continued

Author	Subjects	Setting	Intervention	Scale	Outcome
Stamford, 1972	Exp—9 men, mean age 71.5 yrs, 21 yrs institutionalized Control—8 men, mean age 65.2 years, 22 yrs institutionalized	Psychiatric hospital	5x/wk x 12 wks Treadmill walking program @ 70% age adjusted max HR	Bicycle ergometer and treadmill	Dec HR and SBP response to ex Dec resting SBP
Stamford, 1973	5 men recently hospitalized (RI) (>1 yr), mean age 66.7 yrs 7 men chronically hospitalized (CI) (mean 23.4 yrs), mean age 68.2 yrs Control 7 men, mean age 70 yrs	Psychiatric hospital	5x/wk x 18 wks 15-30' treadmill walking @ 50-60% age adjusted max HR	Bicycle ergometer	Dec ex HR and SBP and inc O2 pulse CI responded most in first 6 weeks; RI in last 6 weeks with inc intensity of training
Badenhop et al, 1983	14 low-intensity exp (LI) 14 high-intensity exp (HI) 4 controls Mean age 67.8 yrs	Community	4x/wk x 9 wks 15' flexibility, 25' cycling, 10' cool down HI—60-75% max HR LI—30-45% max HR	Bicycle ergometer	Max power on ex test inc 25% (LI) and 26% (HI) VO2max inc 16% (LI) and 14.8% (HI) Dec submaximal ventilation 14.6% (LI) and 11.1% (HI)
Sidney & Shephard, 1978	14 men, 28 women aged 60-83 Self-selected exercise groups: high frequency, high intensity (HFHI) n=8; high frequency, low intensity (HFLI) n=14; low frequency, high intensity (LFHI) n=8; low frequency, low intensity (LFLI) n=12	Community	4x/wk x 14 wks 15' warm-up and 30' walking LI—120-130 bpm HI—140-150 bpm	Bicycle ergometer	Inc in VO2max .08 l/min HFHI, .20 l/min LFHI, .58 l/min HFHI; no change LFLI Physical work capacity improved significantly only in HFLI and HFHI groups

Strengthening

Study	Subjects	Setting	Protocol	Type	Results
Aniansson et al., 1980	12 exp, 12 controls 69-74 yrs	Community	3x/wk x 12 wks Dynamic and static ex with body weight as resistance		Significant increases in static and dynamic strength ranging from 8-22%
Frontera et al., 1988	12 men 60-72 yrs	Community	3x/wk x 12 wks 80% 1 RM knee extensors and flexors		1 RM inc 117% (R)knee ext, 107% (L)knee ext, 227% (R) and (L) knee flex; Isokinetic strength inc 8.5-18.5% @ 60°/sec and 14.7-18.2% @ 240°/sec
Moritani & deVries, 1980	5 men, mean age 21.8 yrs 5 men, mean age 69.6 yrs	Community	3x/wk x 8 wks PRE's @ 66% 1 RM for elbow flexors	Isometric	Significant inc in max strength in both old (mean=13.8 lbs) and young (mean=26 lbs) groups; Percent change 23% old, 30% young
Fiatarone et al., 1990	10 subjects Mean age 90.2 yrs	SNF	3x/wk x 8 wks 80% of 1 RM for quads	Dynamic	Mean strength gain 174% 48% inc tandom gait speed; 2 subjects stopped using canes
Fisher et al., 1991	14 subjects Mean age 82 yrs	SNF	3x/wk x 6 wks Isometric and isotonic quad ex		Muscular endurance inc 35%, strength inc 15%; excluding those who did not improve, strength inc 30-150%, velocity 35-90%

continued

25

Table 1.1 Continued

Author	Subjects	Setting	Intervention	Scale	Outcome
Activities of Daily Living					
Breines, 1988	249 subjects 85% >65 yrs Multiple dx	SNF	OT 5x/wk Mean=43 days	Functional Assessment Scale	75% improved a mean of 3.42 levels; 2% declined in function
Applegate et al., 1983	100 subjects Mean age 79 yrs Multiple dx	Geriatric unit of acute rehab	Rehabilitation program Mean=23 days	None	72% improved in grooming; 46% in dressing, 34% in housekeeping, 83% in feeding
Carey et al., 1988	6194 subjects 68% 60 yrs Multiple dx	Acute rehab	Rehabilitation program Mean=32 days	LORS-II	Subjects: 60-69 inc mean 23.1% points 70-76 inc mean 23.3% points 77+ inc mean 22.9% points
Granger et al., 1988	539 subjects Mean age 69 yrs Stroke	Acute rehab	Rehabilitation program Mean=37 days	Barthel	Mean scores inc from 37 at admission to 66 at discharge
Adler et al., 1980	45 subjects <55 yrs 45 subjects 50-65 yrs 45 subjects 66-75 yrs 45 subjects >75 yrs Stroke	Acute rehab	Rehabilitation program Mean=29 days	Gaylord Index	Subjects <55 inc 21.99 points 55-65 inc 19.37 points 66-75 inc 18.95 points >75 inc 14.53 points (not statistically sign.)
Shillam et al., 1983	19 subjects 63% SCI, 21% BI, 10% CVA	Acute hospital	OT bathing training	Bathing section of Klein-Bell	Mean scores pretest 3.6, posttest 17.9

Seating Adaptations and Positioning Strategies

Study	Subjects	Setting	Intervention	Measurement	Results
Borello-France, 1988	Exp—2 groups of 14 Control 13 Mean age 71.3 Stroke	Acute rehab	Seating changes and rehabilitation program 1 group seat boards 1 group seat and back boards		Seat boards only dec lateral pelvic tilt; seat boards and back boards combined dec lateral pelvic tilt, lateral trunk flexion, posterior pelvis tilt and thoracic kyphosis

Positioning Strategies to Reduce Contractures

Study	Subjects	Setting	Intervention	Measurement	Results
Lehmkuhl et al., 1990	25 subjects with BI Ages 3-54 years	Rehab hospital	Serial casting, motor point block and 5 subjects with tendon releases	ROM measurements	Mean measurements Pre Post Elbows −64.9 −29.7 Knees −53.6 −35.4 Ankles −25.9 −13.6
Booth et al., 1983	42 subjects with BI Cortical injury and ankle contracture Brainstem and ankle Cortical and knee Brainstem and knee	Rehab hospital	Serial casting Mean=28 days Mean=39 days Mean=22 days Mean=31 days	ROM measurements	Mean improvements (degrees) −16 pre +.7 post −24 pre +2 post −32 pre −5 post −25 pre −10 post
King, 1982	1 female with intercranial hemorrhage	Rehab hospital	Serial casting x 16 days Night splint x 3 wks	ROM measurements	Contracture improved from −90° to −15°

Cognitive Retraining

Study	Subjects	Setting	Intervention	Measurement	Results
Leer, 1984	40 subjects with stroke	Acute rehab	4 hrs/wk x 3 wks Block design training plus normal stroke rehab program		Higher improvement scores in personal hygiene, dressing, homemaking, and community ADL/vocational skills

continued

Table 1.1 Continued

Author	Subjects	Setting	Intervention	Scale	Outcome
Carter et al., 1983	Acute stroke patients, 16 exp, mean age 70.5 yrs 17 controls, mean age 73.4 yrs Acute CVA	Acute hospital rehab	3x/wk x 3 wks in addition to normal stroke rehab program	Letter cancelation, object matching, estimating 1 minute	Mean improvements (of 100 pts) 　　　　　Exp　Contr Scanning　35.9　3.8 Visual/spatial　31.0　-3.3 Time judgment　24.8　-7.8
Carter et al., 1988	Acute stroke patients, 16 exp, mean age 70.5 yrs 17 controls, mean age 73.4 yrs	Acute hospital rehab	3x/wk x 3 wks in addition to stroke rehab program	Barthel scores	No significant differences in overall scores; significant differences in personal hygiene, toilet transfer, bathing, and dressing scores
Aphasia					
Hagen, 1973	Acute stroke patients, 10 exp, 10 control Age 49-57 yrs	Acute hospital LTC unit	Speech therapy beginning 3 mos after CVA	Minnesota Differential Diagnosis for Aphasia (MDDA)	Improvement in reading comprehension, language formulation, speech production, spelling, and arithmetic in exp versus controls
Wertz et al., 1986	New stroke patients Grp I—29 men, mean age 59 yrs Grp II—36 men, mean age 60 yrs Grp III—29 men, mean age 57 yrs	Outpatient	GRP I—therapy 8-10 hrs/wk x 12 wks with speech therapist, then no treatment x 12 wks GRP II—8-10 hrs/wk x 12 wks therapist designed program done by friend or family, then no treatment x 12 wks GRP III—no treatment x 12 wks, then 8-10 hrs/wk x 12 wks by therapist	Porch Index of Communicative Ability (PICA)	Mean improvement in PICA subscales after 24 weeks: 　　　I　II　III Gest.　21.05　16.77　22.41 Verb.　16.4　15.02　15.48 Graph.　20.17　16.72　16.03

Study	Subjects	Setting	Treatment	Measure	Results
Shewan & Kertesz, 1984	Grp I—24 subjects Grp II—25 subjects Controls—23 subjects Aged 29-85, mean 67.5	Outpatient	3hr/wk x 1 year Grp I—stimulation-facilitation therapy Grp II—stimulation therapy by nurses Control—no treatment	Western Aphasia Battery (WAB)	No significant differences between treated groups Percentage gains made by treatment groups greater than controls by a factor of 1.6 to 25.6 for the various subscales
Basso et al., 1979	162 exp group 119 controls Mean age 50.2 yrs 85% CVA, 11% trauma, 4% other	Not described	Speech therapy 45-50' at least 3x/wk x at least 5 mos		Significant improvement in oral expression, auditory and verbal comprehension, writing and reading versus controls
Lincoln et al., 1984	Acute stroke patients 163 exp group 164 controls	Acute hospital or outpatient	Speech therapy 2hr/wk for 34 wks	PICA, Functional Communication Profile (FCP)	No significant differences on PICA or FCP at 10, 22, 34 weeks 55% of exp subjects received less than half their treatments
Marshall & Phillips, 1983	80 men Mean age 56.5 yrs Left CVA	Acute hospital	Speech therapy for at least 2 months, 2-5x/wk	PICA	Initial severity, time since CVA, auditory comprehension, age, fluency, and general health status correlated with good versus poor terminal speech performance
Holland et al., 1989	50 subjects Mean age 72 yrs New CVA	Acute hospital	Speech therapy 6x/wk at least 15'/session	WAB	Shorter LOS and younger age strongly correlated to recovery Gender, side of lesion, etiology of CVA, and presence of hemiplegia at discharge moderately correlated

continued

Table 1.1 Continued

Author	Subjects	Setting	Intervention	Scale	Outcome
Outcomes of Rehabilitation					
Barnes, 1984	70 subjects Mean age 82 years Recent hip fracture	SNF	Physical therapy		40% regained preambulatory status, 96% became ambulatory Only previous lower extremity fracture and number of PT visits correlated with return to prefracture level of ambulation
Kauffman et al., 1987	18 subjects Mean age 93 Recent hip fracture	SNF	Physical therapy		62.5% regained independence in ambulation 44% returned home 90% still ind in ambulation after 1 yr
Katz et al., 1964	127 subjects 50–98 yrs old Recent hip fracture	Hospital for persons with prolonged illnesses	Rehabilitation program	Katz ADL scale	24% returned to prefracture ambulation status at 6 mos, 43% at 1 yr, 49% at 18 mos, 50% at 2 yrs 63% ind in ambulation at 6 mos, 71% at 2 yrs 53% regained prior level of ADL skill
Jette et al., 1987	75 subjects >50 yrs Recent hip fracture	Acute hospital	Physical therapy vs. comprehensive team rehabilitation	Functional Status Index	No difference between type of rehab program Persons with intertrochanteric fractures: 53% regained prefracture

Study	Subjects	Setting	Program	Results
Steinberg & Freedland, 1990	144 subjects <75 yrs 102 subjects >75 yrs Acute CVA	Acute hospital	Stroke rehabilitation program	ambulation indoors, 54% outdoors, 49% stair climbing, 21% IADL skill With subcapital fractures 79% indoors, 50% outdoors, 54% stairs, 26 IADL skill No significant differences at discharge between groups in walking, transfers, bladder management, bathing, dressing, or LOS Significant differences in bowel management, eating, and place of discharge
Parry, 1983	100 subjects Mean age 87.6 yrs Various diagnoses	SNF	Geriatric rehabilitation program	Significant improvements in 47%, limited improvements in 32% 71% returned to the community, 56% to previous living situation
Ceder et al., 1980	103 subjects Mean age 75 yrs New hip fracture	Acute hospital	Hospital rehabilitation program and home visits after discharge	75% discharged directly home from acute hospital, 82% and 86% at home at 4 and 12 mos
Kaplan & Ford, 1975	1864 subjects 62-99 yrs Various diagnoses	SNF	Geriatric rehabilitation program	61% discharged; 61% of those (37% of total) returned to independent living

continued

Table 1.1 Continued

Author	Subjects	Setting	Intervention	Scale	Outcome
O'Neil et al., 1987	53 subjects Mean age 78 yrs Various diagnoses	Regional rehab center	Slow-stream rehabilitation program		36% discharged to home, 49% to nursing home, 15% died
Snaedal et al., 1984	78 subjects Hip fracture	Hospital for chronic care	Rehabilitation program		At 4 months of 69 survivors 12% had been discharged to community; at 1 yr of 59 survivors 32% were living in the community

NOTE: BI=brain injury; dec=decrease(d); CVA=stroke; dx=diagnoses; ex=exercise; exp=experimental; grp=group; hr=hour; HR=heart rate; inc=increase(d); ind=independent; LOS=Length of stay; LTC=long-term care; mo=month; OT=occupational therapy; PREs=progressive resistive exercises; PT=physical therapy; RH=Retirement home; RHR=resting heart rate; 1-RM=1 repetition maximum; ROM=range of motion; SBP=systolic blood pressure; SNF=skilled nursing facility; VC=vital capacity; wk=week; x=times; yr=year.

2

Improving Medication Use in the Nursing Home

BRADLEY R. WILLIAMS, PHARM.D.
JOHN F. THOMPSON, PHARM.D.
KENNETH V. BRUMMEL-SMITH, M.D.

INTRODUCTION

The risk to elderly persons posed by medications is well documented. The population age 65 and older consumes more medication than any other segment of the population (51), and nursing home (NH) residents are among the most heavily medicated of this population (61). In addition to the risks presented by the use of multiple medications, the danger is compounded by age-related changes in pharmacokinetic and pharmacodynamic variables (58,49) and poor prescribing habits (63). Indicators of the problem include polypharmacy (37), overuse of PRN drug orders (6,32), and high cost of medications (7). Clinical results of the problem include a high prevalence of adverse drug reactions (9), particularly falls and mental confusion (29,68).

Although the medical literature contains a large body of research that discusses drug-related problems in the elderly, a very small segment is devoted to the NH population. Most of the medication-related research on the NH population focuses on a description of problems encountered. However, there is a limited segment that investigates the role of clinicians, particularly pharmacists, in interventions to alter prescribing or drug use patterns.

Three major issues emerge regarding medication use in the NH: (a) the scope and prevalence of drug-related problems in long-term care facilities, (b) specific strategies for monitoring drug use in nursing homes, and (c) the expanded role of nonphysicians to improve medication use. These issues will be the major focus of this chapter.

SCOPE AND PREVALENCE OF DRUG-RELATED PROBLEMS

Studies of drug use in long-term care institutions date back to at least the 1960s. The primary topics of this research have been psychotropic agents, diuretics and cardiovascular drugs, antibiotics, and recently, histamine-2 receptor antagonists. Other drug classes have also been studied, but much less extensively.

Table 2.1 reviews the literature addressing the use of psychotropic agents. Most studies are descriptive in nature and were conducted in skilled nursing facilities; populations range from a very few to several thousand. Many studies assessed the use of psychotropic agents in general and did not focus on a single pharmacologic or therapeutic class. Most included at least neuroleptics, antidepressants, and anxiolytics/sedative-hypnotics; also included in some studies were cerebral vasodilators (56,85), antihistamines (3,2,43,15), lithium (26,8,10,1), analgesics (33,85), and antiparkinsonism agents (33,8).

Some research included very large populations (85,60,50,8,3,1,23,27) and described wide-ranging problems with the prescribing of many psychotropic agents. Among the problems noted are higher frequency of psychotropic drug use among institutionalized as compared to community-dwelling elderly (85,50), high prescribing rates among physicians with large NH practices and in large facilities (60), excessive duration of therapy (8), and use as chemical restraints (3). Similar problems of inappropriately high use extend to the rest home environment (75,77,1). The consistency of results across studies with varying sample size and different levels of care is both notable and disturbing. It is clear that improvements in psychotropic prescribing in these populations are still needed.

Although eloquently describing the inappropriate use of psychotropic agents in the NH, little of the literature focuses on efforts to improve the situation. Ingman et al. (1975), Fottrell et al. (1976), and Marttila et al. (1977) describe interventions that demonstrated an improvement in prescribing, although no long-term follow-up was conducted in any of these studies. Interventions are described, however, in the body of literature that focuses on clinician activities in NHs that will be discussed later.

Literature focusing on the use of cardiovascular agents and diuretics is reviewed in Table 2.2. In contrast to the descriptive nature of the psychotropic literature, the majority of these articles describe interventions to reduce the use of drugs, primarily cardiac glycosides (55,25,44,79) and diuretics (54), and monitor clinical outcomes. Although the populations in these studies are small, the results are consistent. Based on this limited evidence, it appears that digitalis glycosides are frequently employed without any therapeutic benefit in the NH population and can usually be safely discontinued. The results for diuretics are less consistent but indicate general excessive use.

The use of antibiotics is examined in Table 2.3. This is a very small body of descriptive literature conducted primarily among small samples. Consistent findings are poor diagnostic evaluations (81,86,35,40). Only Katz et al. (1990) addressed the issue of clinical outcomes, finding that most patients improved despite poor evaluation and empiric therapy.

Gastrointestinal drug use is described in Table 2.4. The primary focus of this literature is the use of histamine-2 receptor antagonists. The uniform conclusion is that these drugs are used frequently without justification and for periods of time longer than necessary (66,41,52,22). As with most of the other cited classes, clinical outcomes are not addressed.

Tables 2.5 and 2.6 review the use of anticholinergic and nonsteroidal antiinflammatory drugs, respectively. The little research conducted suggests suboptimal use of both classes of drugs.

STRATEGIES FOR MONITORING DRUG USE

The monitoring of drug use in the NH has been the primary role of the pharmacist through the process of drug regimen review (30). Since the landmark study by Cheung and Kayne (1975) a consistent body of literature has demonstrated the effectiveness of the pharmacist in reducing the number of medications used by patients (see Table 2.7).

In a review of several studies that focused on medication use in NHs, Gurwitz et al. (1990) assessed the results generated by three primary designs: controlled trials, time-series studies, and one-group pretest-posttest. The most frequent intervention in these and other reports is the drug regimen review. Unfortunately, these studies vary widely in design, but most important, few have included control groups. Almost all of the studies involved some measurement of physician or nurse response to consultations provided by the pharmacist as part of the drug regimen review process. Virtually none of the studies measure a patient clinical outcome as a result of the medication change. Other methodological deficiencies include the absence of sufficient data collection in the time-series design studies, failure to control for extraneous factors that may influence the study outcomes, the general use of small convenience samples in one or two facilities, and the use of the patient rather than the prescriber as the unit of analysis.

Although it appears that strategies such as drug regimen review or drug use evaluation, when associated with physician feedback and stop order policies, decrease the number of drugs prescribed, it is unknown whether these changes result in any positive clinical outcomes.

Although physicians appear to be responsive to comments from clinical pharmacists in the NH setting, the response to specific educational programs in office settings is much less clear. Two researchers have attempted to influence physician prescribing for NH patients by directly approaching prescribers in their offices rather than indirectly at the NH. Soumerai and Avorn (1987) demonstrated a positive effect of educational visits ("academic detailing") by clinical pharmacists on physician prescribing, but Ray et al. (1987) found no effect after a similar intervention. A number of factors, such as the structure of the educational visit and the drugs being targeted, may have influenced the outcomes. What is clear is that further research employing this methodology is warranted.

EXPANDED ROLE OF NONPHYSICIANS

Very little attention has been paid to the use of nonphysicians in expanded or nontraditional roles to improve drug utilization in the NH (Table 2.8). Perhaps the best-known study is that conducted by Thompson et al. (1984) employing the clinical pharmacist as a prescriber while working under the supervision of a primary care physician. Several patient outcome measures demonstrated positive change. However, if as Gurwitz et al. (1990) indicate, the unit of analysis had been the prescriber rather than the patient, the positive impact of the prescribing clinical pharmacist may have been much less clear. The study by Kane et al. (1989) indicates a positive effect from the utilization of geriatric nurse practitioners, but drug therapy was only one component; thus the improvement in patient outcome due to the improvement in medication use cannot be evaluated separately.

The research published to date indicates a strong likelihood of dependence on individual practitioners (both physicians and non-physicians involved in the studies) rather than all members of a given profession. There are currently no data to indicate that any of the results can be generalized to any group outside the individual facilities (72,39) or corporations (38) where the practitioners are employed.

RESEARCH AGENDA

Research to date has clearly indicated two facts. First, medications, particularly psychotropic medications (Table 2.1), are inappropriately prescribed for NH patients. Second, the pharmacist, through drug regimen review (Table 2.7), can significantly reduce the number and cost of drugs used in this environment. However, neither the clinical effects of more rational prescribing nor the patient outcomes produced by pharmacist-initiated reductions in drugs administered have been adequately assessed. Future research to improve medication use in the NH will require strengthened designs, focus on patient outcome measurements, and innovative interventions.

Design

The majority of studies conducted to date are surveys or of one-group pretest-posttest design. A major flaw of the survey is its point prevalence nature. Additionally, this design precludes any resolution to problems noted. Difficulties associated with the one-group pretest-posttest design, most notably the lack of a control group, have been well reviewed by Gurwitz et al. (1990). Given the challenge of including control groups in NH settings, the utilization of a time-series design is perhaps the most practical solution for all but the largest projects.

The frequent use of the convenience sample also presents significant obstacles to conducting effective research. Because of the proprietary nature of the NH industry and of the practitioners, the prevalence of convenience or volunteer samples is understandable. However, this decreases the likelihood that results, particularly in studies with small populations, can be generalized. Because many of the practitioners in these settings may have inadequate research skills or resources for analysis, many reports become descriptive rather proving the benefit of a particular intervention. Although the teaching NH may increase the caliber of the research, it may reduce the generalizability of any results by raising the standard of practice to that of an academic site.

Outcome Measures

Outcome measures must reflect positive changes in patient conditions. Variables such as medication orders or medication usage by subjects are frequently studied without addressing other pertinent variables such as actual drug administration (of orders) or appropriate indication or change in subject health status. Measurements include number of drugs, prevalence of use, cost of therapy, acceptance of recommendations, plus myriad others, but few reports seem to use the same set, making comparisons of results difficult if not impossible. Robers (1988) has described several other methodological inconsistencies throughout the NH literature.

Much of the descriptive literature regarding medication use has neglected indications for use. Zawadski et al. (1978) and other researchers (60,4,28,8,75,1,23), all of whom researched populations greater than 1,000, did not address the issue of appropriate diagnosis or indications. Only the literature studying the use of histamine-2 receptor antagonists (Table 2.4) consistently focused on this issue.

The problem of diagnosis or indication is addressed in the literature that discusses strategies to improve medication use (Table 2.7). The activities of the clinical pharmacist and others, particularly through the drug regimen review process, have successfully decreased the number and cost of drugs, but the significance of that success in terms of improved patient outcome has not been determined. There appears to be an underlying assumption that a reduction in the number of drugs per se demonstrates improved drug use, whereas a change to a more appropriate medication or the addition of a new drug may produce a positive change in patient condition.

Potential Strategies

Future research must address several issues. There is a need to determine which drugs in fact are more likely to produce a negative clinical outcome among the institutionalized elderly, particularly those age 80 years and older. One strategy to accomplish this would be the development of a quality-controlled prospective adverse drug reaction (ADR) reporting system. All patients with a change in clinical condition would be assessed at the NH or acute hospital for the contribution by a potential ADR to the change in clinical status. The rationale for this strategy is the hypothesis that the old-old have more adverse reactions from common medications than do the young-old and that many of these reactions are interpreted as the result of "aging," stroke, dementia, or other illness.

The effectiveness of strategies to improve drug use in the NH must also be determined. As mentioned, the change in patient outcome resulting from alterations in drug therapy has not been adequately studied. A large-scale controlled trial utilizing consistent methods and measures will largely eliminate problems encountered in previous studies. An ideal setting would be a large corporate chain or a consortium of facilities throughout several states or geographic regions. Such a setting would improve the chance for standardization of methods and allow the incorporation of a control group. An epidemiologic study is required in order to supply a sufficiently large population to identify infrequent problems such as those encountered with certain types of drugs (e.g., NSAID-induced renal complications).

The role of nonphysicians in improving drug use also requires further study. Although pharmacists and others have demonstrated contributions to improvement in drug use, only one study (72) has focused on the pharmacist as a prescriber and one (38) has addressed the role of the nurse practitioner providing direct patient care. Nothing to date has been published regarding the use of the physician assistant as a primary care provider in the NH. A trial to demonstrate a team approach to primary care is needed utilizing the complementary expertise of a nurse practitioner and pharmacist or physician assistant and pharmacist. These combinations would allow for chronic management of stable patients, freeing the physician to concentrate on complex cases requiring greater diagnostic expertise. Such a study would need a large population, studied under controlled conditions for a sufficient period of time to allow an assessment of clinical outcomes.

A final research strategy is the evaluation of a limited drug formulary for use among NH patients. The formulary would be developed by an expert panel. Protocols requiring specified drug monitoring (e.g., physical assessment, laboratory measures) would be coupled with the formulary. Nonformulary drug requests would be reviewed and approved by an outside expert or panel. The effect of the formulary on drug prescribing and patient outcomes would be evaluated through a controlled trial in matched NHs against an open formulary.

Although a large body of literature addresses various aspects of drug use in NHs, the scope and quality of that literature is quite diverse. A number of important issues have been studied, but rarely have the reports approached the "ideal." The recommendations presented in this chapter are intended to suggest broad topics to be addressed in future research efforts. Adequate investigation will require collaborative efforts among academicians, practitioners, and the NH industry. Accomplishing that will in itself be a major step in improving drug use in the NH.

REFERENCES

1. Avorn, J., Dreyer, P., Connelly, K., et al. (1989). Use of psychoactive medication and the quality of care in rest homes. *New England Journal of Medicine, 320,* 227-232.
2. Beardsley, R. S., Larson, D. B., Burns, B. J., et al. (1989). Prescribing of psychotropics in elderly nursing home patients. *Journal of the American Geriatrics Society, 37,* 327-330.
3. Beers, M., Avorn, J., Soumerai, S. B., et al. (1988). Psychoactive medication use in intermediate-care facility residents. *Journal of the American Medical Association, 260,* 3016-3020.
4. Blazer, D. G., Federspiel, C. F., Ray, W. R., et al. (1983). The risk of anticholinergic toxicity in the elderly: A study of prescribing practices in two populations. *Journal of Gerontology, 38,* 31-35.
5. Brodie, D. C., Lofholm, P., & Benson, R. A. (1977). A model for drug use review in a skilled nursing facility. *Journal of the American Pharmaceutical Association, NS17,* 617-623.
6. Brown, C. H., & DeSimone, E. M. (1980). Use of PRN medications in skilled nursing facilities. *Contemporary Pharmacy Practice, 3,* 209-215.
7. Brown, C. H., & Kirk, K. W. (1984). Cost of discarded medication in Indiana long-term care facilities. *American Journal of Hospital Pharmacy, 41,* 698-702.
8. Buck, J. A. (1988). Psychotropic drug practice in nursing homes. *Journal of the American Geriatrics Society, 36,* 409-418.
9. Budden, F. (1985). Adverse drug reactions in long-term care facility residents. *Journal of the American Geriatrics Society, 35,* 449-450.
10. Burns, B. J., & Kamerow, D. B. (1988). Psychotropic drug prescriptions for nursing home residents. *Journal of Family Practice, 26,* 155-160.
11. Cantù, T. G., & Korek, J. S. (1989). Prescription of neuroleptics for geriatric nursing home patients. *Hospital and Community Psychiatry, 40,* 645-647.
12. Carter, B. L., Small, R. E., & Garnett, W. R. (1981). Monitoring digoxin therapy in two long-term facilities. *Journal of the American Geriatrics Society, 29,* 263-268.
13. Cheung, A., & Kayne, R. (1975). An application of clinical pharmacy services in extended care facilities. *California Pharmacist, 23,* 22-43.

14. Chrymko, M. M., & Conrad, W. F. (1982). Effect of removing clinical pharmacy input. *American Journal of Hospital Pharmacy, 39*, 641.
15. Coccaro, E. F., Kramer, E., Zemishlany, Z., et al. (1990). Pharmacologic treatment of noncognitive behavioral disturbances in elderly demented patients. *American Journal of Psychiatry, 147*, 1640-1645.
16. Cooper, J. W. (1985). Effect of initiation, termination, and reinitiation of consultant clinical pharmacist services in a geriatric long-term care facility. *Medical Care, 23*, 84-88.
17. Cooper, J. W., & Bagwell, C. G. (1978). Contribution of the consultant pharmacist to rational drug usage in the long-term care facility. *Journal of the American Geriatrics Society, 26*, 513-520.
18. Cooper, J. W., & Francisco, G. E. (1980). Psychotropic usage in long-term care geriatric patients. *Hospital Formulary, 16*, 407-419.
19. Crossley, K., Henry, K., Irvine, P., et al. (1987). Antibiotic use in nursing homes: Prevalence, cost and utilization review. *Bulletin of the New York Academy of Medicine, 63*, 510-518.
20. Curtis, J. R., Rovner, B. W., Klein, L. E., et al. (1989). Prescribing efficiently in nursing homes. *Psychosomatics, 30*, 198-202.
21. Degelau, J., Somani, S., Cooper, S. L., et al. (1990). Occurrence of adverse effects and high amantadine concentrations with influenza prophylaxis in the nursing home. *Journal of the American Geriatrics Society, 38*, 428-432.
22. Di Giambattista, R. (1990). H-2 antagonist drug-use review in eight long-term care facilities. *Consultant Pharmacist, 5*, 88-92.
23. Doane, K. W., Risse, S. C., Schrempp, C. O., et al. (1989). Prevalence of neuroleptic use in nursing homes. *Consultant Pharmacist, 4*, 367-370.
24. Elzarian, E. J., Shirachi, D. Y., & Jones, J. K. (1980). Educational approaches to promoting optimal laxative use in long-term-care patients. *Journal of Chronic Disease, 33*, 613-626.
25. Fonrose, H. A., Ahlbaum, N., Bugatch, E., et al. (1974). The efficacy of digitalis withdrawal in an institutional aged population. *Journal of the American Geriatrics Society, 22*, 208-211.
26. Fottrell, E., Sheikh, M., Kothari, R., et al. (1976). Long-stay patients with long-stay drugs. *Lancet, 1*, 81-82.
27. Garrard, J., Makris, L., Dunham, T., et al. (1991). Evaluation of neuroleptic drug use by nursing home elderly under proposed Medicare and Medicaid regulations. *Journal of the American Medical Association, 265*, 463-467.
28. Gilleard, C. J., Morgan, K., & Wade, B. E. (1983). Patterns of neuroleptic use among the institutionalized elderly. *Acta Psychiatrica Scandinavica, 68*, 419-425.
29. Granek, E., Baker, S. P., Abbey, H., et al. (1987). Medications and diagnoses in relation to falls in a long-term care facility. *Journal of the American Geriatrics Society, 35*, 503-511.
30. Gurwitz, J. H., Soumerai, S. B., & Avorn, J. (1990). Improving medication prescribing and utilization in the nursing home. *Journal of the American Geriatrics Society, 38*, 542-552.
31. Hood, J. C., Lemberger, M., & Stewart, R. S. (1975). Promoting appropriate therapy in a long-term care facility. *Journal of the American Pharmaceutical Association, NS15*, 32-37.
32. Howard, J. B., Strong, K. E., & Strong, K. E., Jr. (1977). Medication procedures in a nursing home: Abuse of PRN orders. *Journal of the American Geriatrics Society, 25*, 83-84.

33. Ingman, S. R., Lawson, I. R., Pierpaoli, P. G., et al. (1975). A survey of the prescribing and administration of drugs in a long-term care institution for the elderly. *Journal of the American Geriatrics Society, 23,* 309-316.
34. James, D. S. (1985). Survey of hypnotic drug use in nursing homes. *Journal of the American Geriatrics Society, 33,* 436-439.
35. Jones, S. R., Parker, D. F., Liebow, E. S., et al. (1987). Appropriateness of antibiotic therapy in long-term care facilities. *American Journal of Medicine, 83,* 499-502.
36. Jue, S. G., Clark, B. G., & Araki, M. (1985). Inservice teaching and adverse drug reactions in a nursing home. *Drug Intelligence and Clinical Pharmacy, 19,* 483-487.
37. Kalchthaler, T., Coccaro, E., & Lichtiger, S. (1977). Incidence of polypharmacy in a long-term care facility. *Journal of the American Geriatrics Society, 25,* 308-313.
38. Kane, R. L., Garrard, J., Skay, C. L., et al. (1989). Effects of a geriatric nurse practitioner on process and outcome of nursing home care. *American Journal of Public Health, 79,* 1271-1277.
39. Karki, S. D., Mott, P., & Rosato, L. (1991). Impact of a team approach on reducing polypharmacy. *Consultant Pharmacist, 6,* 133-137.
40. Katz, P. R., Beam, T. R., Brand, F., et al. (1990). Antibiotic use in the nursing home: Physician practice patterns. *Archives of Internal Medicine, 150,* 1465-1468.
41. Kreling, D. H., & Schommer, J. C. (1990). Costs of potentially inappropriate psychotropic drug orders for nursing home residents: Method and estimation. *Consultant Pharmacist, 5,* 166-172.
42. Lamy, P. P., & Krug, B. H. (1978). Review of laxative utilization in a skilled nursing facility. *Journal of the American Geriatrics Society, 26,* 544-549.
43. Lantz, M. S., Louis, A., Lowenstein, G., et al. (1990). A longitudinal study of psychotropic prescriptions in a teaching nursing home. *American Journal of Psychiatry, 147,* 1637-1639.
44. Lapierre, G., Pevonka, M. P., Stewart, R. B., et al. (1983). Evaluation of hypertensive therapy in a skilled nursing facility. *Drug Intelligence and Clinical Pharmacy, 17,* 39-44.
45. Lipowski, E. E., Bauwens, S. F., & Collins, T. M. (1988). An examination of histamine-2 receptor antagonist use by Medicaid recipients in Wisconsin long-term care facilities. *Journal of the American Geriatrics Society, 36,* 531-536.
46. Marttila, J. K., Hammel, R. J., Alexander, B., et al. (1977). Potential untoward effect of long-term use of flurazepam in geriatric patients. *Journal of the American Pharmaceutical Association, NS17,* 692-695.
47. Meuleman, J. R., Nelson, R. C., & Clark, R. L. (1987). Evaluation of temazepam and diphenhydramine as hypnotics in a nursing-home population. *Drug Intelligence and Clinical Pharmacy, 21,* 716-720.
48. Milliren, J. W. (1977). Some contingencies affecting the utilization of tranquilizers in long-term care of the elderly. *Journal of Health and Social Behavior, 18,* 206-211.
49. Montamat, S. C., Cusack, B. J., & Vestal, R. E. (1989). Management of drug therapy in the elderly. *New England Journal of Medicine, 321,* 303-309.
50. Morgan, K., & Gilleard, C. J. (1981). Patterns of hypnotic prescribing and usage in residential homes for the elderly. *Neuropharmacology, 20,* 1355-1356.
51. National Center for Health Statistics. (1987). *Health statistics on older persons—United States, 1986* (DHHS Publication Number (PHS) 87-1409). Washington, DC: U.S. Department of Health and Human Services.
52. O'Connor, T. W., Solomon, D. A., & Nicholas, B. A. (1989). Substitution of antacid therapy for inappropriate H-2-antagonist therapy in long-term care facilities. *Consultant Pharmacist, 4,* 643-649.

53. Pink, L. A., Cooper, J. W., & Francis, W. R. (1985). Digoxin-related pharmacist-physician communications in a long-term care facility: Their acceptance and effects. *Nursing Homes, 34,* 25-30.

54. Portnoi, V. A., & Pawlson, L. G. (1981). Abuse of diuretic therapy in nursing homes. *Journal of Chronic Disease, 34,* 363-365.

55. Priddle, W. W., & Rose, M. (1966). Curtailing therapy in a home for the aged, with special reference to digitalis, diuretics and low-sodium diet. *Journal of the American Geriatrics Society, 14,* 731-734.

56. Prien, R. F., Haber, P. A., & Caffey, E. M. (1975). The use of psychoactive drugs in elderly patients with psychiatric disorders: Survey conducted in twelve Veterans Administration hospitals. *Journal of the American Geriatrics Society, 23,* 104-112.

57. Pucino, F., Baumgart, P. J., Strommen, G. L., et al. (1988). Evaluation of therapeutic drug monitoring in a long-term care facility: A pilot project. *Drug Intelligence and Clinical Pharmacy, 22,* 594-596.

58. Pucino, F., Beck, C. L., Seifert, R. L., et al. (1985). Pharmacogeriatrics. *Pharmacotherapy, 5,* 314-326.

59. Ray, W. A., Blazer, D. G., Schaffner, W., et al. (1987). Reducing antipsychotic drug prescribing for nursing home patients: A controlled trial of the effect of an educational visit. *American Journal of Public Health, 77,* 1448-1450.

60. Ray, W. A., Federspiel, C. F., & Schaffner, W. (1980). A study of antipsychotic drug use in nursing homes: Epidemiologic evidence suggesting misuse. *American Journal of Public Health, 70,* 485-491.

61. Robers, P. A. (1988). Extent of medication use in U.S. long-term care facilities. *American Journal of Hospital Pharmacy, 45,* 93-100.

62. Rovner, B. W., David, A., Lucas-Blaustein, M. J., et al. (1988). Self-care capacity and anticholinergic drug levels in nursing home patients. *American Journal of Psychiatry, 145,* 107-109.

63. Segal, J. L., Thompson, J. F., & Floyd, R. A. (1979). Drug utilization and prescribing patterns in a skilled nursing facility: The need for a rational approach to therapeutics. *Journal of the American Geriatrics Society, 27,* 117-122.

64. Seifert, R., Jamieson, J., & Gardner, R. (1983). Use of anticholinergics in the nursing home: An empirical study and review. *Drug Intelligence and Clinical Pharmacy, 17,* 470-473.

65. Shannon, R. C., & DeMuth, J. E. (1984). Application of federal indicators in nursing home drug regimen review. *American Journal of Hospital Pharmacy, 41,* 912-916.

66. Sherman, D. S., Avorn, J., & Campion, E. W. (1987). Cimetidine use in nursing homes: Prolonged therapy and excessive doses. *Journal of the American Geriatrics Society, 35,* 1023-1027.

67. Sloane, P. D., Mathew, L. J., Scarborough, M., et al. (1991). Physical and pharmacologic restraint of nursing home patients with dementia. *Journal of the American Medical Association, 265,* 1278-1282.

68. Sobel, K. G., & McCart, G. M. (1983). Drug use and accidental falls in an intermediate care facility. *Drug Intelligence and Clinical Pharmacy, 17,* 539-542.

69. Soumerai, S. B., & Avorn, J. (1987). Predictors of physician prescribing change in an educational experiment to improve medication use. *Medical Care, 25,* 210-222.

70. Strandberg, L. R., Dawson, G. W., Mathieson, D., et al. (1980). Effect of comprehensive pharmaceutical services on drug use in long-term care facilities. *American Journal of Hospital Pharmacy, 37,* 92-94.

71. Taylor, A. T., & Martell, P. H. (1980). Physician acceptance of clinical pharmacy service in a skilled nursing home. *Journal of the American Geriatrics Society, 28,* 227-229.

72. Thompson, J. F., McGhan, W. F., Ruffalo, R. L., et al. (1984). Clinical pharmacist prescribing drug therapy in a geriatric setting: Outcome of a trial. *Journal of the American Geriatrics Society, 32,* 154-159.

73. Tsai, A. E., Cooper, J. W., & McCall, C. Y. (1982). Pharmacist impact on hematopoietic and vitamin therapy in a geriatric long-term care facility. *Hospital Formulary, 17,* 225-241.

74. Vlasses, P. H., Lucarotti, R. L., Miller, D. A., et al. (1977). Drug therapy review in a skilled nursing facility: An innovative approach. *Journal of the American Pharmaceutical Association, NS17,* 92-94.

75. Weedle, P. B., Poston, J. W., & Parish, P. A. (1988a). Use of hypnotic medicines by elderly people in residential homes. *Journal of the Royal College of General Practitioners, 38,* 156-158.

76. Weedle, P. B., Poston, J. W., & Parish, P. A. (1988b). The use of digoxin in 55 residential homes for elderly people. *Postgraduate Medical Journal, 64,* 292-296.

77. Weedle, P. B., Poston, J. W., & Parish, P. A. (1990). Drug prescribing in residential homes for elderly people in the United Kingdom. *DICP, The Annals of Pharmacotherapy, 24,* 533-536.

78. Wilcher, D. E., & Cooper, J. W. (1981). The consultant pharmacist and analgesic/anti-inflammatory drug usage in a geriatric long-term care facility. *Journal of the American Geriatrics Society, 29,* 429-432.

79. Wilkins, C. E., & Khurana, M. B. (1985). Digitalis withdrawal in elderly nursing home patients. *Journal of the American Geriatrics Society, 33,* 850-851.

80. Williams, B. R. (1991). Risk of NSAID-induced renal toxicity in institutionalized elderly. *Journal of Geriatric Drug Therapy, 5(3),* 47-57.

81. Williams, B. R., Ferraro, R., Nurse, J., et al. (1980). Treatment of urinary tract infections in skilled nursing facility patients. *Contemporary Pharmacy Practice, 3,* 1-5.

82. Williamson, D. H., Cooper, J. W., Kotzan, J. A., et al. (1984). Consultant pharmacist impact on antihypertensive therapy in a geriatric long-term care facility. *Hospital Formulary, 19,* 123-128.

83. Witte, K. W. (1982). Digoxin-use review in a skilled-nursing facility. *American Journal of Hospital Pharmacy, 39,* 1530-1532.

84. Young, L. Y., Leach, D. B., Anderson, D. A., et al. (1981). Decreased medication costs in a skilled nursing facility by clinical pharmacy services. *Contemporary Pharmacy Practice, 4,* 233-237.

85. Zawadski, R. T., Glazer, G. B., & Lurie, E. (1978). Psychotropic drug use among institutionalized and noninstitutionalized Medicaid aged in California. *Journal of Gerontology, 33,* 825-834.

86. Zimmer, J. G., Bentley, D. W., Valenti, W. M., et al. (1986). Systemic antibiotic use in nursing homes: A quality assessment. *Journal of the American Geriatrics Society, 34,* 703-710.

Table 2.1 Psychotropic Agents

References	Subjects Number/Age	Location	Design/Drugs Studied	Methods/Intervention	Conclusions/Outcomes	Limits
Prien et al., 1975	N=1,276 Age≥60	VA hosp (long stay)	Descriptive AD, AP, AX, CV	Chart review of psychoactive drug use in patients with primary psychiatric diagnosis	61% of patients received psychoactive drug Use and dose related to diagnosis and age Choice of drug unrelated to age	Convenience sample survey Unreliability of diagnosis Primarily male subjects
Ingman et al., 1975	N=131 Elderly	ECF	Descriptive, 10-month survey "Neuroactive": AD, AG, AP, AH, TN, AX, SH, Autonomics, "Others"	Pretest-posttest Implementation of a policy to rewrite all orders each month	More neuroactive drugs at baseline for patients with higher cognitive or physical function Reduced prescribing with new policy	Small sample No diagnostic information No assessment of appropriateness of orders
Fottrell et al., 1976	N=200 Adults	Long-stay psychiatric hospital	Quasi-experimental Randomized AD, AP, AX, L, SH	Pre- and posteval-uation of clinical status and mental state after alteration of psychotropic drugs	Approximately 1/2 of patients on psychotropic drugs improved or unchanged with reduced medication	One hospital Nonspecific criteria for drug alteration Unblinded Diagnosis, drug, dose information not stated Psychiatric patients only

continued

Table 2.1 Continued

References	Subjects Number/Age	Location	Design/Drugs Studied	Methods/Intervention	Conclusions/Outcomes	Limits
Marttila et al., 1977	N=750 Elderly	SNF, ICF	Quasi-experimental SH	Chart review of flurazepam orders Presentation of findings to utilization review committee	Adverse reactions correlated with dose and frequency of use Oversedation noted among infrequent users Presentation of findings to committee reduced prescribing	Convenience sample Contribution to other agents not evaluated No follow-up to reduced prescribing
Milliren, 1977	N=131 Elderly	ECF	Descriptive Randomized cross-section of convenience sample Same drugs as Ingman et al., 1975	Secondary analysis of data from Ingman et al., 1975 Correlate major tranquilizer use to patient characteristics	Higher use of "neuroactive" drugs among females, patients with low mental status, patients unfriendly to staff	Small convenience sample One facility
Zawadski et al., 1978	N=2 million Medicaid Age≥60; young	LTCF; community	Descriptive Retrospective survey All prescribed drugs	Review of paid claims data for 15 most frequently prescribed drugs	Aged use more drugs than young; institutionalized aged use more drugs than noninstitutionalized aged Psychotropic drug use is frequent among the institutionalized aged	Expenditures used to determine drug usage No diagnosis information No measure of appropriateness of prescribing

46

Study	Sample	Setting	Design	Purpose	Findings	Limitations
Ray et al., 1980	N=5,902 Medicaid Age≥65	ICF	Descriptive Retrospective review of paid claims data AP	Review 1 year paid claims data for antipsychotic drugs Correlate drug use to facility and prescriber characteristics	9% of antipsychotic users were receiving drug chronically High prescription rates associated with family practice, rural setting, large NH practice, large facility size One MD as primary prescriber associated with high prescription rates	No chart review No diagnosis information Arbitrary definition of "chronic use" for psychotropic drugs
Morgan & Gilleard, 1981	N=1,154 Elderly	Local authority homes	Survey SH	Measure prevalence of use	Use higher than among community elderly Positive correlation between use and age, but none for dose and age No preference for short-acting agents	Descriptive only No reports regarding adverse reactions
Gilleard et al., 1983	N=839 Age≥60	LTCF, acute hospitals, rehab, assessment units	Descriptive Cross-sectional population study AP	Review of patient and medication administrative records for previous 24 hrs Interview of ward staff	Neuroleptic use associated with patients who were confused, weepy, never cheerful, disturbed others at night, use of concurrent hypnotics No correlation with incontinence, immobility Use rates possibly reflect institutional practice rather than patient need	Local sample No dosage analysis Point prevalence design

continued

Table 2.1 Continued

References	Subjects Number/Age	Location	Design/Drugs Studied	Methods/Intervention	Conclusions/Outcomes	Limits
James, 1985	N=765 Elderly	SNF, ICF	Descriptive SH	Survey of volunteer homes	10% using hypnotics; 11% with HS orders for sedative drugs Flurazepam often used >1 yr duration	Convenience sample "Snapshot" variety
Meuleman et al., 1987	N=17 Elderly	VA NH	Randomized, double-blind, crossover-placebo-controlled SH	Temazepam 15 mg vs. diphenhydramine 50 mg, 5-night therapy with 72-hr washout Sleep questionnaire, cognitive and psychomotor testing	Improved sleep latency and prolonged sleep with diphenhydramine Nonsignificant decrease in neurologic function with temazepam Equal effectiveness	Small sample No control of other medications Short term Only neurologic adverse impacts assessed
Buck, 1988	N=19,516 Medicaid Age≥18	SNF, ICF, ICF/MR	Descriptive AP, AD, AX, SH, PK, L, DHE, Methyl-phenidate, Pemoline	Review of Medicaid paid claims data Multiple regression analysis	Age, functional mental illness associated with psychotropic drug use Most treatment >6 mos Little association with facility characteristics	Medicaid population Only primary diagnoses considered in analyses Information obtained solely from paid claims data
Burns & Kamerow, 1988	N=526 Adults	NH	Descriptive Stratified random sample Volunteer NH AP, AD, SH, AX, L	Review of Nat'l NH Survey Pretest data for psychotropic drugs	32% of all patients received psychotropic drugs Prescribing appropriate for 46%; no indication for 30%	Unreliable diagnosis Volunteer sample Limited data available for drug evaluation Not generalizable

48

Study	Sample	Setting	Design/Drugs	Method	Findings	Limitations
Beers et al., 1988	N=850 Adults (4%<65)	ICF	Descriptive AP, AD, SH, AX(BZDP)	1-mo longitudinal survey of medical records	Over 50% received psychoactive medications, often drugs not appropriate for elderly Neuroleptics used in nonpsychiatric patients, high use of psychoactive drugs on a PRN basis. Use patterns consistent with "chemical restraints"	ICF only Exclusively nonpsychiatric facilities
Avorn et al., 1989	N=1,201 Adults	RH	Descriptive Stratified random sample AP	Statewide survey with follow-up of subsample with large psychiatric population or high psychoactive drug use Chart review; resident testing; staff test for drug knowledge	High use of psychoactive medications Minimal professional supervision Need for more regulatory monitoring	Selection of homes with high psychiatric population Lack of diagnostic information, no evaluation of appropriateness of therapy
Doane et al., 1989	N=4,571 Geriatric	NH	Descriptive AP	3-mo survey during drug regimen review	No correlation between neuroleptic use and facility size Use of neuroleptics lower in facilities with dementia units	Convenience sample No diagnosis data No data of PRN use No data presented to compare use of neuroleptics in dementia units

continued

Table 2.1 Continued

References	Subjects Number/Age	Location	Design/Drugs Studied	Methods/Intervention	Conclusions/Outcomes	Limits
Cantú & Korek, 1989	N=100 Age≥65	NH	Descriptive Randomized from convenience sample AP	1-mo retrospective chart review Compare prescribing to NIMH criteria for neuroleptic use	Problems noted with inappropriate diagnosis or target symptoms, unclear or incomplete PRN orders, excessive doses	Small sample One MD wrote 79% or neuroleptic orders. Unvalidated criteria for evaluation of prescribing
Beardsley et al., 1989	N=526 Age≥65	SNF, ICF	Descriptive Stratified random sample of volunteer NH AP, AD, AX, SH	Record review and interview Data from National NH Pretest Survey Analysis of frequency of use	Frequent use of multiple psychotropics. Frequent duplication of therapy 21% with no supporting diagnosis	Unreliable diagnoses Limited data for assessment of appropriateness Drug orders only, no record of administration
Kreling et al., 1990	N=760 Age≥65	LTCF	Descriptive AP, AD, AX, SH	Review 1-mo billing period to estimate direct cost of inappropriate prescribing	80.7% of dollars spent were for inappropriately prescribed medications Most frequent problem was no indication for use	Convenience sample Assumption that no written diagnosis equaled no indication 1983 data, with 1988 cost estimates Cost estimated from brand name for some multisource drugs
Lantz et al., 1990	N=91 Elderly	NH	Descriptive AP, AD, AX, AH	Medical record abstract, 30-day period annually for 5 yrs Analyze use patterns	Episodic use more common than continuous use Need for prospective, longitudinal research assessing efficacy and adverse effects	Teaching NH, atypical facility Stringent definition of continuous use No evaluation of appropriateness of prescribing

Study	Location	Sample	Design	Method	Findings	Limitations
Coccaro et al., 1990	LTCF	$N=59$ Age ≥55	Randomized, double-blind, crossover Haloperidol, exazepam, and diphenhydramine	Washout, 2-wk dosage adjustment, 4-wk therapy for agitation	All three agents equally effective No cognitive effects	Small population No placebo therapy Short-term trial
Sloane et al., 1991	SNF	$N=625$ Elderly	Descriptive Randomized from volunteer NH AP, AD, AX, SH	Observation, interview, questionnaire to compare dementia units with standard SNF	Dementia units reduce physical restraint but not drug use Multiple factors predict choice of restraints	Cross-sectional Short term Possible bias in patient characteristics (unit vs. nonunit)
Garrard et al., 1991	NH	$N=3,191$ Age≥65	Descriptive Nonproportionate, simple random sample AP	Abstract patient health records to evaluate neuroleptic prescribing based on OBRA 1987 criteria for patients on admission and after admission	No correlation with NH characteristics Age ≥85, other mental disorders, and admission from acute hospital predict "ineligible" prescribing	Not all neuroleptics recorded Other psychotropic drugs excluded Record review only

NOTE: Location: ECF—Extended care; ICF—Intermediate care; LTCF—Long-term care; NH—Nursing home; RH—Rest home; SNF—Skilled nursing. Drug: AD—antidepressant; AG—analgesic; AHTN—antihypertensive; AH—antihistamine; AP—antipsychotic; AX—anxiolytic; CV—cerebrovasodilator; L—lithium; PK—parkinsonism; SH—sedative hypnotics.

Table 2.2 Cardiovascular Drugs and Diuretics

Reference	Subjects Number/Age	Location	Design/Drugs Studied	Methods/Interventions	Conclusions/Outcomes	Limits
Priddle & Rose, 1966	N=110 Elderly	NH	Prospective, open trial CG, D, K	In patients with no clear indication, discontinue diuretic and potassium; if no adverse effects, discontinue digitalis.	Therapy altered in 39 of 110 subjects. Periodic review to change drug regimen is warranted	Small population; No control; Single facility; Few data presented
Fonrose et at., 1974	N=31 Elderly	LTCF	Single-blind, placebo-controlled CG	In patients without documented need, replace digitalis with placebo	15 of 31 subjects did not require digitalis after 4 mos. Periodically reevaluate cardiac status for continued need	Small population; Single facility; Few data presented
Carter et al., 1981	N=57 Age≥59	SNF, ICF	Descriptive Retrospective CG	Chart review to examine appropriateness of digitalis use measured against 13 audit criteria	Most subjects met diagnosis criteria; dose and laboratory monitoring criteria not frequently met. Toxicity associated with poor monitoring	Small population; Few prescribers; Arbitrary criteria; Retrospective review
Portnoi & Pawlson, 1981	N=27 Elderly	NH	Prospective Unblinded D	Discontinue diuretic and observe subjects for 6 mos	3 deaths, unrelated to therapy. No problems related to HTN or CHF. Symptomatic improvement in some subjects. Diuretics overused in the NH population	Small population; Study conducted in one facility; Unblinded design

Study	N/Age	Location	Design	Intervention	Findings	Limitations
Witte, 1982	N=23 Elderly	SNF	OGPPT CG	Concurrent DUE	Overuse of serum levels; Improved outcomes with pharmacist monitoring	Small population; Short term; Arbitrary criteria for appropriateness
Lapierre et al., 1983	N=32 Age>60	NH	Prospective Blinded observers CG	Monitoring of ongoing hypertension treatment	Excessive, unnecessary treatment in 9 of 21 drug-treated subjects; Poor documentation in medical records; Frequent review of therapy is warranted	Small population; Study conducted in a single facility
Wilkins & Khurana, 1985	N=26 Elderly	NH	Prospective CG	If subject in normal sinus rhythm, discontinue drug and monitor for 4 mo	19 of 19 subjects did not require digoxin; CHF patients can be safely taken off digitalis; care needed with atrial fibrillation	Small population; Study conducted in a single facility
Weedle et al., 1988b	N=1,888 Age>60	RH	Descriptive Epidemiologic CG	Record review, interview	Digitalis recipients older; Frequent potential drug interactions; Periodic review to confirm continued need is warranted	Retrospective; No clear diagnosis information

NOTE: Location: ICF—Intermediate care; LTCF—Long-term care; NH—Nursing home; RH—Rest home; SNF—Skilled nursing. Design: OGPPT—One-group pretest-posttest. Intervention: DUE—Drug use evaluation. Drug: AH—antihypertensives; CG—cardiac glycosides; D—diuretics; K—potassium supplements.

Table 2.3 Antibiotics

Reference	Subjects Number/Age	Location	Design	Methods/Interventions	Conclusions/Outcomes	Limits
Williams et al., 1980	N=114 Age≥49	SNF	Descriptive	Record review of patients with UTI to assess therapy	Poor diagnosis, drug treatment, and follow-up Medicaid patients less likely to receive appropriate antibiotic therapy	Small population Arbitrary criteria for appropriateness Weak statistical analysis Point prevalence Not outcome based
Zimmer et al., 1986	N=173 Age≥57	SNF, ICF	Descriptive	Chart review of patients with antibiotic therapy within previous 30 days Match treatment against developed criteria	Low use rate Poor documentation, incomplete workups Overall antibiotic treatment frequently inappropriate Infection treatment in SNF an often-neglected problem	Point prevalence Liberal criteria for appropriate therapy Not outcome based
Crossley et al., 1987	N=117 NH	NH	Descriptive	Telephone survey of nursing directors and pharmacy suppliers Compare antibiotic costs and use patterns	Antibiotic costs are higher in NH than in the community	Telephone survey of volunteer participants Survey content not stated Localized to one metropolitan area
Jones et al., 1987	N=96 Adults	NH	Descriptive	Review of abstracted medical records and reports by three reviewers to assess antibiotic therapy	Less than 50% of infections treated appropriately Cephalosporins most often used inappropriately;	Small population Study limited to two nursing homes Interrater reliability not tested Not outcome based

					cotrimoxazole most often used appropriately Antibiotic therapy generally not well managed Physician education, treatment guidelines are needed	
Degelau, 1990	N=98 Age≥63	NH	Open-label, controlled trial	Amantadine 100 mg QD or 200 mg QD for 14 days	Adverse effects in 22%; associated with higher mg/kg doses Large variability in drug serum concentrations Cost, safety, and efficacy of low-dose amantadine requires study	Small population
Katz, 1990	N=720	SNF, ICF	Noncurrent, prospective	Quarterly chart review Clarify prescribing and assess treatment outcome over 1 year	Subjective symptoms, laboratory/physical criteria most common for diagnosis Poor or questionable documentation for antibiotic use Most patients were clinically better despite empiric treatment	Limited to two nursing homes Number of prescribers not indicated

NOTE: Location: ICF—Intermediate care; NH—Nursing home; SNF—Skilled nursing.

Table 2.4 Gastrointestinal Agents

Reference	Subjects Number/Age	Location	Design/Drugs Studied	Methods/Interventions	Conclusions/Outcomes	Limits
Lamy & Krug, 1978	N=73 Age not stated	SNF	Descriptive LAX	Chart review to determine use patterns	50 of 73 patients receiving laxatives Overall use pattern was appropriate Insufficient attention paid to diet	Small population Convenience sample No diagnosis noted No criteria stated for determining appropriateness
Elzarian et al., 1980	N=87 Elderly	NH	Pre- and posttest	In-service education	Decreased laxative use	Small population Not outcome based
Sherman et al., 1987	N=60 Age≥63	NH	Descriptive Cimetidine	Record review to assess use patterns	60 of 3,042 patients received cimetidine Generally excessive treatment duration Poor justification Assessment of risk/benefit of continued therapy is needed	Point prevalence Not outcome based
Lipowski et al., 1988	N=1,046 Age not stated	NH	Descriptive H2	Record review; paid claims data review; questionnaire	Frequent multiple therapies Excessive duration No indication in 49% General pattern of inappropriate prescribing	Medicaid population Point prevalence

O'Connor et al., 1989	N=1,630 Age not stated	LTCF	Cost analysis survey H2	Review medical records; assess cost savings by substituting antacids when appropriate	42% of H2-antagonist therapy inappropriate Potential savings of up to $345,000 by antacid substitution	Convenience sample during drug regimen review Point prevalence
Di Giambattista, 1990	N=74 Adults	SNF, ICF	Descriptive H2	Chart review	Appropriate diagnosis in 65% Excessive duration in all subjects	Convenience sample Number of prescribers not stated

NOTE: Location: ICF—Intermediate care; LTCF—Long-term care; NH—Nursing home; SNF—Skilled nursing. Drugs: H2—histamine-2-receptor antagonists; LAX—laxatives.

Table 2.5 Anticholinergic Agents

Reference	Subjects Number/Age	Location	Design	Methods/Interventions	Conclusions/Outcomes	Limits
Blazer et al., 1983	N=5,902 Age≥65	SNF	Descriptive	Retrospective review of paid claims files	59% received anticholinergic drugs Higher toxicity risk than in comparable ambulatory group More SNF patients taking multiple drugs	Medicaid population No diagnosis data or assessment of appropriateness Estimates only of use patterns
Seifert et al., 1983	N=83 Age≥55	SNF	Descriptive	Evaluation of mental status, anticholinergic drug use, and dosage in confused and nonconfused patients	Nonsignificantly higher doses among confused patients	Small population No measures of appropriateness Unclear evaluation methods for confusion
Rovner et al., 1988	N=22 Elderly	ICF	Prospective	Correlate serum levels of anticholinergic drugs with self-care skills in demented patients	Higher serum levels associated with lower self-care skills	Small population Specific drugs and doses not indicated Medications were not stopped and skills not retested

NOTE: Location: ICF—Intermediate care; SNF—Skilled nursing.

58

Table 2.6 Nonsteroidal Antiinflammatory Drugs

Reference	Subjects Number/Age	Location	Design	Methods/Interventions	Conclusions/Outcomes	Limits
Wilcher & Cooper, 1981	N=143 Elderly	SNF, ICF	OGPPT	Concurrent DUE	Decrease in use of codeine, acetaminophen Increased use of NSAID More use of scheduled analgesics for chronic pain	Small population No data on prevalence of use before or after intervention Number of prescribers is not stated
Williams, 1991	N=357 Age≥65	SNF	Descriptive	Chart review for prevalence of NSAID use and assessment of renal function	11% using NSAIDs Poor documentation of reasons for use Nonsignificantly higher prevalence of hypertension among users 20% of NSAID users monitored for renal function More research needed to determine risk of renal complications in SNF	Small population Limited to two facilities Arbitrary criteria for renal function monitoring

NOTE: Location: ICF—Intermediate care; SNF—Skilled nursing; Design: OGPPT—One-group pretest-posttest; Intervention: DUE—Drug use evaluation; NSAID—Nonsteroidal antiinflammatory drug.

Table 2.7 Strategies to Improve Medication Use

Reference	Subjects	Location	Design	Intervention	Conclusions/Outcomes	Limits
Cheung & Kayne, 1975	N=517	SNF	OGPPT	DRR	18% reduction in prescriptions; Reduction in drug administration errors, adverse drug reactions; Reduced costs to health care system	Number of prescribers not stated; Patient outcomes not stated
Hood et al., 1975	N=40	SNF	NR-CT	DRR	11% reduction in medications	No group data to compare compatibility
Brodie et al., 1977	N=55	SNF	OGPPT	DRR	32% reduction in prescriptions	Number of prescribers not stated; Patient outcomes not stated
Vlasses et al., 1977	N=116	SNF	OGPPT	DRR	71% of communications answered by prescriber; 53% of pharmacist recommendations implemented	Small population; Number of prescribers not stated; Patient outcomes not indicated
Cooper & Bagwell, 1978	N=116	SNF	OGPPT	DRR	34% reduction in average drugs/patient; 46% reduction in PRN medications; 19% reduction in routine medications	Study conducted in one facility; Number of prescribers not stated; Automatic stop orders begun concurrently

Study	N	Setting	Design	Intervention	Results	Comments
Strandberg et al., 1980	N=401	SNF, ICF	Time series	DRR, DUR, Stop orders	No change in mean drugs/patient Decreased total doses/patient/month 19% decrease in number of prescriptions per patient/month 32% decrease in number of nonprescription drugs/patient/month	Number of prescribers not stated Patient outcomes not indicated
Taylor & Martell, 1980	N=92	SNF	OGPPT	Pharmacist participation in patient care conferences	75.8% acceptance rate of pharmacist recommendations	Single facility Number of prescribers not stated No clinical outcome data
Cooper & Francisco, 1980	N=104	SNF	OGPPT	DRR	Reduced psychotropic drug orders from 90% to 36% of patients	No data on actual consumption Single facility Number of prescribers not stated
Young et al., 1981	N=25	SNF	Time series	DRR	Reduced average number of drugs/patient from 6.0 to 4.2 Reduced administered doses by 18.5% Cost savings of $0.40/patient day	Single facility Small population Number of prescribers not indicated No patient outcome data

continued

Table 2.7 Continued

Reference	Subjects	Location	Design	Intervention	Conclusions/Outcomes	Limits
Chrymko & Conrad, 1982	$N=21$	LTCU	OGPPT	Effect of loss of consultant pharmacist	19% increase in prescriptions	No patient outcome data Small population
Tsai et al., 1982	$N=53$	NH	OGPPT	DRR	42% increase in iron supplements and vitamins after intervention	Inadequate clinical data on patients
Shannon & DeMuth, 1984	$N=1,132$	SNF, ICF	Survey	Review drug orders and check against federal indicators	Medications similar in SNF and ICF Significantly more drug administration errors in facilities where indicators not applied	No patient outcome data
Williamson et al., 1984	$N=30$	LTCF	NR-CT	DRR	Increased systolic BP, decreased adverse reaction risk in experimental group	Control group not receiving antihypertensive therapy No data on how adverse drug reactions were measured
Cooper, 1985	$N=72$	LTCF	OGPPT	Initiation, termination, and reinstitution of consultant pharmacist	Drug use reduced by 46.1% and 42.7% Higher hospitalization and fewer deaths	LTCF was facing closure—number of prescribers not indicated

Study	N	Location	Design	Intervention	Results	Comments
Jue et al., 1985	N=173	SNF	NR-CT	DRR, In-service	10.8% incidence of potential adverse drug reactions Nonsignificant decrease in study facility In-service ineffective in increasing nursing staff ability to report adverse drug reactions	Presence of nurse practitioner in control facility may have confounded the results
Pink et al., 1985	N=83	LTCF	OGPPT	DRR	Reduced digoxin use in consulted patients	No clinical data on cardiac outcomes
Ray et al., 1987	N=200 (MDs)	MD office	NR-CT	Academic detailing	No decrease in medication orders for psychotropic drugs	Education to physicians only
Soumerai & Avorn, 1987	N=319 (MDs)	MD office	R-CT	Academic detailing	18% reduction in orders for targeted drugs (cephalexin, cerebral vasodilators, propoxyphene)	Education to physicians only
Curtis et al., 1989	N=175	SNF	OGPPT	Recommend changes in number of doses/day or time of administration	Medication administration time reduced 19% cost savings for drug administration	Appropriateness of therapy not addressed

NOTE: Location: ICF—Intermediate care; LTCF—Long-term care; LTCU—Long-term care unit; NH—Nursing home; SNF—Skilled nursing. Design: NR-CT—Nonrandomized, controlled trial; OGPPT—One-group pretest-posttest; R-CT—Randomized, controlled trial. Intervention: DRR—Drug regimen review.

Table 2.8 Role of Nonphysicians

Reference	Subjects	Location	Design	Intervention	Conclusions/Outcomes	Limits
Thompson et al., 1984	$N=152$	SNF	PPT-CT	Drug management by clinical pharmacists	Reduced number of drugs Reduced hospitalization More discharges to lower care levels Fewer deaths Potential cost savings	Patient, not prescriber, as unit of analysis Subjects not randomly assigned Select academic pharmacists as prescribers Unclear role of MD No clinical outcomes No cost analysis
Pucino et al., 1988	$N=28$	SNF	OGPPT	Pharmacist ordering and interpretation of trough drug levels	50% of measured levels subtherapeutic 50% positive response by MD to recommendations Inadequate use of drug serum level monitoring	
Kane et al., 1989	$N=9,738$	SNF	Quasi-experimental	Geriatric nurse practitioner provided patient care	Reduced drug use among long-stay patients Fewer hospitalizations More discharges to home	Volunteer homes Medications small part of study GNP role established prior to study
Karki et al., 1991	$N=113$	ICF	NR-CT	Weekly DRR by multidisciplinary team	Reduced average drugs/patient Reduced drug costs	Single facility No clinical outcomes

NOTE: Location: ICF—Intermediate care; SNF—Skilled nursing. Design: NR-CT—Nonrandomized, controlled trial; OGPPT—One-group pretest-posttest; PPT-CT—Pretest-posttest controlled trial. Intervention: DRR—Drug regimen review.

3

Infections and Infection Control

SANTIAGO DELEON TOLEDO, M.D.
ARIANE AN, PHARM.D.
FAWN TAKEMOTO, PHARM.D.
DEAN C. NORMAN, M.D.

BACKGROUND

Infections are a major cause of morbidity and mortality and a leading cause of acute care hospitalization for nursing home (NH) residents (29,25,59). Over 1.5 million infections occur annually in the long-term care setting, and the risk of acquiring an infection in a NH approaches that of an acute care hospital (27). Despite the magnitude of this problem, the existing literature is relatively sparse and problematic. This is because standard methods for both defining and reporting infections have not been clearly established and accepted. Similarly, clinically detailed process criteria for the management of infections in NHs also have not been established.

Other problems further complicate evaluation of the existing NH infection literature. First, surveillance periods vary, and it becomes difficult to interpret the literature because of seasonal variations in illnesses (e.g., influenza outbreaks in NHs tend to occur in the late fall and winter). Second, prevalence rates are often not clearly distinguished from incidence rates and each rate may be reported in a different fashion. For example, incidence may be reported as infections per 100 patients at risk, infections per 100 patient months, infections per 1,000 patient care days, or in other units. Finally, many of the published studies have reported infections in a predominantly male population of Veterans Administration NHs and the results may not be applicable to the general population.

Despite the shortcomings of existing studies, it can be determined that the most important NH infections are (a) lower respiratory infections, which are associated with a high mortality rate; (b) urinary tract infections, of which indwelling bladder catheters cause a significant number of symptomatic infections; and (c) skin and soft tissue infections (see Table 3.1 and 60,63,53). Outbreaks of respiratory illness (e.g., viral influenza, respiratory syncytial virus, tuberculosis), gastrointestinal illness (e.g., bacterial, protozoan, and viral enteritis), ectoparasite infection (e.g., scabies), and colonization and infection with multidrug-resistant bacteria (e.g., methicillin-resistant *Staphylococcus aureus*) are also important problems in NHs. These potentially preventable infection outbreaks necessitate the development and implementation of infection control programs tailored to meet the needs of the individual NH's existing resources.

REVIEW AND TABLES OF RECENT RESEARCH

In this section we concentrate on literature published during the past several years. The discussion is *not* intended to be comprehensive, and the reader is referred to the textbooks given as references above that review essentially all of the existing studies done on NH infections and infection control. We have selected many of the articles we consider to exemplify the best work being done in various areas. Some of the articles cited in this section could not easily be abstracted in table form and do not appear in the tables.

At the current time, the vast majority of the research on infections and infection control in NHs is descriptive, with relatively few intervention/outcome studies. The set of references shown in Table 3.1 are representative of basic general epidemiology studies on NH infections. Garibaldi et al. (1981) published the classic paper on the prevalence of NH infections (16.2%), identifying risk factors for infections and pointing out that the clustering of cases of upper respiratory and other similar site infections suggested that localized outbreaks were occurring frequently. Moreover, this point prevalence study also identified high employee turnover and lack of attention to infection control as important factors in explaining the high prevalence of infection. Magaziner et al. (1991) recently published an impressive prevalence study, looking at 4,259 residents in 53 Maryland NHs. This study found the prevalence of infection to be as high as 32% for residents with a combination of skin ulcers, urethral catheters, and bedfast status. If none of the three markers was present, then the prevalence was only 2%.

Recently, efforts have been made to accurately determine the incidence of infection in NHs. In one recent study, moderately intensive surveillance revealed an infection incidence rate of 9.45 per 1,000 patient days on a unit containing very debilitated residents (16). In another recent prospective study, Jackson et al. (1992) employed nurse practitioners to intensively survey infections in a 300-bed NH over a period of 3 years. This study found an incidence of 7.1 infections per 1,000 patient care days—higher than most of the previous reported incidence rates, which range from 3.0 to 6.7 per 1,000 patient days. According to Jackson, many of these infections would not have been recognized by persons less skilled than nurse practitioners, and their use in the survey may account for the data. This study should serve as a model for future studies because of the excellent design and clear definitions for the various types of infections.

Two important studies have established the incidence of bacteremia in NHs to be between 0.20 and 0.36 episodes per 1,000 patient care days (52,40). The urinary tract is the source for the majority of bacteremia episodes in NHs, differing from the acute care hospital setting where intravenous catheters are the source of the majority of bacteremia episodes. The incidence and severity of bacteremia in NHs are dependent on the level of severity of underlying illness.

The studies shown in Table 3.2 are representative of studies on the problem of antibiotic resistance in NHs, specifically methicillin-resistant *Staphylococcus aureus* (MRSA). In a questionnaire survey of 395 responding Minnesota NHs, it was reported that 12% of these facilities had residents colonized with MRSA (58). Furthermore, policies on MRSA varied widely between the homes, with 40% stating that persons with MRSA would not be accepted. This study emphasizes the need to develop uniform policies for the control of MRSA in long-term care facilities. Colonization rates of MRSA in studies of single institutions vary from 13% to 23% (4,41,42). Moreover, Murphy et al. (1992) found a significant number of admissions from acute care hospitals already colonized with MRSA. Symptomatic staphylococcal infection occurs in a variable percentage of MRSA carriers (6%-25%). It is not clear from the existing studies whether or not MRSA is any more virulent than methicillin-susceptible *S. aureus* (MSSA), and higher rates of staphylococcal infection observed in MRSA carriers may be because risk factors for colonization with MRSA (e.g., generalized debility) may be the same for actual infection with staphylococci. Further studies are needed to resolve this issue. Moreover, studies are needed to define infection control policies to deal with this problem. Given the limited resources of NHs and difficulties with eradication of the carrier state, MRSA will continue to be a problem.

The six studies shown in Table 3.3 are representative of work done on viral respiratory infection in the NH. Viruses are an important cause of acute respiratory illnesses in the institutionalized elderly (20). Influenza is the most important viral pathogen causing epidemics of acute respiratory illness in chronic care facilities. Interventions shown to be effective in controlling influenza include vaccination, early recognition of outbreaks and isolation, and prophylaxis with amantadine (13). Amantadine use is associated with adverse reactions if the dose is not adjusted for renal dysfunction (54). Moreover, amantadine resistance is becoming a problem, which makes it even more imperative to rapidly and effectively isolate cases (39,17). Respiratory syncytial virus may also cause moderate to severe influenzalike illness in NHs (48) and more studies are needed to develop management strategies for this pathogen. Similarly, nonviral pathogens such as the bacterium *Bordetella pertussis* may cause influenzalike symptoms (1). Thus it is important to thoroughly investigate outbreaks of respiratory illness in NHs in order to institute appropriate infection control programs to limit morbidity.

Bacterial pneumonia is associated with the highest mortality of all the common infections encountered in long-term care facilities (see above). There are several excellent reviews of this subject (64,46,47). Tuberculosis is not covered in this chapter and the reader is referred to a review of the pioneering work done by Stead and Dutt (1991). Table 3.4 shows abstracts of a few important articles on bacterial respiratory infection. In the classic study by Marrie et al. (1986), it was found that NH-acquired pneumonia (NHAP) differed significantly from community-acquired pneumonia (CAP) in the elderly: (a) mortality for NHAP was 40.5%, versus 28% for CAP; (b) NHAP was more likely to be associated with dementia and cerebrovascular disease with aspiration whereas CAP was more likely to be associated with chronic obstructive pulmonary disease; and (c) NHAP was more likely to be treated with aminoglycosides. The study by Hirata-Dulas et al. (1991) is an example of recent studies evaluating various antibiotic regimens for the treatment of NHAP. Some of these regimens allow a portion of the therapy to be with an oral or intramuscular agent, which may enable certain mildly to moderately ill patients with NHAP to be easily treated in long-term care facilities, thus avoiding the stress and expense of acute hospitalization, or at least decreasing the number of days spent in the acute care facility.

Urinary tract infection is certainly one of the most common infections in NHs and has been extensively reviewed (18). Examples of a few recent descriptive studies are shown in Table 3.5. In general, bacteriuria increases with increasing age, debility, chronic diseases, and abnormalities of the genitourinary tract. Therefore, bacteriuria is very common in NH residents. Whether or not bacteriuria is a marker for chronic disease or actually increases mortality remains in controversy, although the general opinion is now leaning toward bacteriuria simply being a marker. Symptomatic urinary tract infections are common and are a frequent complication of indwelling bladder catheters (49).

Outbreaks of gastrointestinal illness are common in institutions and may be especially severe in NHs (8). The articles shown in Table 3.6 are representative of some of the studies reporting these diseases. Many of these outbreaks can be prevented by proper food-handling techniques and other simple infection control procedures (8,62,15). Thomas et al. (1990) have shown that *Clostridium difficile* colonization may result in up to a third of cases of NH residents treated with antibiotics. Moreover, colonization with this pathogen may lead to increased morbidity/mortality. Thus, appropriate use of antibiotics in NHs is an important factor in limiting this pathogen.

The nontreatment of fever in the NH in general is associated with a high mortality rate (5). However, Fabiszewski et al. (1990) pointed out that aggressive management of certain subpopulations of residents may not be associated with improved survival. This study, abstracted in Table 3.7, looked at the effect antibiotic therapy had on febrile episodes in patients with dementia of the Alzheimer's type (DAT). During a 34-month observation period, it was found that antibiotic therapy for fever improved survival in patients with mild DAT but did not alter survival in those with severe DAT when compared to a control group of DAT patients who only received comfort measures for fever episodes. This is an important study because it brings up ethical and other issues regarding treatment of infections in severely impaired residents.

Castle et al. (1991) hypothesized that many NH residents with an apparently blunted fever response may actually have a significant change in temperature that is not recognized because of a low baseline temperature (see Table 3.7). This was confirmed by a retrospective review of charts for cases of infection defined by criteria that deliberately excluded fever. Moreover, the study provided data suggesting that (a) a change in temperature of 2.4°F from baseline is highly suggestive of infection, and (b) perhaps in the setting of a change in functional status, the threshold for a significant fever should be lowered to 100°F and possibly 99°F. The results of this study have been confirmed in a prospective study to be submitted by the same authors (12).

RESEARCH ON ANTIBIOTIC USE IN NURSING HOMES

The prevalence and characteristics of antibiotic use in NHs have been reviewed in several large population studies. At any point in time, 5%-10% of NH patients are on systemic antibiotics, while over a 1-year period, about 50% of NH patients may expect to receive a course of antibiotics (36,65,61,33). In a study by Zimmer et al. (1986), systemic antibiotic use was examined in 42 skilled nursing facilities and 11 intermediate care facilities in Rochester, New York. On the day of the survey, 7.7% of the patients were on systemic antibiotics from a random sample of 2,238 out of 4,378 beds. Magaziner et al. (1991) determined the prevalence of NH-acquired infections to be 4.4% among the 4,259 residents of 53 NHs in Maryland. Based on data from the 1985 National Nursing Home Survey, these 4,259 patients were demographically and functionally representative of patients in U.S. NHs. Warren et al. (1991) surveyed the same group of NHs over a 1-year period and determined that of the final cohort consisting of 3,899 patients from 52 homes, 54% received at least one antibiotic course. Katz et al. (1990) reviewed systemic antibiotic usage every 4th month for 1 year in two New York NHs comprising 720 beds. Approximately one of every four residents was treated with a systemic antibiotic.

Beta lactams were the most frequently prescribed antibiotics, followed by sulfonamides, erythromycins, and tetracyclines (61,33,31,65). The use of these antibiotics corresponded well with the most common sites of infections observed: urinary tract, skin, and respiratory tract. About 90% of infections were treated by a single antibiotic. The most frequently self-identified medical specialty of the primary care physicians prescribing antibiotics was internists (58%), followed by geriatricians (23%), family practitioners (13%), and generalists (6%) (33). Criteria for initiation of systemic antibiotics in NHs were found not to be as stringent as those used in tertiary care facilities. Examination of medical records revealed a frequent lack of documentation, incomplete workups, and missing objective evidence for identifying the suspected site of infection (65,61,33). Although empiric prescribing of antibiotics in NHs was generally associated with favorable clinical outcomes, the absence of standard minimum diagnostic criteria for initiating antibiotics may lead to unnecessary treatment, development of antibiotic-resistant bacterial strains, adverse drug effects, and increased medical care costs.

RESEARCH ON PROCESS OF CARE FOR INFECTION IN NURSING HOMES

One study that looked at quality of care in NHs with and without nurse practitioners has been further evaluated to look at the management of fever in 60 NHs with 8,800 residents (Buchanan, personal communication, 1991). Fever was identified by an oral or equivalent rectal temperature of 100°F or more for 12 hours or more. Residents were observed for varying lengths of time, ranging from 6 weeks to 2 years. During this study, 37% of the residents had at least one episode of fever (21% had only one episode, 9% had two episodes, and 7% had three or more febrile episodes). A physician was notified roughly 86% of the time but only about 40% of patients had a chest examination, only 13% had a chest radiograph ordered, and only 30% had a urinalysis. Thus, this study suggests that quality of care for infection may be poor in NHs.

In another NH study looking at the nursing process in managing fever, it was documented that when fever was detected (the criterion of a fever being any temperature equal to or exceeding 100.2°F), no physician was contacted 35% of the time in a hospital-based NH and 38% of the time in a community-based NH (23). Moreover, this same study found that the median time from the onset of fever to physician contact ranged from a timely 4 hours in the hospital-based NH to a discouraging 12.5 hours in the community-based NH. This same group published another study, this time documenting that nurses in different types of NHs were indifferent when it came to contacting a physician regarding any fever unless the temperature was higher than 102°F (34).

FUTURE RESEARCH NEEDS

As described above, much of the research done thus far in NHs has been largely descriptive in nature. Thus, although much has been learned about the epidemiology of infections in the long-term care setting, specific interventions to decrease the incidence of infections in this setting have been limited predominantly to immunoprophylaxis, specifically vaccines for the prevention of certain viral (e.g., influenza) and bacterial (e.g., *Streptococcus pneumoniae*) respiratory illness. Future research should focus on interventions to deal with all aspects of infection and infection control in NHs.

There is no question that NH patients are at increased risk for serious infections compared to noninstitutionalized elderly. The risk and severity of infection are proportional to the inoculum and virulence of the specific pathogens and inversely proportional to the integrity of host defenses. For example, the risk of developing pneumonia is proportional to the amount of aspirate—which may be increased by diseases that affect swallowing, such as cerebrovascular disease, or the misuse of sedating medications—and the type of the pathogens in the aspirate and the virulence of the pathogens. For example, certain gram-negative bacilli and *Staphylococcus aureus* are more likely to be present in debilitated patients and in those recently exposed to antibiotics. Pulmonary host defenses such as the cough reflex are compromised to some degree by normal aging but are further compromised by long-standing respiratory diseases such as chronic obstructive pulmonary disease and lung cancer (64).

From the above discussion it can easily be seen that risk factors associated with infection in the elderly include (a) limited reserve capacity to respond adequately to stress because of biologic changes with age and underlying chronic diseases; (b) abnormalities in host defenses; (c) delay in diagnosis and institution of treatment; (d) generally higher morbidity from invasive procedures; (e) poorer clinical response to treatment; and (f) greater risk for adverse drug reactions.

Research should be focused on interventions to reduce risk factors for infection, such as reducing the morbidity and impact from chronic diseases. For example, in the case of pneumonia, education and treatment strategies to reduce the incidence of smoking at all ages and studies to evaluate methods to reduce or minimize aspiration in order to lessen this problem are needed. Further, educational interventions should be established to improve compliance with known effective infection control methods that are relatively easy to carry out. Some of these include up-to-date isolation procedures, infection and antibiotic use surveillance, vaccination and amantadine usage, enforcement of strict hand-washing procedures, screening patients and staff for tuberculosis, careful food-handling techniques, and universal precautions. These education interventions must take into account the level of education and turnover of nursing aides.

Research strategies would also include better ways to identify patients with impaired immune function. Castle et al. (1991) are working on the role of skin testing and in vitro blood tests to evaluate immune function in NH residents. This type of work should be encouraged. Further, the prevalence of malnutrition is high in NH patients, also compromising immune function and host defenses. Thus, more research should be directed at interventions to improve the nutritional status of NH residents, perhaps through serial nutritional assessments and aggressive nutritional therapy.

Research strategies for reducing the delay in initiating appropriate therapy should be developed. At our institution we are engaged in several projects looking at ways to improve detection of fever in NH patients and at the process of care for febrile illness in the NH. To determine the actual number of febrile episodes in a NH, we are employing a simple method utilizing a tympanic membrane instrument that will allow daily monitoring of temperatures on all NH residents. Some of these data are in press (11).

We have also begun pilot studies to develop clinically detailed process criteria for the management of episodes of infection. These are essential because inappropriate care of the infected elderly NH resident may result in unnecessary morbidity, mortality, and resource expenditures. In any event, education intervention studies are indicated to educate NH staff and physicians about research findings that impact on their patients. For example, the findings of Castle et al. (1991) suggest that any change in functional status associated with an oral temperature of 99°F or greater is likely to indicate a serious infection.

More studies are needed to improve the appropriateness of antibiotic usage in NHs. Studies looking at the appropriateness of antimicrobial therapy have found that approximately 8.0% of patients in the NH are on antibiotics (see above). However, chart review documented an indication for antimicrobial therapy in only 62% of these cases (see above section on antibiotic use). There may have been indications for antimicrobial therapy that were not recorded for some of the remaining 38% of the cases. However, even if the actual figure for inappropriate antibiotic use is somewhat lower, the cost and quality implications for NH residents as a whole are considerable. We estimate that in any given year up to 210,000 NH patients may receive inappropriate antimicrobial therapy. Improper use of antibiotics has several potential consequences. Unnecessary costs are one of them. A 10-day course of an oral antibiotic may cost as little as $50. However, a 10-day course of a parenteral third-generation cephalosporin, a type of drug that is often used for empiric antibiotic therapy, costs several hundred dollars. Thus, a course of antibiotics can range as high as $1,000. Quality deficits such as these could significantly add to national health care costs. Further, the inappropriate use of antibiotics may result in costly drug toxicity, the emergence of resistant pathogens, and unnecessarily increased risk of antibiotic-induced diarrhea.

In summary a list of what we consider to be research priorities include:

Relevant to All Infections:

1. Encourage studies that will enable easy identification of patients at risk for serious infection. In particular, research should focus on quantitative assessment of host defenses, especially immune function. Studies to develop better methods for early detection of infection should also be encouraged.
2. Encourage studies developing clinically detailed process criteria for the prevention and management of infections in NHs. These process criteria should be linked to quality of care (e.g., outcome) measures.
3. Encourage studies to reduce the inappropriate use of antimicrobial therapy. Studies are needed to establish optimal doses, routes, and duration of antimicrobial therapy for infected NH patients whether they are cared for in the NH or in the acute care setting.
4. Encourage intervention studies for improvement of NH staff compliance in carrying out current recommendations for infection control and management.

Relevant to Some Specific Infections:

1. Develop simple and inexpensive tests to determine the precise etiology of pneumonia and infected pressure ulcers, and to rapidly diagnose tuberculosis. Newer methods in molecular biology hold the most promise.
2. Establish methods to determine if and when catheter-related bacteriuria has a significant clinical effect, as opposed to simple colonization. Along the same line, research is needed to develop strategies to minimize the use of bladder catheters in NHs. In many cases, some catheter use is appropriate, but more research is needed on establishing methods to reduce colonization and infection associated with this use.
3. Develop better influenza and pneumonia vaccines and methods to increase the immune response to these vaccines. Again, more studies to develop methods to improve compliance with existing vaccination and infection control programs in NHs are needed.

4. Encourage studies to determine interventions to reduce the risk of post-herpetic neuralgia. The varicella-zoster vaccine looks promising and should be studied to see if the vaccine will reduce both the incidence of herpes zoster and post-herpetic neuralgia (35).

REFERENCES

1. Addiss, D. G., Davis, J. P., Meade, B. D., et al. (1991). A pertussis outbreak in a Wisconsin nursing home. *Journal of Infectious Diseases, 164,* 704-710.
2. Alvarez, S., Shell, C. G., Woolley, T. W., et al. (1988). Nosocomial infections in long-term facilities. *Journal of Gerontology, 43*(1), M9-17.
3. Bloom, H. G., & Bottone, E. J. (1990). Aeromonas hydrophila diarrhea in a long-term care setting. *Journal of the American Geriatrics Society, 38,* 804-806.
4. Bradley, S. F., Terpenning, M. S., Ramsey, M. A., et al. (1991). Methicillin-resistant *Staphylococcus aureus:* Colonization and infection in a long-term care facility. *Annals of Internal Medicine, 115,* 417-422.
5. Brown, N. K., & Thompson, D. J. (1979). Nontreatment of fever in extended-care facilities. *New England Journal of Medicine, 300,* 1246-1250.
6. Bryant, H. E., & Athar, M. A. (1989). Risk factors for escherichia coli 0157:H7 infections in an urban community. *Journal of Infectious Diseases, 160,* 858-864.
7. Buchanan, J. L., Bell, R. M., Arnold, S. B., et al. (1990). Assessing cost effects of nursing home-based geriatric nurse practitioners. *Health Care Financing Review, 11*(3), 67-78.
8. Carter, A. O., Borczyk, A. A., Carlson, J. A. K., et al. (1987). A severe outbreak of *Escherichia coli* 0157:H7-associated hemorrhagic colitis in a nursing home. *New England Journal of Medicine, 317,* 1496-1500.
9. Castle, S. C., Norman, D. C., Perls, T. T., et al. (1990). Analysis of cutaneous delayed-type hypersensitivity reaction and T cell proliferative response in elderly nursing home patients: An approach to identifying immunodeficient patients. *Gerontology, 36,* 217-229.
10. Castle, S. C., Norman, D. C., Yeh, M., et al. (1991). Fever response in elderly nursing home residents: Are the older truly colder? *Journal of the American Geriatrics Society, 39,* 853-857.
11. Castle, S. C., Toledo, S. D., Daskal, L., et al. (1992a). The equivalency of infrared tympanic membrane thermometry in nursing home residents. *Journal of the American Geriatrics Society,* in press.
12. Castle, S. C., Yeh, M., Toledo, S. D., et al. (1992b). *Prospective study of diurnal variation of temperature and fever response in nursing home residents.* Manuscript submitted for publication.
13. Cate, T. R. (1991). Influenza in the elderly. In M. S. Niederman (Ed.), *Respiratory infections in the elderly* (pp. 99-121). New York: Raven.
14. Chiaramonte, M., Floreani, A., & Naccarato, R. (1982). Hepatitis B virus infection in homes for the aged. *Journal of Medical Virology, 9,* 247-255.
15. Choi, M., Yoshikawa, T. T., Bridge, J., et al. (1990). Salmonella outbreak in a nursing home. *Journal of the American Geriatrics Society, 38,* 531-534.
16. Darnowski, S. B., Gordon, M., & Simor, A. E. (1991). Two years of infection surveillance in a geriatric long-term care facility. *American Journal of Infection Control, 19*(4), 185-190.

17. Degelau, J., Somani, S. K., Cooper, S. L., et al. (1992). Amantadine-resistant influenza A in a nursing facility. *Archives of Internal Medicine, 152,* 390-392.
18. Dontas, A. S. (1990). Urinary tract infection in nursing home residents. In A. Verghese & S. L. Berk (Eds.), *Infections in nursing homes and long-term care facilities* (pp. 126-143). New York: Karger.
19. Fabiszewski, K. J., Volicer, B., & Volicer, L. (1990). Effect of antibiotic treatment on outcome of fevers in institutionalized Alzheimer patients. *Journal of the American Medical Association, 263*(23), 3168-3172.
20. Falsey, A. R., Treanor, J. J., Betts, R. F., et al. (1992). Viral respiratory infections in the institutionalized elderly: Clinical and epidemiologic findings. *Journal of the American Geriatrics Society, 40*(2), 115-119.
21. Farber, B. F., Brennen, C., Puntereri, A. J., et al. (1984). A prospective study of nosocomial infections in a chronic care facility. *Journal of the American Geriatrics Society, 32,* 499-502.
22. Finnegan, T. P., Austin, T. W., & Cape, R. D. T. (1985). A 12-month fever surveillance study in a veterans' long-stay institution. *Journal of the American Geriatrics Society, 33*(9), 590-594.
23. Franson, T. R., Schicker, J. M., LeClair, S. M., et al. (1988). Documentation and evaluation of fevers in hospital-based and community-based nursing homes. *Infection Control and Hospital Epidemiology, 9,* 447-450.
24. Garibaldi, R. A., Brodine, S., & Matsumiya, S. (1981). Infections among patients in nursing homes. *New England Journal of Medicine, 305*(15), 731-735.
25. Gordon, W. Z., Kane, R. L., & Rothenberg, R. (1985). Acute hospitalization in a home for the aged. *Journal of the American Geriatrics Society, 33,* 519-523.
26. Gross, P. A., Rodstein, M., LaMontagne, J. R., et al. (1988). Epidemiology of acute respiratory illness during an influenza outbreak in a nursing home. *Archives of Internal Medicine, 148,* 559-561.
27. Haley, R. W., Culver, D. H., White, J. W., et al. (1985). The nationwide nosocomial infection rate: A need for vital statistics. *American Journal of Epidemiology, 121,* 159-167.
28. Hirata-Dulas, C. A. I., Stein, D. J., Guay, D. R. P., et al. (1991). A randomized study of ciprofloxacin versus ceftriaxone in the treatment of nursing home-acquired lower respiratory tract infections. *Journal of the American Geriatrics Society, 39,* 979-985.
29. Irvine, P. W., Van Buren, N., & Crossley, K. (1984). Causes for hospitalization of nursing home residents: The role of infection. *Journal of the American Geriatrics Society, 32,* 103-107.
30. Jackson, M. M., Fierer, J., Barrett-Connor, E., et al. (1992). Intensive surveillance for infections in a three-year study of nursing home patients. *American Journal of Epidemiology, 135*(6), 685-696.
31. Jones, S. R., Parker, D. F., Liebow, E. S., et al. (1987). Appropriateness of antibiotic therapy in long-term care facilities. *American Journal of Medicine, 83,* 499-502.
32. Kane, R. L., Garrard, J., Skay, C. L., et al. (1989). Effects of a geriatric nurse practitioner on process and outcome of nursing home care. *American Journal of Public Health, 79*(9), 1271-1282.
33. Katz, P. R., Beam, T. R., Brand, F., et al. (1990). Antibiotic use in the nursing home: Physician practice patterns. *Archives of Internal Medicine, 150,* 1465-1468.
34. LeClair, S. M., Schicker, J. M., Duthie, E. H., et al. (1988). Survey of nursing personnel attitudes towards infections and their control in the elderly. *American Journal of Infection Control, 16,* 159-166.

35. Levin, M. J., Murray, M., Rotbart, H., et al. (1992). Immune response of elderly individuals to a live attenuated varicella vaccine. *Journal of Infectious Diseases, 166,* 253-259.

36. Magaziner, J., Tenney, J. H., DeForge, B., et al. (1991). Prevalence and characteristics of nursing home-acquired infections in the aged. *Journal of the American Geriatrics Society, 39,* 1071-1078.

37. Magnussen, M. H., & Robb, S. S. (1980). Nosocomial infections in a long-term care facility. *American Journal of Infection Control, 8*(1), 12-17.

38. Marrie, T. J., Durant, H., & Kwan, C. (1986). Nursing home-acquired pneumonia: A case study. *Journal of the American Geriatrics Society, 34,* 697-702.

39. Mast, E. E., Harmon, M. W., Gravenstein, S., et al. (1991). Emergence and possible transmission of amantadine-resistant viruses during nursing home outbreaks of influenza A (H3N2). *American Journal of Epidemiology 134,* 988-997.

40. Muder, R. R., Brennen, C., Wagener, M. M., et al. (1992). Bacteremia in a long-term-care facility: A five-year prospective study of 163 consecutive episodes. *Clinical Infectious Diseases, 14,* 647-654.

41. Muder, R. R., Brennen, C., Wagener, M. M., et al. (1991). Methicillin-resistant staphylococcal colonization and infection in a long-term care facility. *Annals of Internal Medicine, 114,* 107-112.

42. Murphy, S., Denman, S., Bennett, R. G., et al. (1992). Methicillin-resistant staphylococcus aureus colonization in a long-term care facility. *Journal of the American Geriatrics Society, 40,* 213-217.

43. Nicolle, L. E., Brunka, J., McIntyre, M., et al. (1992). Asymptomatic bacteriuria, urinary antibody, and survival in the institutionalized elderly. *Journal of the American Geriatrics Society, 40,* 607-613.

44. Nicolle, L. E., Henderson, E., Bjornson, J., et al. (1987). The association of bacteriuria with resident characteristics and survival in elderly institutionalized men. *Annals of Internal Medicine, 106,* 682-686.

45. Nicolle, L. E., McIntyre, M., Zacharias, H., et al. (1984). Twelve-month surveillance of infections in institutionalized elderly men. *Journal of the American Geriatrics Society, 32,* 513-519.

46. Niederman, M. S. (1991). Nosocomial pneumonia in the elderly. In M. S. Niederman (Ed.), *Respiratory infections in the elderly* (pp. 207-239). New York: Raven.

47. Nunley, D., Verghese, A., & Berk, S. L. (1990). Pneumonia in the nursing home patient. In A. Verghese & S. L. Berk (Eds.), *Infections in nursing homes and long-term care facilities* (pp. 95-114). New York: Karger.

48. Osterweil, D., & Norman, D. (1990). An outbreak of an influenza-like illness in a nursing home. *Journal of the American Geriatrics Society, 38,* 659-662.

49. Ouslander, J. G., Greengold, B., & Chen, S. (1987). Complications of chronic indwelling urinary catheters among male nursing home patients: A prospective study. *Journal of Urology, 138,* 1191-1195.

50. Ryan, C. A., Tauxe, R. V., Hosek, G. W., et al. (1986). Escherichia coli 0157:H7 diarrhea in a nursing home: Clinical, epidemiological, and pathological findings. *Journal of Infectious Diseases, 154*(4), 631-638.

51. Scheckler, W. E., & Peterson, P. J. (1986). Infections and infection control among residents of eight rural Wisconsin nursing homes. *Archives of Internal Medicine, 146,* 1981-1984.

52. Setia, U., Serventi, I., & Lorenz, P. (1984). Bacteremia in a long-term care facility. *Archives of Internal Medicine, 144,* 1633-1635.

53. Smith, P. W. (Ed.). (1989). *Infection control in long-term care facilities.* New York: John Wiley.

54. Stange, K. C., Little, D. W., & Blatnik, B. (1991). Adverse reactions to amantadine prophylaxis of influenza in a retirement home. *Journal of the American Geriatrics Society, 33,* 700-705.
55. Stead, W. W., & Dutt, A. K. (1991). Tuberculosis in elderly persons. *Annual Review of Medicine, 42,* 267-276.
56. Terpenning, M. S. (1992). Hepatitis B, hepatitis C, and immunodeficiency syndrome (AIDS): Anticipating long-term care needs. *Journal of the American Geriatrics Society, 40,* 295.
57. Thomas, D. R., Bennett, R. G., Laughon, B. E., et al. (1990). Postantibiotic colonization with clostridium difficile in nursing home patients. *Journal of the American Geriatrics Society, 38,* 415-420.
58. Thurn, J. R., Belongia, E. A., & Crossley, K. (1991). Methicillin-resistant *Staphylococcus aureus* in Minnesota nursing homes. *Journal of the American Geriatrics Society, 39,* 1105-1109.
59. Tresch, D. D., Simpson, W. M., & Burton, J. R. (1985). Relationship of long-term and acute-care facilities. The problem of patient transfer and continuity of care. *Journal of the American Geriatrics Society, 33,* 819-826.
60. Verghese, A., & Berk, S. L. (Eds.). (1990). *Infections in nursing homes and long-term care facilities.* New York: Karger.
61. Warren, J. W., Palumbo, F. B., Fitterman, L., et al. (1991). Incidence and characteristics of antibiotic use in aged nursing home patients. *Journal of the American Geriatrics Society, 39,* 963-972.
62. White, K. E., Hedberg, C. W., Edmonson, L. M., et al. (1989). An outbreak of giardiasis in a nursing home with evidence for multiple modes of transmission. *Journal of Infectious Diseases, 160*(2), 298-304.
63. Yoshikawa, T. T., & Norman, D. C. (1987a). Infections in the nursing home population. In T. T. Yoshikawa & D. C. Norman (Eds.), *Aging and clinical practice: Infectious diseases* (pp. 108-127). New York: Igaku-Shoin.
64. Yoshikawa, T. T., & Norman, D. C. (1987b). Pneumonia. In T. T. Yoshikawa & D. C. Norman (Eds.), *Aging and clinical practice: Infectious diseases* (pp. 73-85). New York: Igaku-Shoin.
65. Zimmer, J. G., Bentley, D. W., Valenti, W. M, et al. (1986). Systemic antibiotic use in nursing homes: A quality assessment. *Journal of the American Geriatrics Society, 34,* 703-710.

Table 3.1 General Epidemiology

Reference Location Institution	Type of Facility	Study Design	Subjects Patient Age	Type of Infection/Pathogen	Statistical Reports	Mortality/ Adverse Outcomes	Factors Associated With Mortality/Adverse Outcome and Other Findings
Magnussen & Robb, 1980 VAMC Pittsburgh, PA	2-mo survey of the VAMC LTC institution (Oct-Nov 78) 2 levels of care: a. nursing home b. intermediate care	Retrospective 2-mo survey (Oct-Nov 78)	N=398 veterans ($\bar{x}$ age 71.3 yrs) 39% over 75 yrs Mean age of infected patients is 70.5 yrs	81 infections identified and 72 were nosocomial —UTI 71.6% —Respiratory tract 13.5% —Skin 11.1% —Bacteremia 2.5% —Other infections 1.3%	Total infection rate is 20.5% NH-acquired infection rate is 18.2%	NR	1. No significant difference in infection rate between the 2 levels of care. 2. UTI was the predominant infection and opportunistic pathogens were the principal organism instead of E. coli.
Garibaldi et al., 1981 Farmington, CT	7 skilled-care NH homes in Salt Lake City (5 proprietary, 2 nonproprietary)	Series of 1-day prevalence surveys (point prevalence study)	N=532 patients (193 M, 339 F) Median age 81 yrs 19% ≥90 yrs N=97 infections in 86 patients (16% of population surveyed)	NH-acquired infections —Decubitus ulcers —Conjunctivitis —Symptomatic UTI —Lower RTI	Prevalence among 532 patients is 16.2% (women 20%, men 12%)	NR	Contributory factors to high prevalence of infections in NH: 1. Advanced age 2. Underlying diseases 3. Immobility 4. Fecal incontinence 5. Indwelling urethral catheters

continued

Table 3.1 Continued

Reference Location Institution	Type of Facility	Study Design	Subjects Patient Age	Type of Infection/Pathogen	Statistical Reports	Mortality/ Adverse Outcomes	Factors Associated With Mortality/Adverse Outcome and Other Findings
							High prevalence of infectious diseases and clustering of cases reflect increased susceptibility to infection, lack of attention to infection control practices
Setia et al., 1984 Bergen Pines County Hospital, Paramus, NJ	Long-term care (LTC) facility 571-bed	Prospective study 2-year period (81-82)	N=460 patients (118 M, 342 F) 1. Control population ($\bar{x}$ age 76.9 yrs) 88% more than 60 yrs 2. Bacteremic population ($\bar{x}$ age 79.0 yrs) 94% more than 60 yrs	Bacteremia	—Gram (+) 24% —Gram (−) 67% —Polymicrobial 9% Bacteremia rate 0.3 per 1,000 patient days.	Overall mortality was 35% —Gram (+) 50% died —Gram (−) 25% died —Polymicrobial 67% died	1. Sources of bacteremia: —Urinary tract 56% —Skin, subcutaneous 14% —Respiratory tract 10% 2. Most common Gram (+) *Staph. aureus*, most common Gram (−) *E. coli, Proteus* species, and *Klebsiella enterobacter* group

Source	Setting	Study design	Population	Infection findings	Rate/Incidence	Deaths	Conclusions
Farber et al., 1984 VAMC-Univ. of Pittsburgh Pittsburgh, PA	Chronic care facility in Aspinwall (432 beds) A. 228-bed NH B. 161 intermediate care beds C. 43 medical beds	Prospective study (Dec 82 to Dec 83)	A. NH N=43 x̄ age 68 yrs B. Intermediate care N=68 x̄ age 68 yrs	NH-acquired infections: Pneumonia and UTI accounted for 49% of all infections	*Infection rate:* A. NH 0.67 infections per 100 patient days B. Intermediate care 1.35 infections per 100 patient days	A. NH n=7 deaths B. Intermediate care n=33 deaths	3. 50% of deaths occurred within 24 hours of diagnosis. Infection rates in chronic care facilities vary with: 1. Level of care 2. Adequacy of infection control practices 3. Quality of nursing care
Nicolle et al., 1984 Calgary, Alberta, Canada	2 long-term wards of a veterans hospital in Winnipeg	Prospective surveillance (12-mo)	N=68 males (x̄ age 79 yrs) n=50 residents with infections (111 episodes identified)	NH-acquired infections: —Lower respiratory tract 32% —Febrile episode 23% —Skin, soft tissue 19% —Gastroenteritis 17% —Upper respiratory tract 2.7% —Urinary tract 2.7% —Osteomyelitis 2.7% —Others 1.8%	*Incidence* of 192.7 infections per 100 patient years	Mortality rate from infection of 10.3 per 100 residents per year 7/19 (37%) resident deaths were due to infection; these 7 deaths represented 6.3% of all infection episodes	Resident characteristics that correlated with infection: 1. Bladder incontinence 2. Bowel incontinence Only pneumonia was associated with significant mortality Mental status or degree of mobility did not correlate with infection

continued

Table 3.1 Continued

Reference Location Institution	Type of Facility	Study Design	Subjects Patient Age	Type of Infection/Pathogen	Statistical Reports	Mortality/ Adverse Outcomes	Factors Associated With Mortality/Adverse Outcome and Other Findings
Finnegan et al, 1985 London, Ontario, Canada	Veterans' Care Center (VCC) 258-bed continuing care hospital	Prospective study over 12 mos (Feb 81 to Jan 82) of fever episodes	N=98 patients (12 patients c̄ 14 episodes of fever refused) N=86 subjects enrolled in the study	NH-acquired infections: —128 episodes of fever (≥38.5°C rectally or >38.0°C orally on 2 occasions at least 1 hour apart)	*Incidence of fever:* 1.0 episode per 24 patient months in hospital	16% mortality associated with febrile episodes	1. Lower respiratory tract infections (32%) and urinary tract infections (23%) 2. *Strep. pneumoniae* was most common pathogen in chest infection and *Proteus mirabilis* in UTI 3. 35% had *no* evidence of any infection
Scheckler & Peterson, 1986 Madison, WI	8 rural nonproprietary NH in Wisconsin	1. Initial prevalence survey (Jan-Feb 84) 2. Comprehensive 6 consecutive mo prospective surveillance	Prevalence survey: N=403 residential (97 M, 306 F) (x̄ age 83.4 yrs) 6-mo surveillance N=265 *episodes of acute infection*	NH-associated infections	*Prevalence of infections:* 56 (13.9%) infections in 52 (12.9%) residents 6-mo *incidence of 10.7 infections per 100 resident months*	84 deaths during surveillance period Only a few due to infection	Clusters of infection by site, pathogens, or month of onset were uncommon, possibly due to active infection control programs

Study	Setting	Methods/Sample	Type of infection	Results	Deaths	Comments
Alvarez et al., 1988 VAMC Johnson City, TN	1. Skilled-care units Ward A 60 beds Ward B 59 beds 2. NH care unit Ward C 61 beds	2 phases: Retrospective: 1. 4-year routine surveillance (Jan 80–Dec 83) Prospective: 2. 1-day a month prevalence study for 12 mos. *Prevalence study:* N=132 male patients x̄ age 68.2 yrs *Incidence study:* 853 infection episodes identified over 4 yrs	NH-acquired infections	*Prevalence study:* *Total infection rate 6.6% (46 episodes identified in 689 patients at risk)* *Incidence study:* *Global infection rate of 3.86 per 1,000 patient care days*	NR	The high incidence of infections in chronic care facilities correlates well with the poor functional status
Jackson et al., 1992 UCSD, San Diego, CA —Supported by NIA	Proprietary 300-bed skilled nursing facility (SNF)	Prospective study of intensive surveillance over a 3-yr period (Aug 84 to May 87); used nurse practitioners to assess patients for infection on regular basis. 666 of 714 (93%) of eligible subjects enrolled —75% females (x̄ age 81.6 yrs) (788 episodes of NHAI identified)	NH-associated infections (NHAI)	Overall incidence of NHAI was 7.1 infections per 1000 patient days —47% in the respiratory tract —25% in soft tissues —18% symptomatic UTI —2% bacteremia —9% other infections	—29% died during study period —infection associated with 12% of the deaths	Prior studies probably underestimate incidence of infection because of lack of in-service surveillance

continued

Table 3.1 Continued

Reference Location Institution	Type of Facility	Study Design	Subjects Patient Age	Type of Infection/Pathogen	Statistical Reports	Mortality/ Adverse Outcomes	Factors Associated With Mortality/Adverse Outcome and Other Findings
Magaziner et al., 1991 Baltimore, MD —Supported by NIH —Univ. of MD School of Medicine	53 licensed LTC facilities in Maryland	Case finding then review of records of 4,259 patients in stratified random sample of 53 NHs	4,259 case records of patients ≥65 yrs	NH-acquired infections	Prevalence —4.4% a. Skin infection —35% b. Fever of uncertain source —13% c. Symptomatic urinary tract infection (UTI)—12% d. Lower respiratory tract (LRTI) —12%	NR	Risk factors include: a. Skin ulcers b. Urethral catheters c. Bedfast status d. Tracheotomy, lung disease
Darnowski et al., 1991 Baycrest Center for Geriatric Care Toronto, Ontario, Canada	1. Unit A—Home for the Aged (350-bed SNF) 2. Unit B—Chronic care hospital (300 beds)	Prospective surveillance (June 87 to May 89)	1. Unit A: N=47 (70% F) x̄ age 89 yrs 2. Unit A: N=32 (60% F) x̄ age 77 yrs	1. Major sites of infection: a. Urinary tract b. Lower respiratory c. Skin d. Soft tissue 2. Epidemics 2° to respiratory virus, TB, MRSA, and E. coli	Infection rate per 1,000 patient days: 1. Unit A 1.77 2. Unit B 9.45	16 deaths: 1. 6 (37%) primarily due to infection: —5 due to pneumonia —1 due to urosepsis 2. 10 unrelated to infection	1. Higher infection rate in Unit B is probably due to more debilitated patient population 2. Goals of surveillance in LTC facilities are: a. Facilitate early

| Muder, et al., 1992 Pittsburgh, PA | 432-bed long-term care (LTC) facility —204 intermediate care —228 nursing home care | Prospective study over 5 yrs (85-89) | N=144 patients (21-95 yrs x̄ age 68.6) —163 episodes of bacteremia | Bacteremia | Rate of bacteremia increased from 0.20 to 0.36 cases per 1,000 patient days from 1985-89 and complicated 6.5% of infections | Overall mortality 21.5% | detection of outbreaks b. Identify preventable endemic infections 1. Majority of isolates were Gram (–); *Providencia stuartii, E. coli,* and *Proteus sp.* were most common 2. *Staph. aureus* was the most frequent Gram (+) isolate (33% MRSA) 3. Bacteremia was polymicrobial in 36 episodes (22%) with mortality 29%–50% depending on origin of bacteremia 4. Portals of entry included urinary tract (55%), respiratory tract (11%), and soft tissue (9%) |

continued

Table 3.1 Continued

Reference Location Institution	Type of Facility	Study Design	Subjects Patient Age	Type of Infection/Pathogen	Statistical Reports	Mortality/ Adverse Outcomes	Factors Associated With Mortality/Adverse Outcome and Other Findings
							5. Mortality was associated with: —Residence on intermediate care unit —Change in mental status —Relatively recent admission

NOTE: MRSA=Methicillin-resistant *Staph. aureus*. MSSA=Methicillin-susceptible *Staph. aureus*. UTI=Urinary tract infection. RTI=Respiratory tract infection. NHAI=Nursing home associated infection. NR=Not reported. *=Statistically significant.

Table 3.2 Methicillin-Resistant *Staphylococcus Aureus*

Reference Location Institution	Type of Facility	Study Design	Subjects Patient Age	Type of Infection/Pathogen	Statistical Reports	Mortality/ Adverse Outcomes	Factors Associated With Mortality/Adverse Outcome and Other Findings
Bradley et al., 1991 Ann Arbor, MI Dept of VAMC	LTC facility attached to acute care VAMC	Prospective monthly surveillance for 1-yr	N=341 ($\bar{x}$ age 63.9 yrs)	Methicillin-resistant *Staph. aureus* (MRSA)	Monthly *prevalence* MRSA colonization rate is 23%	No mortality/ 3% of total population had MRSA infection.	Colonization risk factors: 1. Poor functional status 2. 25% already colonized with MRSA at admission 3. 10% newly admitted acquired MRSA Only 3% acquired MRSA from roommate
Thurn et al., 1991 Minnesota St. Paul-Ramsey Med. Ctr.	All LTC facilities in MN.	12-question survey of categorical responses (for directors of LTC and director of nursing)	N=445 LTCF	MRSA	Only 88% of NH responded 12% of NH had residents colonized/infected with MRSA 40% would not accept patients with MRSA	NR	Problems identified: 1. Policies regarding admission of patients colonized or infected with MRSA are not uniform 2. MRSA in LTC facilities is widespread and underrecognized
Muder et al., 1991	2 NH units	Prospective cohort study	N=197 patients:	MRSA carriers n=32	—25% of MRSA carriers	MRSA carriers: 53% died	Persistent MRSA carriage was

continued

Table 3.2 Continued

Reference Location Institution	Type of Facility	Study Design	Subjects Patient Age	Type of Infection/Pathogen	Statistical Reports	Mortality/ Adverse Outcomes	Factors Associated With Mortality/Adverse Outcome and Other Findings
VAMC Pittsburgh, PA		using monthly and bimonthly surveillance Jan 86–Dec 88 (3 yrs)	NH 1 99—interme-diate nursing unit (mean age 64.8 yrs) NH 2 98—nursing home care unit (mean age 70.7 yrs)	MSSA carriers n=44 Noncarriers n=88	had staph infections —4% of MSSA carriers had staph infections —4.5% of non-carriers had staph infections *Rate* of de-velopment of *infection* is 15% for every 100 days of MRSA carriage	MSSA carriers: 29% died	most significant predictor of staphylocal infection
Murphy et al., 1992 Baltimore, MD Johns Hopkins U. School of Med. Div. of Geriatrics	University-affilia-ted LTC facility 233 beds (2 adjacent nursing units): 1. Chronic care 2. Skilled/ intermediate care	Retrospective cross-sectional surveillance culture survey over a 4-mo period	Long-term: 1. Chronic care medical unit N=38 2. Inter-mediate care unit N=67 Admissions: 1. Chronic medical ad-missions N=55 2. Admitted to other units N=63 (x̄ age=69.1 yrs)	MRSA	MRSA colonization *prevalence* in chronic care unit vs. intermedi-ate care unit is 52.6% vs. 4.5% MRSA colo-nization *prevalence* in chronic medical admis-sions vs. adm. to other units 43.6% vs. 9.5%	NR	Colonization at admission risk factors: 1. Male 2. More listed Dx incl. pressure sores 3. Previous (+)/MRSA culture 4. Urinary incontinence

MRSA=Methicillin-resistant *Staph. aureus*. MSSA= Methicillin-susceptible *Staph. aureus*.

Table 3.3 Respiratory Viruses

Reference Location Institution	Type of Facility	Study Design	Subjects Patient Age	Type of Infection/Pathogen	Statistical Reports	Mortality/ Adverse Outcomes	Factors Associated With Mortality/Adverse Outcome and Other Findings
Gross et al., 1988 Hackensack Med. Ctr. Hackensack, NJ	525-bed Jewish home and hospital for the aged (JHHA) in New York	Surveillance (Nov 82 to Apr 83)	N=138 residents	Influenza A/Arizona/82 (H3N2)	75/138 (54%) residents had acute and convalescent sera with ≥ 4-fold rise in titers	NR	1. 59% of residents immunized before the outbreak of influenza; outbreak begins in Nov., peaks in Feb. and disappears in April 2. Significant level of herd immunity accounted for slow progression in NH
Mast et al., 1991 Bureau of Community Health and Prevention, Wisconsin Div. of Health, Madison, WI	2 NH units	Retrospective cohort study (Jan 1988) using chart review for evaluating influenza vaccination program and amantadine prophylaxis	NH 1. 60% vaccinated NH 2. 79% vaccinated	Influenza A (H3N2)	*Point estimate of vaccine efficacy in preventing influenzalike illness is 33%*	—9% of vaccinated pts. died —26% of *unvaccinated* died	Need to determine how frequently and under what circumstances the isolation of resistant viruses associated with the use of antiviral agents

continued

Table 3.3 Continued

Reference Location Institution	Type of Facility	Study Design	Subjects Patient Age	Type of Infection/Pathogen	Statistical Reports	Mortality/ Adverse Outcomes	Factors Associated With Mortality/Adverse Outcome and Other Findings
Stange et al., 1991 Cleveland, OH	Retirement home	Retrospective cohort study	N=79 residents accepted the amantadine prophylaxis (mean age 87 yrs) (17 residents refused)	Amantadine complications	41% who received amantadine had attributable adverse reactions (22% classified as severe reactions)	Mortality not reported	Variables associated with severe adverse reactions: 1. Residence in the assisted living section of the facility 2. Greater number of underlying diagnoses 3. Congestive heart failure 4. High serum creatinine
Degelau et al., 1992 Minnesota St. Paul-Ramsey Med. Ctr.	2 NH units: Facility A Facility B	Prospective surveillance program over 1-yr period using: —Case isolation —Rapid index case treatment —Prophylaxis with aman-tadine	Facility A N=148 Facility B N=133	Influenza A	Facility A: —No isolation —18/22 (82%) cases despite amantadine initiation Facility B: —Day 1 isolation plus amantadine No outbreak	NR	Inadequate case isolation may promote further influenza A infection in a NH facility

Source	Setting	Design	Sample	Focus	Results	Mortality	Conclusions
Falsey et al., 1992 Rochester, NY	591-bed NH	Prospective, descriptive, without intervention (Dec 89-Mar 90)	N=133 residents —149 episodes of illnesses (84% were female) mean age 88 yrs	Viral respiratory infections	Viral etiology was documented in 62/149 (42%) illnesses: —RSV 27% —Rhinovirus 7% —Parainfluenza 6% —Influenza 1%	2/40 (5%) with RSV died	1. Viruses are an important cause of acute respiratory infections in elderly institutionalized patients 2. RSV was associated with more severe disease 3. Nosocomial transmission was suggested by clustering of specific viral infections
Osterweil & Norman, 1990 Jewish Home for the Aging Reseda, CA	231-bed multilevel long-term care facility	Surveillance program (Oct 85-Feb 86)	N=196 residents (36 M, 160 F) Mean age 88 yrs (73-102 yrs)	Respiratory syncytial virus (RSV)	—57/196 (29%) had met criteria for acute respiratory illness —14 had acute and convalescent sera with confirmatory titers of Ab against RSV —Attack rate: 29%	—Mortality in 2% —Pneumonia in 5% —Prolonged malaise and anorexia in 46%	1. RSV may be an important cause of respiratory illness in NH 2. Rapid diagnostic tests and ribavirin therapy against RSV warrant further clinical trials

Table 3.4 Bacterial Respiratory Infection

Reference Location Institution	Type of Facility	Study Design	Subjects Patient Age	Type of Infection/Pathogen	Statistical Reports	Mortality/Adverse Outcomes	Factors Associated With Mortality/Adverse Outcome and Other Findings
Addiss et al., 1991 Wisconsin Division of Health	110-bed intermediate care NH	Retrospective chart review (Jul-Nov 85)	N=105 residents (35-101 yrs) 116 employees (16-70 yrs)	Bordetella pertussis (influenzalike illness)	—38/105 (36.2%) of residents were seropositive; 6 seropositive and had clinical pertussis, and 4 were culture (+). —8/104 (7.7%) employees were seropositive but none was culture (+).	No deaths occurred in residents with clinical or laboratory evidence of pertussis	Higher attack rate for residents and clustering of clinical cases were consistent with ongoing transmission within the NH
Marrie et al., 1986 Dalhouise Univ. Victoria General Hosp. Halifax, Nova Scotia, Canada	NH groups Community groups	Case control	NH N=74 (36M, 38F) Comm N=73 (36M, 37F) $\bar{x}$ age 74 yrs	NH-acquired pneumonia vs. CA pneumonia	NH: Aspiration pneum. 31% c̄ sputum culture 63.5% unknown etiol.	NHAP—40.5% mortality CAP—28% mortality	1. NH: Higher incidence of dementia and CVA; patients received cloxacillin and aminoglycosides more frequently

Source	Setting	Design	Sample	Condition	Results	Outcomes	Comments
Hirata-Dulas et al., 1991 Hennepin County Med. Ctr. Minneapolis, MN	Extended care NHs affiliated c̄ teaching hospital	Prospective randomized trial	N=50 patients ≥60 yrs admitted to a hospital 24: ciprofloxacin IV, then PO 26: ceftriaxone IV, then IM	Lower respiratory tract infection (LRTI)	Comm: Hemophilus influenzae 39% c̄ sputum culture 63.5% unknown etiol. Successful outcome in: —50% of patients on ciprofloxacin —54% of patients on ceftriaxone	8% died in each treatment group 8% of ceftriaxone treated had myalgia and high fever	2. Comm: More likely smokers and c̄ COPD; patients received erythromycin more frequently Recurrent oropharyngeal aspiration is a risk factor for antibiotic failure

Table 3.5 Urinary Tract Infection

Reference Location Institution	Type of Facility	Study Design	Subjects Patient Age	Type of Infection/Pathogen	Statistical Reports	Mortality/ Adverse Outcomes	Factors Associated With Mortality/Adverse Outcome and Other Findings
Ouslander et al., 1987 VAMC UCLA School of Med., CA	VAMC-NH	Prospective study	N=54 male c̄ chronic indwelling bladder catheters 106 episodes of symptomatic infection	Symptomatic UTI	106 episodes during 514 patient months or an incidence of 0.21 per patient month at risk	NR	Age, nutritional status, stool incontinence, diabetes mellitus, catheter blockage, and chronic suppressant antimicrobial therapy were not associated with the development of symptomatic UTI
Nicolle et al., 1987 Calgary, Alberta, Canada	Skilled nursing facility	Prospective surveillance over 3-yr period	N=91 elderly male veterans (mean age 79 yrs)	A. Bacteriuria: 1. Continuously bacteriuric 2. Intermittently bacteriuric B. Nonbacteriuric	—Nonbacteriuric 42% —Intermittently bacteriuric 34% —Continuously bacteriuric 25%	UTI caused or contributed to only 2.9% deaths	1. Bacteriuric residents were more frequently confused or demented 2. Bacteriuria was significantly associated with incontinence of bladder and bowel

| Nicolle et al., 1992 Winnipeg, Manitoba, Canada | Long-term care (LTC) facility | —Retrospective review (1987) —Cohort after 3 yrs | N=63 (45 M, 18 F) mean age 78.8 yrs | A. Bacteriuria: 1. *Persistent* n=38 (60%) 2. Infrequent *n*=12 (19%) B. Nonbacteriuric: *n*=13 (21%) | a. *18/38 (47%)* had persistently elevated urine antibody b. *20/38 (53%)* had normal urinary antibody | a. 3/18 (17%) were alive b. 11/20 (55%) were alive | 3. No differences in survival among the 3 groups at 6 years Elderly institutionalized subjects with persistent bacteriuria and elevated urine antibody have decreased survival |

Table 3.6 Gastrointestinal Infection

Reference Location Institution	Type of Facility	Study Design	Subjects Patient Age	Type of Infection/Pathogen	Statistical Reports	Mortality/ Adverse Outcomes	Factors Associated With Mortality/Adverse Outcome and Other Findings
Ryan et al., 1986 Omaha, Nebraska	101-bed intermediate care NH	Case summary (Sept 84)	N=101 residents (mean age 86 yrs)	E. coli 0157:H7 gastrointestinal infection	34/101 (34%) developed diarrheal illness	4/101 (4%) died	Infection with E. coli 0157:H7 can cause a wide range of severe manifestations with elderly and may resemble ischemic colitis
Carter et al., 1987 Laboratory Center for Disease Control Ottawa, Ontario, Canada	NH	Retrospective case review (Sept 1-Oct 18, 1985)	N=169 elderly NH residents	E. coli 0157:H7-associated hemorrhagic colitis	55/169 (33%) affected 12/55 (22%) developed hemolytic-uremic synd.	19/55 (35%) died 11/12 (92%) with hemolytic-uremic synd. died	1. Incubation period of 4-9 days (mean 5-7 days) 2. Older age and previous gastrectomy increased the risk. Outbreak may have been related to poor food handling

| Chiaramonte et al., 1982 Padova, Italy | 3 different institutions for the aged: A: house-hotel B: 2 different homes for the aged | Seroepidemiological study | A: N=83 (17 M, 66 F) (63-94 yrs x̄ age 82) B: N=108 (47 M, 61 F) (65-93 yrs x̄ age 75) | Hepatitis B | Cumulative *prevalence* of HBV in A and B is higher than noninstitutionalized aged group 71.2% vs 37.6% | NR | 1. HBs Ag ± anti HBc: A—18.0% B—8.3% Noninstitutionalized 1.8% 2. Anti HBs ± anti-HBc: A—33.7% B—50.9% Noninstitutionalized—26.0% 3. Institutionalized aged had increased serological evidence of HBV c̄ respect to their noninstitutionalized counterparts 4. HBs Ag asymptomatic carrier rate was much higher than expected 5. Most symptomatic carriers were also positive for HBe Ag |

continued

Table 3.6   Continued

Reference Location Institution	Type of Facility	Study Design	Subjects Patient Age	Type of Infection/Pathogen	Statistical Reports	Mortality/ Adverse Outcomes	Factors Associated With Mortality/Adverse Outcome and Other Findings
White et al., 1989 Minnesota Dept of Health	NH with a child day care center located in the premises	Surveillance using questionnaire and stool collection (April-June 86)	115 residents, 122 employees, 46 children enrolled	Giardia lamblia (diarrheal illness)	Giardiasis cases identified in: —35 residents —38 employees —15 school children	NR	Multiple modes of transmission: 1. Food borne 2. Person-to-person Awareness of potential problem and techniques of disease control in facilities that combine child care and care for elderly
Choi et al., 1990 VAMC UCLA Sch. of Med. West LA, CA JHA	Community NH	Retrospective review of charts Feb-May 87	N=199 NH residents	Salmonella gastroenteritis (S. heidelberg) outbreak	Prevalence of diarrhea before outbreak was 1% 44/199 had diarrhea; 19 cases were positive of S. heidelberg	NR	1. Clinical spectrum of salmonella gastroenteritis is variable 2. NH outbreaks of salmonella impose a high economic burden

Thomas et al., 1990 Johns Hopkins Univ. Sch. of Med. Baltimore, MD	233-bed LTC facility	Prospective study	N=108 patients (150 courses of antibiotics over 6 mos)	Clostridium difficile Pseudomonas colitis (postantibiotic diarrhea)	Stool specimens from 36 (33%) of patients following the first course of Ab'c antibiotic tx and 12 (33%) were infected c̄ C. difficile	12-mo surveillance showed 83% mortality in infected px vs. 50% in the noninfected px	Postantibiotic C. difficile serves as a marker for death in NH patients This may be related in part to clinically unrecognized C. difficile colitis or absorption of toxins from gut lumen to systemic circulation

Table 3.7 Miscellaneous Publications

Reference Location Institution	Type of Facility	Study Design	Subjects Patient Age	Type of Infection/Pathogen	Statistical Reports	Mortality/ Adverse Outcomes	Factors Associated With Mortality/Adverse Outcome and Other Findings
Bloom & Bottone, 1990 St. Luke's / Roosevelt Hospital, New York, NY Mt. Sinai School of Med., NY	Hebrew Home for the Aged (784-bed LTC facility)	Case report 3-day period mid-Aug 88	N=17 patients (x̄ age 87.0 yrs)	Aeromonas hydrophilus diarrheal outbreak	—36% had (+) stool cultures —76% had <48-hr illness —76% had 2-4 loose stools —88% afebrile	1/17 (6%) fatality	Usually mild and self-limited, but fatal if protracted dehydration
Fabiszewski et al., 1990 Bedford, MA Boston, MA	LTC facility	Prospective study over 34 mos 3 fever groups: 1. No fever observed 2. Antibiotic (fever episode evaluated and treated with antibiotic if indicated) 3. Palliative (supportive therapy only)	N=104 patients (97% male) —75 patients with 172 episodes of fever —29 patients had no fever	Fever episodes in patients with Alzheimer's dementia		Fever treated with antibiotic group: —9 died —83 recovered Palliative group: —19 died —61 recovered	1. Incidence of fever was similar in Antibiotic and Palliative groups 2. Treatment of fever with antibiotics does not alter the outcome of fever in patients c̄ advanced Alzheimer's dementia

| Castle et al., 1991 VAMC UCLA Sch. of Med., CA NHCU | Retrospective study over 20 mos 3 groups: 1. Fever responders 2. Non-responders 3. Mixed | N=26 residents (mean age 78.0 yrs) —69 episodes of infection N=50 residents prospectively followed for fever response | Fever episodes in elderly NH residents | —25/53 (47%) of all infections had a Tmax <101°F or a "blunted" fever response —14/53 (26%) had a Tmax<100°F —6/53 (11%) had a Tmax <99°F —18/53 (34%) had a ΔT <2.4°F | NR | 1. Of the "blunted" fever responses, 25% demonstrated adequate change from baseline temperature ($\Delta T°$ $\geq 2.4°F$) 2. Most infections had a Tmax >99°F 3. Establishing a NH patient's basal T° and monitoring for ΔT and/or lowering the threshold for recognition of fevers in NH residents with a change in function should assist in early recognition of infections |

4

Pressure Ulcers in the Nursing Home

DAN R. BERLOWITZ, M.D., M.P.H.
SPENCER VAN B. WILKING, M.B., B.S.,
M.P.H.

INTRODUCTION

The past several years have witnessed a growing interest and awareness on the topic of pressure-induced skin injury. Pressure ulcers are
now appropriately recognized as a complex problem whose prevention
and treatment challenges the entire interdisciplinary team including
physician, nurse, nutritionist, physical therapist, and pharmacist. In
addition, pressure ulcers are being used by administrative and quality assurance personnel to monitor the process and outcome of care.
Despite this broad interest, substantial deficits in knowledge about
pressure ulcers exist, which a rapidly expanding research literature
is just beginning to address. This literature spans such diverse medical topics as the evaluation of prediction rules, high-technology
beds, and genetically engineered tissue growth factors. Recent reviews have examined some of the clinical (1,47) and methodological
(95) implications of this literature. These reviews, though, have not
dealt with the unique aspects of pressure ulcers in the nursing home
(NH) setting. In this chapter, we will perform such a detailed review
of the existing literature on pressure ulcers with specific regard for
its implications to NHs. Our goal is not only to assist clinicians
practicing in NHs but to help identify methodological problems that
arise in studying pressure ulcers and specific knowledge gaps that
would benefit from further research. Specific topics include: pres-

Dr. Berlowitz is supported by a Department of Veterans Affairs, HSR&D Research Associate
Career Development Award.

sure ulcer classification, epidemiology, pathophysiology, clinical risk factors, prediction rules, prevention, treatment, outcomes, and health services implications.

Definition and Classification

Pressure ulcers are localized areas of tissue necrosis that tend to develop when soft tissue is compressed between a bony prominence and an external surface for a prolonged period of time. Numerous classification schemes to define the extent of these ulcers have been developed for use in the clinical and research setting. The most commonly used staging instrument was that proposed by Shea (1975). Recently, a consensus conference sponsored by the National Pressure Ulcer Advisory Panel (NPUAP) (1989) proposed a modified version of this instrument in an attempt to develop a widely accepted and standardized classification system. Differences between the classification schemes are outlined in Table 4.1. Limited data exist as to the interrater reliability of these methods. Yarkony et al. (1990) addressed this issue when they compared the performance of two registered rehabilitation nurses using both the Shea classification and a system developed by the authors. This system relies on the direct observation of specific tissue types, such as subcutaneous fat, muscle, or bone, rather than on anatomical terms such as epidermis or dermis. Of 72 pressure ulcers evaluated by two nurses, only 68% of the ratings were identical using the Shea classification, whereas 85% agreement was achieved using the Yarkony Scale. Insufficient data exist as to which classification scheme should presently be recommended. Given the broad consensus leading to its development, the NPUAP scheme will probably be extensively used in the future. Nevertheless, due to the limited information on interrater reliability, both clinical communications and research reports relying on a classification scheme must be interpreted with caution unless suitable efforts were made to standardize the assessment process.

Epidemiology

Despite these difficulties in classifying pressure ulcers, numerous studies have attempted to document the extent of the pressure ulcer problem among NH patients. Typically, these studies have relied on measures of the incidence or prevalence of pressure ulcers. Estimates derived from these studies have been shown to vary widely, however. In part, this variation may be explained by differences in the

Table 4.1 Classification System

Stage	Shea	NPUAP	Yarkony/Kirk
1.	Soft tissue erythema, swelling, and induration that may be associated with superficial ulceration limited to the epidermis.	Nonblanchable erythema of intact skin.	A. Red area present longer than 30 minutes but less than 24 hours. B. Red area present longer than 24 hours.
2.	Full thickness ulcer extending to the underlying subcutaneous fat.	Partial thickness skin loss involving epidermis and/or dermis.	Epidermis and/or dermis ulcerated with no subcutaneous fat observed.
3.	Full thickness skin defect extending into subcutaneous fat but limited by the deep fascia.	Full thickness skin loss involving damage or necrosis of subcutaneous tissue that may extend down to but not through underlying fascia.	Subcutaneous fat observed, but no muscle.
4.	Penetration of the deep fascia and extending down to bone.	Full thickness skin defect with extensive destruction; tissue necrosis; or damage to muscle, bone, or supporting structures.	Fascia or muscle observed, but not bone.
5.			Bone observed, no joint space involvement.
6.			Involvement of joint space.

NH population under study. However, differing methodologies also plays a role. Standardized methods to ascertain pressure ulcer status have not been employed. Given the difficulties in detecting Stage 1 ulcers, many studies have elected not to include them. Finally, many of the studies have been small and confined to a single institution. For the purposes of this review, we have limited the analysis to those studies involving more than 100 patients.

Incidence and prevalence studies have certain inherent limitations for a chronic condition such as pressure ulcers. Incidence studies are usually performed by analyzing patients initially without a pressure ulcer and determining how many have an ulcer at some future point in time. Thus, interval ulcers may be missed by incidence studies if the pressure ulcer heals or if the patient dies prior to the specified time period. No data exist to suggest what is the optimal duration for this time period. However, if complete ascertainment of all pressure ulcers is desired, experience suggests that repeated determinations of pressure ulcer status at 1- to 2-week intervals would be required. Prevalence studies may also lead to biased estimates of the pressure ulcer burden in NHs. As these studies typically look at only a single time point, large pressure ulcers that are present for several months will tend to be overrepresented whereas small, rapidly healing ulcers will be underrepresented. More accurate determinations of pressure ulcer prevalence may be obtained by alternate methods. For example, one recent preliminary study has described prevalence as the number of days with a pressure ulcer per 1,000 patient care days (35).

Study results documenting the prevalence of pressure ulcers in NHs are presented in Table 4.2. These studies are divided into two groups, those that examine prevalence at the time of patient admission and those from some random time post admission. Pressure ulcers are extremely common at admission, with a prevalence ranging from 17.4% to 34.7%. It should be noted that the majority of these ulcers are either Stage 1 or 2. However, approximately 15% of the ulcers are Stage 4. Most patients were admitted from an acute care facility, with a range from 81% in Brandeis et al. (1990) to 100% in Reed (1981). The importance of the acute care facility to the problem of pressure ulcers in the NH is also supported by data from Tresch et al. (1985) demonstrating that 30% of patients returning to the NH had new or worse ulcers. Certain limitations of these data should be mentioned. The study reported by Reed (1981) was performed at six extended care facilities, type not specified, whereas Berlowitz and Wilking (1989) used data from a chronic care hospital. The latter study excluded Stage 1 ulcers; the former did not report on the mix of ulcers. Finally, both Spector et al. (1988) and Brandeis et al. (1990) used information from the same data base. It appears that all of the patients in the report by Spector were included by Brandeis et al.

Prevalence rates for pressure ulcers following admission to the NH vary widely with a reported range from 2.5% to 28.7%. Two studies reported very low rates. Petersen and Bittmann (1971) reported on all pressure ulcers in one Danish county. Cases were identified via questionnaires sent to all general practitioners in the county. Significant underreporting is to be expected. Hing (1981) presented results from a national survey that was considered representative of all NH residents. The presence of an ulcer in the surveyed patients was determined by a nurse in conjunction with the medical record. However, criteria for "bedsores" were not specified,

Table 4.2 Prevalence Rate of Pressure Ulcers

Study	Year of Data	Number of NHs	Number of Patients	Prevalence	Percent at Stage				Comment
					1	2	3	4	
On Admission									
Reed, 1981	1977	6	472	21.0%					
Shepard et al., 1987	1984	1	118	34.7%	49	—	—	14	% Stage 2 and 3 not specified
Spector et al., 1988	1984	51	4,951	10.1%	36	36	16	13	Includes patients of Spector (1988)
Brandeis et al., 1990	1984-85	51	14,345	17.4%	35	36	15	14	
Berlowitz & Wilking, 1989	1985-86	1	301	33.0%	—	60	23	17	Excluded Stage 1 ulcers
Post-Admission									
Petersen & Bittmann, 1971	1970		1,930	2.5%					Excluded Stage 1 ulcers
Reed, 1981	1977	6	1,023	10.0%					
Hing, 1981	1977		1,303,100	2.7%					
Pinchcofsky-Devin & Kaminski, 1986		2	232	7.3%					
Brandeis et al., 1990	1984-85	51	5,544	8.9%	24	41	22	13	
Scheckler & Peterson, 1986	1984-85	8	403	9.7%					
Dimant & Francis, 1988		1	326	15.3%					Preeducation program
Dimant & Francis, 1988		1	326	8.9%					Posteducation program
Weiler et al., 1990	1988	4	373	28.7%	60	36	4	1	
Department of Veterans Affairs	1991		12,055	20.0%	57	21	13	9	Unpublished

suggesting that many Stage 1 and 2 ulcers may not have been reported. In addition, the survey included facilities that provided domiciliary care with minimal nursing care so that case mix may have been less severe in these institutions. Two studies reported high prevalence rates. Weiler et al. (1990) did not ascertain pressure ulcer status on NH residents who refused to be examined. This reliance on an examination also led to the detection of mostly Stage 1 ulcers that may have been missed in other studies. The Department of Veterans Affairs (VA) (36) has unpublished data on pressure ulcers resulting from its semiannual survey of all long-term care patients. Once again, the high prevalence of pressure ulcers appears to be due to the reporting of additional Stage 1 ulcers.

Data on the incidence rate for pressure ulcers is only available from three large studies (Table 4.3). All three studies defined a new pressure ulcer as Stage 2 or greater. Berlowitz and Wilking (1989) demonstrated in one chronic care hospital that 10.8% of new admissions developed an ulcer within 3 weeks. These ulcers were all Stage 2. Only 15% of these ulcers progressed to Stage 3 at any time during the subsequent hospitalization. Brandeis et al. (1990) looked at both a new admission group and a resident group with pressure ulcer status measured at 3-month intervals. Approximately 5% of patients in the admission cohort and 2.5% in the resident cohort had a new ulcer at 3 months. Of the patients still in the NH after 2 years, the rate for the two groups had equalized at 21%. Although there are data from the acute care hospital to suggest that most pressure ulcers develop soon after admission (7), Brandeis et al. (1990) provide the only evidence to suggest that the incidence rate for patients in NHs may also be higher immediately following admission. Unpublished data from the VA has shown that 4% of veterans in a NH will have a new ulcer at 6 months. The stage of the incident ulcers is unavailable from both the Brandeis et al. and the VA studies.

PATHOPHYSIOLOGY

Traditional research on pressure ulcer pathophysiology has stressed the significant individual and cumulative contributions of pressure, shear, friction, and moisture (79). Recent works have begun to further elucidate how these factors may actually induce tissue injury. In addition, the interaction of these traditional factors with other elements such as circulatory changes arising as a result of acute illness, as well as the role of nutritional deficiencies contributing to tissue ischemia, is being emphasized.

Table 4.3   Incidence Rate of Pressure Ulcers

Study	Year of Data	Number of NHs	Number of Patients	Monitoring Interval	Incidence	Comment
Berlowitz & Wilking, 1989	1985-86	1	185	3 weeks	10.8% at 3 weeks	
Brandeis et al., 1990	1984-85	51	11,849	3 months	13.2% at 1 year	Admission group
Brandeis et al., 1990	1984-85	5	5,050	3 months	9.5% at 1 year	Resident group
Department of Veterans Affairs	1991			6 months	4% at 6 months	Unpublished

Certainly since the time of Paget an appropriate emphasis has been placed on the role of vertical pressure over a bony surface as the major culprit in pressure ulcer formation (22). Early work on the effects of pressure on dermal blood flow suggested that pressures in excess of the capillary arteriolar pressure of 32 mmHg might markedly compromise oxygenation and microcirculation. These observations were supported in experiments by Kosiak (1959) and Daniel et al. (1981) that reflect the presence of an inverse time-pressure curve such that ulcer formation occurs rapidly with high occlusive pressures or slowly with low occlusive pressures. Both researchers demonstrated impaired tissue circulation at relatively low compression pressures, with local damage due to edema and necrosis occurring rapidly with pressures in excess of 70 mmHg. Pressures as high as 150 mmHg may be encountered when patients lie on a standard hospital mattress. Further important observations regarding the significance of occlusive pressures emerges in work by Nola and Vistness (1980) and Barth et al. (1984). Their work demonstrates that the highest interstitial pressures are found at the bone-muscle interface, with relative sparing noted in the epidermal-dermal layers. This confirms that extensive, deep tissue trauma can occur subdermally with little or no evidence of superficial damage to warn caregivers. Although further research on the effects of occlusive pressure on different tissue strata and microcirculation would be beneficial, this area remains challenging due to difficulties in calibrating transdermal pressures (14).

Less appreciated and more poorly measured by researchers is the contribution of shear to the pathogenesis of pressure ulcers. This phenomenon, caused by the relative displacement of adjacent lamellar surfaces, causes resultant angulation deformity to local blood vessels and lymphatics. V. Alterescu (1989) presents the theoretical underpinnings that show the effect of a process whereby movement of bone against surrounding muscle and subcutaneous tissue with concomitant fixation of epidermis and dermis leads to profound tissue compromise. Work by L. Bennett et al. (1969) supports the additive effect of pressure and shear together, particularly on the deeper tissues, thus contributing to a more dramatic ulcerative process. Unfortunately, full calibration of shear as a physical entity and its relative contribution when evaluated with varying pressure loads has yet to be performed. Nevertheless, identification of shear provides an important first step in research to appreciate its relative contribution to ulcer pathophysiology.

Friction is a process whereby a relative portion of the protective epidermis is abraded, thus compromising the barrier function of outermost skin. Studies addressing friction note that it causes the initial breach of the epidermis, allowing more extensive superficial damage. However, V. Alterescu and K. Alterescu (1988) note that friction does not in itself produce the necrosis or inflammatory changes associated with deep muscle injury. In fact, the epidermis may be more susceptible to the erosive effects of friction if it lies over a zone of swollen, deep tissue damage. On the basis of these observations, it is suspected that friction plays a more tangential role in pressure ulcer pathophysiology than do shear and pressure.

Long-term exposure to moisture in the form of sweat, feces, or urine serves to deplete protective skin oils and leads to skin maceration. Although this factor has been traditionally associated with pressure ulcer formation, little definitive information exists as to the magnitude of moisture's contribution, though it may play a role in the overall destructive process, particularly in the formation of superficial ulcers.

Histopathological studies have described a cascade effect of pressure-induced ischemia leading to edema and additional tissue hypoxia. Witkowski and Parish (1982) describe this chain reaction by showing that small dermal vessels become dilated and porous, followed by interstitial edema, perivascular round cell infiltration, platelet aggregation, and eventually perivascular hemorrhage. Epidermal changes are not seen until late in the course of this process, giving support to the finding that the initial ulceration may occur beneath the skin surface. Krouskop (1983) has stressed the effects of hypoxia on the tissue ecosystem by noting its deleterious effect on collagen production and lymphatic drainage, resulting in cell lysis and liberation of degradative enzymes that cause further necrosis and local tissue damage. Seiler and Stahelin (1986) have demonstrated decreased fibrinolytic activity in tissues adjacent to pressure ulcers and suggested that this may lead to thrombus formation in small vessels. The interaction of these events with nutritional deficiencies as manifested by vitamin C deficiency leading to vessel wall fragility is discussed by Taylor et al. (1974). So too hypoalbuminemia, by disrupting osmotic gradients, may lead to edema with resultant hypoxia. This supports the importance of nutritional factors as contributors to a tissue milieu that becomes more susceptible to pressure-induced injury.

The role of acute medical illness in the development of pressure ulcers is being increasingly recognized. A recent editorial (39) goes so far as to state that "Pressure sores are not irremediable afflictions of longstay patients but a sign of acute illness." Contributing factors have been postulated to include hypotension; dehydration; vasomotor failure; and vasoconstriction secondary to shock, heart failure, or medications. Several studies have directly evaluated the relationship between blood pressure and pressure ulcers. Gosnell (1973), in a small sample of 30 patients, showed that pressure ulcers developed only in patients with a diastolic blood pressure less than 60. Schubert (1991) noted a lower systolic blood pressure among 30 geriatric patients with ulcers compared to 100 without. Among a group of spinal cord injury patients, Mawson et al. (1988) demonstrated a significant inverse association between systolic blood pressure and the subsequent development of a pressure ulcer. However, alternate hypotheses may explain the role of acute illness in pressure ulcer formation. Versluysen (1986) has emphasized that prolonged immobilization on hard surfaces occurring at home, in the emergency room, or in the operating room, along with sedation and dehydration, is the norm for elderly patients with hip fractures. It is likely that patients with other illnesses, when cared for in an environment where staffs' primary concern is the stabilization of the acute condition, will remain at high risk for pressure ulcer development.

These results suggest that there may be a dual process in the development of pressure ulcers such that deep penetrating ulcers are produced in acute illness situations where high occlusive pressures are present, with broad, but superficial ulcers more frequent in settings where abrasion and maceration due to chronic moisture are common. These results clearly imply that the acute hospital setting will remain the source for many of the large ulcers encountered in NHs. Ulcers that do develop in the NH will tend to be smaller and superficial. Clearly, more extensive evaluations of the differences in pressure ulcers based on care settings are required.

CLINICAL RISK FACTORS

Although considerable efforts have been devoted to investigating the pathophysiology of pressure ulcer development, this information has not been readily translated into a greater understanding of the clinical factors involved. A large number of such potential risk factors have been identified. A recent review of 100 randomly selected articles on pressure ulcers found 126 different items listed as risk factors (51). A review of all these factors is beyond the scope of this article. Complicating any review of risk factors is the fact that many of these items have been identified through either clinical observations of small numbers of pressure ulcer patients or studies investigating only one or two factors. This raises the possibility that any demonstrated associations are not causal but instead arise as a result of confounding with some unmeasured item that is a true risk factor. Recognizing these limitations, a number of recent studies have employed large data bases and multivariate modeling to identify those characteristics that appear to be independently associated with pressure ulcers.

Allman et al. (1986) performed the first such study, comparing pressure ulcer patients at an acute care hospital with a control group felt to be at risk for pressure ulcer development on the basis of being bed or chair bound. Three factors, a low serum albumin, fecal incontinence, and a recent fracture, were found to be associated with the presence of a pressure ulcer. Additional cross-sectional studies have subsequently been performed in the NH population. Spector et al. (1988) demonstrated that older age, male sex, nonwhite race, dependence in bathing and transferring, presence of a urinary catheter, fecal incontinence, being bed or chair bound, and absence of rehabilitation potential were all associated with the presence of a pressure ulcer on admission to a NH. Using a larger sample from the same data base, preliminary results from Brandeis et al. (1989) additionally demonstrated that malnutrition, urinary incontinence, insulin or narcotic therapy, and Parkinson's disease were associated with an ulcer. Among patients at one NH, Weiler et al. (1990) identified the presence of an infection, hypertension, poor dietary intake, a decreased level of consciousness, and unwelcome visitors as being associated with the presence of an ulcer. Cross-sectional studies, as listed above, are limited in that they identify factors associated with the presence of a pressure ulcer. Consequently, these studies may identify factors resulting from the ulcer rather than contributing to its development. Berlowitz and Wilking (1989) performed a cohort study to identify factors present on admission to a chronic care hospital that would predict pressure ulcer development. Being bed or chair bound, a history of a cerebrovascular accident, and impaired nutritional intake were all significant predictors. Their data further suggested that hypoalbuminemia, rather than leading to the development of an ulcer, may arise as a result of the ulcer. No subsequent, large, cohort studies have been published in the NH population. A limitation of all these studies is that although the absence or presence of a potential risk factor can be easily determined, means of quantitating that factor are not generally available. In analyzing these data, it is important to note not only what factors were associated with pressure ulcers, but also what commonly assumed factors were shown not to be associated. The power of these studies to detect a significant difference has generally not been addressed.

Among individual characteristics, immobility appears to be the prerequisite for pressure ulcer development. Immobility may be permanent, as in the result of a cerebrovascular accident, or transient, as during an acute illness. Using a device to measure bodily movements in bed, Exton-Smith and Sherwin (1961) demonstrated a high correlation between a lack of spontaneous nocturnal movements and pressure ulcer development. Unfortunately, means of measuring immobility are not available in most clinical settings. As a result, investigators have often relied on alternate clinical characteristics to serve as a marker for immobility. Ambulatory status has been considered as a separate factor that is closely related to immobility. The large studies by Spector et al. (1988), Brandeis et al. (1989), and Berlowitz and Wilking (1989) have all identified being bed or chair bound as an independent risk factor for pressure ulcers. Similarly, an altered level of consciousness, as may arise from severe dementia or delirium, is often cited as a risk factor for pressure ulcers. Immobility, or the failure to recognize immobility, appears to be the primary mechanism of ulcer development in these patients. Interestingly, Barbenel et al. (1986) demonstrated that the use of sedation reduced the number of spontaneous nocturnal movements among elderly hospitalized patients.

Although moisture, as previously noted, may have an important role in skin maceration, the role of urinary incontinence as a risk factor for pressure ulcers remains unclear. Many studies have demonstrated that incontinent patients are at greater risk for pressure ulcers. Lowthian (1976), for example, reported a fivefold increase in the incidence of pressure ulcers among incontinent patients. These studies have generally not taken into account the strong correlation between incontinence and immobility, however. Data from a national survey of NH discharges (Zappolo, 1981) demonstrated that 94% of incontinent pressure ulcer patients were either bed or chair bound. When studies have been performed using multivariate techniques, urinary incontinence is rarely noted as a significant predictor. Of interest, use of a urinary catheter, at least on univariate testing, has consistently been associated with pressure ulcers. Although this finding may arise from the use of these catheters to promote dryness in pressure ulcer patients, a similar association was demonstrated in the prospective study of Berlowitz and Wilking (1989). This further suggests that it is not moisture that is important, but rather the immobility of many incontinent patients.

The importance of nutritional factors in the healing of wounds is well recognized. The role of these nutritional parameters in predicting the future development of pressure ulcers has yet to be clarified. Cross-sectional studies have consistently shown strong associations. Mulholland et al. (1969), Allman et al. (1986), Berlowitz and Wilking (1989), and Breslow et al. (1991) have all shown that patients with pressure ulcers are much more likely to have hypoalbuminemia than control patients. Pinchofsky-Devin and Kaminski (1986) evaluated a large number of nutritional parameters, including albumin, and demonstrated that all 17 patients with pressure ulcers were severely malnourished. This has led to the hypothesis that hypoalbuminemia, as a result of interstitial edema, predisposes to tissue hypoxia and skin breakdown (1,55). Prospective data has not confirmed this hypothesis. Stotts (1987) demonstrated that a wide range of nutritional parameters were not predictive of the future development of an ulcer in a cohort of 387 patients admitted to an acute care hospital for elective surgery. Of note, baseline nutritional parameters were normal in this sample. The data of Berlowitz and Wilking (1989) demonstrating that poor nutritional intake, but not hypoalbuminemia or total lymphocyte count, was associated with pressure ulcer development were previously cited. These data suggest that in evaluating an individual patient's risk, it may be more important to see how well the patient is eating and whether nutritional needs are presently being met than to measure specific nutritional parameters.

These results point to two major areas of future development. First, additional cohort studies need to be performed in the NH population. Second, reliable and valid measures of immobility should be developed. Only then will accurate statements on the clinical risk factors for pressure ulcer development be possible.

PREDICTION RULES FOR PRESSURE ULCER DEVELOPMENT

One reason for identifying clinical risk factors for pressure ulcer development is that this information may be used to prospectively identify high-risk patients. A number of such prediction rules have been developed and tested in NH residents. The most frequently cited of these instruments is the Norton Scale (73). This scale rates patients on four grades in five different areas including general physical condition, mental state, activity, mobility, and incontinence. A score of 14 or below indicates at-risk patients. Numerous modifications have been proposed. Several investigators (49,98) have operationalized the items in the Norton Scale so as to reduce the ambiguity of such terms as good, fair, poor, or very bad used in describing physical condition. Gosnell (1973), in addition, added a category for nutrition. Goldstone and Roberts (1980), based on work done on an orthopedic ward, suggested that only the activity and mobility scale used by Norton were necessary. Other proposed predictions rules include the Braden Scale (17), the Knoll assessment tool (103), the Waterlow method (107), and the Anderson Scale (7).

Criteria for the evaluation of prediction rules have been described (106). Most of the prediction rules cited above fail these criteria on several counts. None has been derived prospectively from large patient populations; instead they have relied on clinical judgments. The predictive factors have often been poorly defined. Consequently, interrater reliability may vary widely, with reported values as low as 12% and as high as 90% (17,50). Bergstrom et al. (1987a) have demonstrated that the training and experience of the evaluators are important predictors of interrater reliability. Outcome events are also often poorly defined in that the time frame for the development of an ulcer must be specified. Finally, blinding of the assessments must be ensured.

Ultimately, the judgment of any prediction rule must be based upon how well it performs. The sensitivity and specificity of the various instruments have been recently reviewed (D. M. Smith et al., 1991). Data from NHs are quite limited, however. Gosnell (1973), in a study of her scale in 30 patients, demonstrated a sensitivity of 50%

and specificity of 73%; the Knoll instrument, in a study involving 60 residents, showed a sensitivity of 86% and a specificity of 56% (103). These values are within the range reported in other settings. Prediction rules may also be judged by their positive predictive value (18). Using a 5% incidence rate for ulcers and the sensitivity and specificity results from the Knoll instrument, Bayes's theorem allows the calculation of the positive predictive value as 9.3%. This means that fewer than 1 in 10 patients identified as high risk will go on to develop an ulcer.

No specific recommendations can be made as to which prediction rule should be utilized in NHs. Any of the instruments may fulfill a role in educating staff as to risk factors for pressure ulcer development. However, the low sensitivity, specificity, and positive predictive value appear to limit their clinical utility. Considerable resources are required to reassess patients at 2- to 3-week intervals as required by these instruments. Finally, the performance of these prediction rules may be no better than experienced clinicians. Additional testing in a variety of settings is clearly indicated. Such extensive testing is currently under way with the Braden Scale.

Prevention of Pressure Ulcers

The ultimate goal of these prediction rules is to identify high-risk patients so that appropriate preventive measures are implemented in a timely manner. Preventive measures have traditionally focused on interventions designed to relieve pressure, as well as to limit exposure to shear, friction, and moisture. Although such efforts are beneficial, it is also being recognized that the prevention of pressure ulcers must involve not only the entire NH staff, but also patients and families. As a result, educational means for increasing staff recognition of high-risk patients and to heighten patient self-awareness are being emphasized.

The first step in pressure ulcer prevention is the correction of potentially reversible risk factors. Although no study has directly examined this, efforts to increase mobility, promote dryness, and ensure adequate nutritional intake are all likely to be beneficial. Many residents, however, will remain at risk for pressure ulcers despite these attempts. In these patients, pressure relief is critical.

Pressure relief has two major components, proper positioning of patients and appropriate use of pressure-reducing devices. Frequent turning of patients—at 2- to 3-hour intervals—is often recommended and has been shown by Norton et al. (1975) to reduce the incidence of pressure ulcers. Unpublished work by Crumpton et al. (Berecek, 1975) has confirmed the efficacy of such a turning regime. Recent studies have also investigated the benefit of small, unscheduled, shifts in body position, such as adjusting the position of a limb. Two small studies were unable to show any benefit from this approach (29,94). Seiler and Stahelin (1985) emphasized the importance of positioning patients in the 30-degree right or left oblique position, as this avoids placing pressure on the common ulcer sites. Using a historical control group, they documented that such positioning, in combination with supersoft supports, led to a decrease in ulcers. Elevation of the head of the bed beyond 30 degrees should also be avoided as this predisposes to excess shearing forces. Pressure-induced ischemic injury, however, may develop within 2 to 3 hours. Consequently, efforts at positioning patients must be combined with use of a pressure-reducing device. Although a large number of such devices exist, they can generally be divided into two types: static and dynamic. Static devices include gel, foam, and water mattresses. A number of clinical trials, as outlined by D. M. Smith et al. (1991), have demonstrated that these specialized mattresses and pads reduce the incidence of pressure ulcers when compared to standard mattresses in the acute care setting. It is likely that similar benefits exist within the NH. Studies have not yet conclusively demonstrated which of these static devices provide the greatest benefit. For example, Lazzara and Buschmann (1991) showed no differences between a gel mattress and an air-filled overlay in a study to evaluate the prevention of pressure ulcers over a 6-month period. Specialized pads are also available for use with wheelchairs. Their efficacy has been extensively studied in patients with spinal cord injuries. Dynamic devices are motor powered and include air-fluidized beds as well as other types of specialized beds (111). Once again, although these devices have not been tested as preventive tools in NHs, there is little reason to doubt their efficacy.

Related to the wide range of pressure-relieving devices are those preventive strategies intended to address shear, friction, and moisture. Sheepskin fleeces to ankles, elbows, and sacrum have been examined in NHs by Denne (1979). It is proposed that such devices not only relieve pressure but prevent shear and may help keep the patient dry by virtue of the rapid evaporation characteristics of the material. Use of draw sheets for turning, or the addition of a large, firm pillow at the end of the bed to prevent slippage and shear are mentioned in various reviews but no extensive studies have tested their usefulness.

Several studies have evaluated the efficacy of educational programs involving multidisciplinary teams and intervention protocols for high-risk patients. Moody et al. (1988) established that in an acute care hospital such a program significantly reduced the incidence of pressure ulcers and led to a savings of $74,000 over 1 year in expenses related to specialized beds. In the long-term care setting, several studies have documented the beneficial effects of staff education as part of a quality assurance program (37,23). Educational efforts may also be targeted toward patients, although this literature has been based primarily on patients with spinal cord injuries. In this population, various techniques, especially when combined with alarms to notify patients of excessive time in one position, have been found to be useful in pressure ulcer prevention (31). Barnes (1987) has outlined the development of a patient and family educational program dealing particularly with out-patients at risk for pressure ulcers. Whether similar efforts to empower NH residents to care for themselves can be successful is open to study.

These data have obvious implications for the development of preventive programs within the NH. The low positive predictive value of existing prediction instruments suggests that a small group of high-risk patients cannot be identified. Thus the accurate targeting of potentially very effective, but also very expensive interventions, such as air-fluidized beds, is not possible. Further, the wide variety of clinical problems encountered in the NH, ranging from hemiplegic patients in a wheelchair to comatose, bed-bound patients, means that no single intervention will always be appropriate. Clearly a wide-ranging approach is required that combines state-of-the-art knowledge of the different preventive measures with a dedicated NH staff that can motivate the entire organization, including patients, to work toward a common goal. Further research to specifically identify those preventive measures that are most effective in a given situation is indicated.

OUTCOMES OF PRESSURE ULCER PATIENTS

Complication of pressure ulcers is well known, including osteo-myelitis, pyarthroses, bacteremia, and amyloidosis (79). For many clinicians, experience with pressure ulcers has centered around a few unfortunate individuals with large ulcers and prolonged hospitalizations. This has led to the impression that pressure ulcers rarely heal and are usually associated with poor health outcomes. Frequently cited data from acute care hospitals support this view. Pressure ulcers often cause bacteremia, and this bacteremia is associated with a 50%

mortality (30,43). Osteomyelitis is also a frequent occurrence, found in approximately one third of nonhealing ulcers (99). Recent articles have given a different picture of the outcome of NH patients with pressure ulcers, however.

Several articles have suggested that pressure ulcers may be a major source of infection in the NH. Garibaldi et al. (1981), in a prevalence study of 532 patients residing in seven NHs, demonstrated that 6% of the population had an infected pressure ulcer and an additional 10.2% had some other infection. A similar study (85) among 403 residents of eight NHs demonstrated rates of 4% for infected ulcers and 9.9% for other infections. During 6 months of follow-up, an additional 265 infections developed in this population, of which only 14 were infected pressure ulcers. Criteria for infection in these studies was the presence of a purulent exudate. The significance of these infections is unclear, especially when one considers the high overall prevalence of infection. A large study of 1,256 residents of nine extended care facilities suggests that pressure ulcers are an uncommon cause of fever in this population (28). The 1-year rate of hospitalization is also not increased in pressure ulcer patients (25). Pressure ulcers are the source of infection in 7%-14% of bacteremic NH patients (90,83), however. Pressure ulcers may also serve as a reservoir for highly resistant organisms that may infect other patients. The presence of a pressure ulcer is significantly associated, with an odds ratio of 2.9, to the colonization of patients with methicillin-resistant *Staphylococcus aureus* (70). A second study showed a nonsignificant trend relating the presence of a pressure ulcer to colonization with multiply resistant gram-negative bacilli among NH patients admitted to an acute care hospital (45). (See Chapter 3.)

Another important outcome for pressure ulcers is whether or not the wound heals. An early study by Michocki and Lamy (1976) suggested that ulcer healing is uncommon. Only 5 of the 54 pressure ulcers detected in 22 patients ever healed. The stages of the ulcers were not specified. However, this appears to be a highly unusual population, as 17 patients died during the short follow-up period. These results conflict with experience in other patient care settings. For example, among paraplegic patients on a plastic surgery service, 50%-70% of ulcers healed with nonsurgical interventions (33). Recent studies have confirmed this improved prognosis. Berlowitz and Wilking (1990), during a 6-week follow-up period, showed that 42% of the pressure ulcers present on admission to a chronic care hospital healed and an additional 37.7% showed some improvement. Similarly, in their large study, Brandeis et al. (1990) demonstrated a

6-month healing rate of 74% in Stage 2 ulcers, 59% in Stage 3 ulcers, and 33% in Stage 4 ulcers. With longer follow-up, over 95% of Stage 2 and 3 ulcers and over 75% of Stage 4 ulcers healed. Caution must be used in interpreting this data due to the high dropout rate of patients in the study. Of note, in both of these studies, treatment of the pressure ulcer involved standard wound care methods but no aggressive surgery or use of specialized beds.

The data of Michocki and Lamy (1976) showing a high mortality among pressure ulcer patients raise the issue as to whether the pressure ulcer may cause this increased mortality rate. Pressure ulcers are frequently noted in the terminal stage of disease (Howell, 1969). In the study of Berlowitz and Wilking (1990), the relative risk of dying within 6 weeks was 1.9 in patients with an ulcer present on admission, 3.1 in patients who developed a new ulcer, and 3.3 in patients whose ulcer failed to improve. The 1-year mortality was also significantly increased among patients with pressure ulcers in the study by Brandeis et al. (1990). There is evidence from Berlowitz and Wilking's study that pressure ulcers are not the cause of this increased mortality rate. The risk of dying was the same for Stage 2 ulcers as for Stage 3 and 4 ulcers. Pressure ulcers were not independently associated with patient death in multivariate models including diagnoses and functional status. Finally, all pressure ulcers that developed were Stage 2 and consequently unlikely to cause a tripling in the risk of dying.

Overall, these data seem to suggest that the outcome of pressure ulcers in the NH is not as poor as noted in the acute care hospital. Although localized infection is common, fever and hospitalizations are rare. The majority of ulcers will heal with conservative therapies. Although pressure ulcer patients have an increased mortality, this is likely due to severe co-morbid conditions. This should not imply that pressure ulcers are a benign condition that can be ignored. The good outcome of many pressure ulcer patients may be related to the close attention and care they receive. Important health outcomes, such as quality of life, have never been determined for this population. Finally, for a small minority of patients, pressure ulcers remain a life-threatening condition.

TREATMENT OF PRESSURE ULCERS

The above data suggest that pressure ulcers can be successfully managed in the NH environment, but this does not necessarily allow the determination of the optimal means of treatment. Complicating such a determination is the wide variety of interventions, ranging from topical sugar, gold leaf, and electric lamps (16) to air-fluidized beds and platelet-derived growth factor (80), that have been advocated as effective therapies. Numerous reviews of these different treatment modalities have been recently published (95,47,101). It has been appropriately recognized that only through well-designed, randomized, controlled, clinical trials can accurate statements as to the optimal treatment of pressure ulcers be made. Unfortunately, relatively few such studies have been performed and their interpretation is often open to question due to biases in the study design.

Methodological problems with clinical trials of pressure ulcer therapy have long been recognized (41). Difficulties with quantitating the extent of disease, including size of the ulcer, whether or not it is infected, and whether necrotic tissue is present, suggest that treatment groups may be dissimilar and also raise questions as to what features of the pressure ulcer are being treated. For example, certain topical therapies, such as wet-to-dry dressings, may be very effective in the presence of necrotic tissue but harmful to a well-granulating wound. Failure to standardize interventions other than the ones under study implies that the different treatment groups may be receiving a variety of differing therapies. Thus, beneficial effects arising from sham therapy are probably the result of the increased turning and mobilization accompanying the use of that device (41). Blinding as to which treatment a patient is receiving is rarely possible. Co-morbid conditions will contribute to a high dropout rate. Finally, outcome measures for the clinical trial are usually not standardized. Although healing of the wound is often evaluated, a more appropriate outcome measure would be time to healing. Serial measurements of pressure ulcer size, including area (102) and volume have rarely been employed and have yet to be critically evaluated.

Despite the limitations of the existing literature, it is clear that appropriate therapy of pressure ulcers should consist of two major components, correction of the underlying risk factors and proper attention to basic wound care. Several observational studies have demonstrated improved outcomes with the correction of risk factors. For example, Allman et al. (1987) demonstrated improved healing in pressure ulcer patients with higher protein nitrogen intake, whereas Berlowitz and Wilking (1990) showed that patients who remain bed or chair bound are less likely to have an improvement in their ulcer. Pressure relief, obtained either through frequent repositioning or the use of a pressure-reducing device, is a critical component of therapy. Features of the different pressure-reducing devices are discussed in the previously cited reviews. Treatment of the wound must include the control of infection, removal of necrotic tissue, and provision of a moist environment. Pressure ulcers with greater than 10^6 bacteria per milliliter rarely heal (75), nor do ulcers with anaerobic flora (84,89). Thus, clinical trials have shown a benefit with topical gentamicin (12), silver sulfadiazine (59), and oral metronidazole (8). Use of topical disinfectants, such as acetic acid, povidone-iodide, and Dakin's solution remain controversial as they are cytotoxic to fibroblasts and may impair healing. The removal of necrotic tissue may be accomplished with wet-to-dry dressings, enzymatic agents, hydrophilic polymers, or surgery. Once the ulcer is clean and granulating well, the use of occlusive or semiocclusive dressings will promote a moist environment and epithelialization of the wound (61). Four clinical trials have demonstrated improved healing with this approach to dressings (74,87,48,4).

Despite the success of these therapies, NH staff frequently must address the question of when more aggressive, and usually more expensive, interventions are required. These may include use of an air-fluidized bed or surgical techniques including grafts, flaps, or wound excision. Allman et al. (1987), in a randomized clinical trial, showed that an air-fluidized bed does lead to an increased rate of healing among pressure ulcers in acute care patients. However, R. G. Bennett et al. (1989), in their retrospective analysis on the use of air-fluidized beds at one NH, point to several limitations. Although significant improvements can result, prolonged therapy of at least 2 to 4 months is usually required. Due to death or clinical deterioration, many patients will not receive the intervention for a sufficient length of time to show a benefit. Recommendations for the use of air-fluidized beds in the NH are presented by these authors. Further studies would help clarify these indications.

Surgical reconstruction of pressure ulcers has a high rate of initial success in selected patients, but concerns remain as to its long-term efficacy (38). Recognizing the limitations of the existing data, Siegler and Lavizzo-Mourey (1991) recently performed a decision analysis to evaluate the use of a myocutaneous flap procedure in moderately demented residents with a Stage 3 pressure ulcer. These results suggest that surgery is the preferred approach when its success rate is greater than 30% or the rate of healing with conservative measures is less than 40%. An economic analysis revealed that surgery was $17,000 more expensive, although much of this difference was due to additional survival in the surgery group. Care must be taken in interpreting these results, as very limited data exist with which to calculate the probabilities of various outcome events.

Ultimately, in determining which treatments to employ, we strongly endorse the approach of Moss and LaPuma (1991). Treatment of the pressure ulcer must be consistent with overall therapeutic goals. For those patients who would demonstrate marked improvement in health outcomes with healing of the ulcer, interventions such as surgery and air-fluidized beds would be appropriate. Other NH patients will show little improvement in quality of life despite healing of the ulcer, so more conservative therapies would be indicated. In a minority of patients where comfort is the sole concern, even interventions such as turning and dressing changes may be contraindicated.

HEALTH SERVICES IMPLICATIONS

Pressure ulcers have important implications for the delivery of health services within the NH. They are significant contributors to the cost of care. Much of this research relating to cost estimates for pressure ulcers arises from the acute care setting. For example, Brody (1986) observed that depending on the severity of the ulcer and the degree of intervention, costs ranging from $5,000 to $40,000 per patient *per annum* could be generated. Allman et al. (1986) demonstrated that the median hospital cost per admission for pressure ulcer patients was $27,000, as compared to $13,000 in a control group of at-risk patients. A more complete analysis of cost variables in the acute care setting has been carried out by V. Alterescu (1989), in which she includes estimates of room and board, laundry costs, professional services, and special therapies such as air-fluidized beds to arrive at a cost of $80 per patient per day.

Estimates from NHs may be more difficult to calculate. Most services in this setting do not generate a bill and length of hospitalization tends not to be affected by the presence of an ulcer. Also, in instances where severe ulcers are present, costs may be shared with other institutions, as patients are often transferred for hospital level of care. Clearly pressure ulcer patients do require increased services. Roddy et al. (1987), using a time-motion evaluation of nursing services, determined that 29 minutes per day were required for the multiple dressing changes and treatment adjustments performed by staff. One study, by Frantz et al. (1991), did deal directly with costs. They retrospectively reviewed expenses incurred by an 830-bed long-term care facility over a 5-year period. One hundred fifty-five subjects with a total of 240 pressure ulcers were treated at an estimated cost of $116,416. This sum included approximations of nursing time, materials, medications related to therapy, and laboratory services, but did not include fees for other caregivers such as doctors or nutritionists. This amount is markedly lower than estimates of cost for ulcer care obtained from the acute hospital setting, but may merely reflect the wide variations in how costs are assessed.

The consensus statement of the National Pressure Ulcer Advisory Panel (1989) summarizes the current problems regarding accurate cost estimates and recommends that the scope of future inquiries should be broad enough to include not only the added costs caused uniquely by ulcers but also those more subtle related expenses pertaining to such issues as nutritional improvement and full management of co-morbid conditions. These recommendations should provide the stimulus and framework for further research intended to provide a specific estimate of pressure ulcer costs in the NH.

Pressure ulcers may also serve as a marker of the quality of care within the NH. Although no study has directly demonstrated a link between poor-quality care and pressure ulcers, anecdotal evidence certainly suggests that such a relationship exists. Traditionally, quality assessment has relied on measures of the structure, process, and outcome of care. Structural features, such as the number and training of nursing staff, are likely to be important in the prevention and treatment of pressure ulcers, but this has yet to be examined. Process criteria deal with whether specific items of care for ulcers have actually been performed. These studies have included efforts to document the care given to pressure ulcer patients (66) and the development of an extensive criteria map for evaluating the potential for skin breakdown (21). Process criteria are often difficult to use in NHs, however. Much of the care tends to be performed routinely and is poorly documented. For example, the medical record will not contain information on the number of times a bed-bound patient was actually turned. Consequently, there has recently been a strong emphasis on assessing quality through the outcomes of long-term care (56,54). Indeed, pressure ulcers have frequently been advocated as such a readily measurable outcome (54,82). Quality assessment reviews may then focus on the frequency with which patients develop a new ulcer, as has been done in the VA, or on the percentage of ulcers that heal within a given time period. However, great care is required in interpreting these data. Unless the outcome measure is risk adjusted on the basis of case mix, it will not be clear whether poor outcomes are secondary to poor care or just care of a sicker population. No efforts have yet been made to develop risk-adjusted models of outcomes for pressure ulcers.

In using the development of a new pressure ulcer as an outcome measure, it is also important to ask whether there is a baseline rate that is acceptable or if the development of even a single ulcer represents a lapse in care. Current HCFA guidelines addressed to state Physician Review Organizations have detailed the need to assess each pressure ulcer in the quality assurance process. These instructions recommend the determination of whether the ulcer was preventable and further observation as to the potential or presence of adverse effects (63). Whether this approach can lead to improved care has yet to be demonstrated. Given the difficulty in identifying all high-risk patients, as well as current trends to admit sicker patients, it appears, however, that some new pressure ulcers will always be encountered in NHs. Experience suggests that ongoing attempts to reduce this rate are likely to be successful no matter how low it may initially be. This implies that present efforts toward continuous quality improvement, in which the entire health care organization is motivated to improve the quality of care, are likely to be particularly successful when dealing with pressure ulcers. The previously cited works by Blom (1985) and Dimant and Francis (1988) certainly reflect initial steps in that direction.

CONCLUSIONS

Pressure ulcers, as with most clinical conditions encountered in the NH, pose a unique set of challenges that are distinct from those arising in other clinical settings. Although recent research has led to significant advances in our understanding of this problem, considerable gaps remain. This situation is compounded by the many methodological problems in the existing literature, which raise doubts as to the validity of results obtained. Ample opportunities clearly exist for the performance of high-quality research by clinicians, health services researchers, and clinical epidemiologists. Only then will definitive answers be produced that will further limit the problem of pressure ulcers in the NH.

REFERENCES

1. Allman, R. M. (1989). Pressure ulcers among the elderly. *New England Journal of Medicine, 320,* 850-853.
2. Allman, R. M., Laprade, C. A., Noel, L. B., et al. (1986). Pressure sores among hospitalized patients. *Annals of Internal Medicine, 105,* 337-342.

3. Allman, R. M., Walker, J. M., Hart, M. K., et al. (1987). Air-fluidized beds or conventional therapy for pressure sores. *Annals of Internal Medicine, 107,* 641-648.
4. Alm, A., Hornmark, A. M., Fall, P. A., et al. (1989). Care of pressure sores: A controlled study of the use of hydrocolloid dressings compared with wet saline gauge compresses. *Acta Dermato-Venereologica Supplementum, 149,* 1-10.
5. Alterescu, V. (1989). The financial costs of inpatient pressure ulcers to an acute care facility. *Decubitus, 2,* 14-23.
6. Alterescu, V., & Alterescu, K. (1988). Etiology and treatment of pressure ulcers. *Decubitus, 1,* 28-35.
7. Andersen, K., Jensen, O., Kvorning, S., et al. (1982). Prevention of pressure sores by identifying patients at risk. *British Medical Journal, 284,* 1370-1371.
8. Baker, P. G., & Haig, G. (1984). Metronidazole in the treatment of chronic pressure sores and ulcers: A comparison with standard treatments in general practice. *Practitioner, 225,* 569-573.
9. Barbenel, J. C., Ferguson-Pell, M. W., & Kennedy, R. (1986). Mobility of elderly patients in bed: Measurement and association with patient condition. *Journal of the American Geriatrics Society, 34,* 633-636.
10. Barnes, S. H. (1987). Patient/family education for the patient with a pressure necrosis. *Nursing Clinics of North America, 22,* 463-474.
11. Barth, P., Le, K., Madsen, B., et al. (1984). *Pressures profiles in deep tissues.* Proceedings of the 37th annual conference on Engineering in Medicine and Biology, Los Angeles.
12. Bendy, R. H., Nuccio, P. A., Wolfe, E., et al. (1964). Relationship of quantitative wound bacterial counts to healing of decubiti: Effect of topical gentamicin. *Antimicrobial Agents and Chemotherapy, 1,* 147-155.
13. Bennett, L., Kauner, D., Lee, B. Y., et al. (1969). Shear vs. pressure as causative factors in skin blood flow occlusion. *Archives of Physical Medicine and Rehabilitation, 60,* 309-314.
14. Bennett, L., & Lee, B. Y. (1988). Vertical shear existence in animal pressure threshold experiments. *Decubitus, 1,* 18-24.
15. Bennett, R. G., Bellantoni, M. F., & Ouslander, J. G. (1989). Air-fluidized bed treatment of nursing home patients with pressure sores. *Journal of the American Geriatrics Society, 37,* 235-242.
16. Berecek, K. H. (1975). Treatment of decubitus ulcers. *Nursing Clinics of North America, 10,* 171-210.
17. Bergstrom, N., Braden, B., Laguzza, A., et al. (1987a). The Braden scale for predicting pressure sore risk. *Nursing Research, 36,* 205-210.
18. Bergstrom, N., Demuth, P., & Braden, B. (1987b). A clinical trial of the Braden scale for predicting pressure sore risk. *Nursing Clinics of North America, 22,* 417-429.
19. Berlowitz, D. R., & Wilking, S. V. B. (1989). Risk factors for pressure sores: A comparison of cross-sectional and cohort-derived data. *Journal of the American Geriatrics Society, 37,* 1043-1050.
20. Berlowitz, D. R., & Wilking, S. V. B. (1990). The short-term outcome of pressure sores. *Journal of the American Geriatrics Society, 38,* 748-752.
21. Black, M., Green, E., Van Berkel, C., et al. (1989). Criteria map: Potential for skin breakdown—A quality assurance tool for use in any setting. *Quality Review Bulletin, 15,* 340-346.
22. Bliss, M. R. (1992). Acute pressure area care: Sir James Paget's legacy. *Lancet, 339,* 221-223.

23. Blom, M. F. (1985). Dramatic decrease in decubitus ulcers. *Geriatric Nursing, 6*, 84-87.
24. Brandeis, G. H., Morris, J. N., Lipsitz, L. A., et al. (1989). Correlates of pressure sores in the nursing home. *Decubitus, 2*, 60.
25. Brandeis, G. H., Morris, J. N., Nash, D. J., et al. (1990). The epidemiology and natural history of pressure ulcers in elderly nursing home residents. *Journal of the American Medical Association, 264*, 2905-2909.
26. Breslow, R. A., Hallfrisch, J., & Goldberg, A. P. (1991). Malnutrition in tubefed nursing home patients with pressure sores. *Journal of Parenteral and Enteral Nutrition, 15*, 663-668.
27. Brody, J. (1986, August 6). Personal health. *New York Times*.
28. Brown, N. K., & Thompson, D. J. (1979). Nontreatment of fever in extended-care facilities. *New England Journal of Medicine, 300*, 1246-1250.
29. Brown, M. M., Boosinger, J., Black, J., et al. (1981, May). Nursing innovation for prevention of decubitus ulcers in long term care facilities. *Journal of Plastic and Reconstructive Surgical Nursing*, pp. 51-55.
30. Bryan, C. S., Dew, C. E., & Reynolds, K. L. (1983). Bacteremia associated with decubitus ulcers. *Archives of Internal Medicine, 143*, 2093-2095.
31. Carlson, C. E., & King, R. B. (1990). Prevention of pressure sores. *Annual Review of Nursing Research, 8*, 35-56.
32. Daniel, R. K., Priest, D. L., & Wheatley, D. C. (1981). Etiologic factors in pressure sores: An experimental model. *Archives of Physical Medicine and Rehabilitation, 62*, 492-498.
33. Dansereau, J. G., & Conway, H. (1964). Closure of decubiti in paraplegics: Report on 2000 cases. *Plastic and Reconstructive Surgery, 33*, 474.
34. Denne, W. A. (1979). An objective assessment of the sheepskins used for decubitus prophylaxis. *Rheumatology and Rehabilitation, 18*, 23-29.
35. Denman, S., Murphy, S., & Kramer, J. (1990). *An analysis of pressure sore incidence, prevalence, and healing rates in a teaching hospital.* Abstract presented at the 43rd annual scientific meeting of the Gerontological Society of America, Boston.
36. Department of Veterans Affairs. (1991). Unpublished data from Office for Quality Management.
37. Dimant, J., & Francis, M. E. (1988). Pressure sore prevention and management. *Journal of Gerontological Nursing, 14*, 18-25.
38. Disa, J. J., Carlton, J. M., & Goldberg, N. H. (1992). Efficacy of operative cure in pressure sore patients. *Plastic and Reconstructive Surgery, 89*, 272-278.
39. Editorial. (1990). Preventing pressure sores. *Lancet, 335*, 1311-1312.
40. Exton-Smith, A. N., & Sherwin, R. W. (1961). The prevention of pressure sores: Significance of spontaneous bodily movements. *Lancet, 2*, 1124-1126.
41. Fernie, F. R., & Dornan, J. (1976). The problems of clinical trials with new systems for preventing or healing decubiti. In R. M. Kenedi, J. M. Cowden, & J. T. Scales (Eds.), *Bedsore biomechanics* (pp. 315-320). Baltimore, MD: University Park Press.
42. Frantz, R. A. (1991). The cost of treating pressure ulcers in a long-term care facility. *Decubitus, 4*(3), 37-45.
43. Galpin, J., Ghow, A., Bayer, A., et al. (1976). Sepsis associated with decubitus ulcers. *American Journal of Medicine, 61*, 346-350.
44. Garibaldi, R. A., Brodine, S., & Matsumiya, S. (1981). Infections among patients in nursing homes. *New England Journal of Medicine, 305*, 731-735.
45. Gaynes, R. P., Weinstein, R. A., Chamberlin, W., et al. (1985). Antibiotic-resistant flora in nursing home patients admitted to the hospital. *Archives of Internal Medicine, 145*, 1804-1807.

46. Goldstone, L. A., & Roberts, B. V. (1980). A preliminary discriminant function analysis of elderly orthopaedic patients who will or will not contract a pressure sore. *International Journal of Nursing Studies, 17,* 17-23.
47. Goode, P. S., & Allman, R. M. (1989). The prevention and management of pressure ulcers. *Medical Clinics of North America, 73,* 1511-1525.
48. Gorse, G. J., & Messner, R. L. (1987). Improved pressure sore healing with hydrocolloid dressings. *Archives of Dermatology, 123,* 766-771.
49. Gosnell, D. (1973). An assessment tool to identify pressure sores. *Nursing Research, 22,* 55-59.
50. Gosnell, D. J. (1989a). Pressure sore risk assessment: Part 1. A critique of the Gosnell scale. *Decubitus, 2,* 32-38.
51. Gosnell, D. J. (1989b). Pressure sore risk assessment: Part 2. Analysis of risk factors. *Decubitus, 2,* 40-43.
52. Hing, E. (1981). *Characteristics of nursing home residents, health status and care received; National Nursing Home Survey, United States, May-Dec 1977.* Hyattsville, MD: U.S. Department of Health and Human Services; Public Health Service; Office of Health Research, Statistics, and Technology; National Center for Health Statistics.
53. Howell, T. H. (1969). Some terminal aspects of disease in old age: A clinical study of 300 patients. *Journal of the American Geriatrics Society, 17,* 1034-38.
54. Institute of Medicine. (1986). *Improving the quality of care in nursing homes.* Washington, DC: National Academy Press.
55. Kaminski, M. V., Jr., Pinchcofsky-Devin, G., & Williams, S. D. (1989). Nutritional management of decubitus ulcers in the elderly. *Decubitus, 2,* 20-30.
56. Kane, R. L. (1990). Rethinking long-term care. *Journal of the American Geriatrics Society, 38,* 704-709.
57. Kosiak, M. (1959). Etiology and pathology of ischemic ulcers. *Archives of Physical Medicine and Rehabilitation, 40,* 60-69.
58. Krouskop, T. A. (1983). A synthesis of the factors that contribute to pressure sore formation. *Medical Hypotheses, 4,* 37-39.
59. Kucan, J. O., Robson, M. C., Heggers, J. P., et al. (1981). Comparison of silver sulfadiazine, povidoneiodine and physiologic saline in the treatment of chronic pressure ulcers. *Journal of the American Geriatrics Society, 29,* 232-235.
60. Lazzara, D. J., & Buschmann, M. T. (1991). Prevention of pressure ulcers in elderly nursing home residents: Are special support surfaces the answer? *Decubitus, 4,* 42-48.
61. Lidowski, H. (1988). NAMP: A system for preventing and managing pressure ulcers. *Decubitus, 1,* 28-37.
62. Lowthian, P. T. (1976). Underpads in the prevention of decubiti. In R. M. Kenedi, J. M. Cowden, & J. T. Scales (Eds.), *Bedsore biomechanics* (pp. 141-145). Baltimore, MD: University Park Press.
63. Massachusetts Physician Review Organization. (1992). *Massachusetts physician reviewer instruction manual.* Waltham, MA: Author.
64. Mawson, A. R., Biundo, J. J., Jr., Neville, P., et al. (1988). Risk factors for early occurring pressure ulcers following spinal cord injury. *American Journal of Physical Medicine and Rehabilitation, 67,* 123-127.
65. Michocki, R. J., & Lamy, P. P. (1976). The problem of pressure sores in a nursing home population: Statistical data. *Journal of the American Geriatrics Society, 24,* 323-328.
66. Miller, T. V., & Rantz, M. (1989). Quality assurance: Guaranteeing a high level of care. *Journal of Gerontological Nursing, 15,* 10-15.

67. Moody, B. L., Fanale, J. E., Thompson, M., et al. (1988). Impact of staff education on pressure sore development in elderly hospitalized patients. *Archives of Internal Medicine, 148,* 2241-2243.
68. Moss, R. J., & La Puma, J. (1991). The ethics of pressure sore prevention and treatment in the elderly: A practical approach. *Journal of the American Geriatrics Society, 39,* 905-908.
69. Mulholland, J. H., Tui, C., Wright, A. M., et al. (1943). Protein metabolism and bed sores. *Annals of Surgery, 118,* 1015-1023.
70. Murphy, S., Denman, S., Bennett, R. G., et al. (1992). Methicillin-resistant *Staphylococcus aureus* colonization in a long-term-care facility. *Journal of the American Geriatrics Society, 40,* 213-217.
71. National Pressure Ulcer Advisory Panel. (1989). Pressure ulcers prevalence, cost and risk assessment: Consensus development conference statement. *Decubitus, 2,* 24-28.
72. Nola, G. T., & Vistness, L. M. (1980). Differential response of skin and muscle in the experimental production of pressure sores. *Plastic and Reconstructive Surgery, 66,* 728-733.
73. Norton, D., McLaren, R., & Exton-Smith, A. N. (1975). *An investigation of geriatric nursing problems in hospital.* London: Churchill Livingston.
74. Oleske, D. M., Smith, S. P., White, P., et al. (1986). A randomized clinical trial of two dressing methods for the treatment of low-grade pressure ulcers. *Journal of Enterostomal Therapy, 13,* 90-98.
75. Parish, L. C., & Witkowski, J. A. (1989). The infected decubitus ulcer. *International Journal of Dermatology, 28,* 643-647.
76. Petersen, N. C., & Bittmann, S. (1971). The epidemiology of pressure sores. *Scandinavian Journal of Plastic and Reconstructive Surgery, 5,* 62-66.
77. Pinchcofsky-Devin, G. D., & Kaminski, M. V., Jr. (1986). Correlation of pressure sores and nutritional status. *Journal of the American Geriatrics Society, 34,* 435-440.
78. Reed, J. W. (1981). Pressure ulcers in the elderly: Prevention and treatment utilizing the team approach. *Maryland State Medical Journal, 30,* 45-50.
79. Reuler, J. B., & Cooney, T. G. (1981). The pressure sore: Pathophysiology and principles of management. *Annals of Internal Medicine, 94,* 661-666.
80. Robson, M. C., Thomason, A., Phillips, L. G., et al. (1992). Platelet-derived growth factor BB for the treatment of chronic pressure ulcers. *Lancet, 339,* 23-25.
81. Roddy, P. C., Lir, K., & Meiners, M. R. (1987). *Resource requirements of nursing home patients based on time and motion studies* (Publication 87-3408). Washington, DC: U.S. Department of Health and Human Services.
82. Rudman, D., Abbasi, A. A., Tourky, G. M., et al. (1990). Easily measurable adverse outcome indicators in a Veterans Affairs nursing home. *Quality Review Bulletin, 16,* 257-263.
83. Rudman, D., Hontanosas, A., Cohen, Z., & Mattson, D. E. (1988). Clinical correlates of bacteremia in a Veterans Administration extended care facility. *Journal of the American Geriatrics Society, 36,* 726-732.
84. Sapico, F. L., Ginunas, V. J., Thornhill-Joynes, M. T., et al. (1986). Quantitative microbiology of pressure sores in different stages of healing. *Diagnostic Microbiology and Infectious Disease, 5,* 31-38.
85. Scheckler, W. E., & Peterson, P. J. (1986). Infections and infection control among residents of eight rural Wisconsin nursing homes. *Archives of Internal Medicine, 146,* 1981-1984.
86. Schubert, V. (1991). Hypotension as a risk factor for the development of pressure sores in elderly subjects. *Age and Ageing, 20,* 255-261.

87. Sebern, M. D. (1986). Pressure ulcer management in home health care: Efficacy and cost effectiveness of moisture vapor permeable dressing. *Archives of Dermatology, 67,* 726-729.
88. Seiler, W. O., & Stahelin, H. B. (1985). Decubitus ulcers: Preventive techniques for the elderly patient. *Geriatrics, 40,* 53-60.
89. Seiler, W. O., & Stahelin, H. B. (1986). Recent findings on decubitus ulcer pathology: Implications for care. *Geriatrics, 41,* 47-60.
90. Setia, U., Serventi, I., & Lorenz, P. (1984). Bacteremia in a long-term care facility: Spectrum and mortality. *Archives of Internal Medicine, 144,* 1633-1635.
91. Shea, J. D. (1975). Pressure sores: Classification and management. *Clinical Orthopaedics and Related Research, 112,* 89-100.
92. Shepard, M. A., Parker, D., & DeClercque, N. (1987). The under-reporting of pressure sores in patients transferred between hospital and nursing home. *Journal of the American Geriatrics Society, 35,* 159-160.
93. Siegler, E. L., & Lavizzo-Mourey, R. (1991). Management of stage III pressure ulcers in moderately demented nursing home residents. *Journal of General Internal Medicine, 6,* 507-513.
94. Smith, A. M., & Malone, J. A. (1990). Preventing pressure ulcers in institutionalized elders: Assessing the effects of small, unscheduled shifts in body position. *Decubitus, 3,* 20-24.
95. Smith, D. M., Winsemius, D. K., & Besdine, R. W. (1991). Pressure sores in the elderly: Can this outcome be improved? *Journal of General Internal Medicine, 6,* 81-93.
96. Spector, W. D., Kapp, M. C., Tucker, R. J., et al. (1988). Factors associated with presence of decubitus ulcers at admission to nursing homes. *Gerontologist, 28,* 830-834.
97. Stotts, N. A. (1987). Nutritional parameters at hospital admission as predictors of pressure ulcer development in elective surgery. *Journal of Parenteral and Enteral Nutrition, 11,* 298-301.
98. Stotts, N. (1988). Predicting pressure ulcer development in surgical patients. *Heart & Lung, 17,* 641-647.
99. Sugarman, M., Hawes, S., Musher, D. M., et al. (1983). Osteomyelitis beneath pressure sores. *Archives of Internal Medicine, 143,* 683-688.
100. Taylor, T. V., Rimmer, S., & Day, B. (1974). Ascorbic acid supplementation in the treatment of pressure sores. *Lancet, 2,* 544-546.
101. The Medical Letter. (1990). Treatment of pressure ulcers. *Medical Letter, 31,* 17-18.
102. Thomas, A. C., & Wysocki, A. B. (1990). The healing wound: A comparison of three clinically useful methods of measurement. *Decubitus, 3,* 18-25.
103. Towey, A. P., & Erland, S. M. (1988). Validity and reliability of an assessment tool for pressure ulcer risk. *Decubitus, 1,* 40-48.
104. Tresch, D. D., Simpson, W. M., & Burton, J. R. (1985). Relationship of long-term and acute-care facilities. *Journal of the American Geriatrics Society, 33,* 819-826.
105. Versluysen, M. (1986). How elderly patients with femoral fracture develop pressure sores in hospital. *British Medical Journal, 292,* 1311-1313.
106. Wasson, J., Sox, H., Neff, R., et al. (1985). Clinical prediction rules applications and methodological standards. *New England Journal of Medicine, 313,* 793-799.
107. Waterlow, J. (1991, February). A policy that protects: The Waterlow pressure sore prevention/treatment policy. *Professional Nurse,* 258-264.
108. Weiler, P. G, Franzi, C., & Kecskes, D. (1990). Pressure sores in nursing home patients. *Aging, 2,* 267-275.

109. Witkowski, J. E., & Parish, L. C. (1982). Histopathology of the decubitus ulcer. *Journal of the American Academy of Dermatology, 6*, 1014-1021.
110. Yarkony, G. M., Matthews, K., Carlson, C., et al. (1990). Classification of pressure ulcers. *Archives of Dermatology, 126*, 1218-1219.
111. Young, J. B. (1990). Aids to prevent pressure sores. *British Medical Journal, 300*, 1002-1004.
112. Zappolo, A. (1981). *Discharges from nursing homes (1977) National Nursing Home Survey* (Publication #PHS S81-1715). Hyattsville, MD: U.S. Department of Health and Human Services.

5

Assessment, Treatment, and Management of Urinary Incontinence in the Nursing Home

JOSEPH G. OUSLANDER, M.D.
JOHN F. SCHNELLE, PH.D.

INTRODUCTION

Urinary incontinence (UI) is one of the most prevalent, disruptive, and costly conditions that occur in the nursing home (NH) setting. A recent National Institutes of Health (NIH) Consensus Conference (1989) indicated that UI is "epidemic" in NHs and that more needs to be done to assess and manage this condition effectively (52,72). New regulations for NH care under the federal Omnibus Budget Reconciliation Act (1987) include specific standards and recommendations for the assessment and treatment of UI designed to improve the quality of care that incontinent NH residents receive (26,27). Recent studies, summarized later in this chapter, suggest that UI can in fact be managed effectively in a substantial proportion of NH residents.

Although the NIH Consensus Conference, OBRA regulations, and recent clinical trials are certainly steps in the right direction, it will be some time before these developments are translated into clinical practice in the NH setting. At the present time most incontinent NH residents are managed by diapering, and in some cases, scheduled toileting (82,90). Although appropriate for some NH residents, these techniques do not pay sufficient attention to the potentially reversible and rehabilitative aspects of UI. The purpose of this chapter is to review and synthesize research on the assessment, treatment, and management of UI in the NH setting and to make recommendations for clinical practice and future research. For a more clinically oriented approach to UI in NH residents, readers are referred elsewhere (65,37). First the epidemiology, consequences, and pathophysiology of UI in the NH will be briefly reviewed.

PREVALENCE, INCIDENCE, AND ASSOCIATED FACTORS

Studies of the prevalence of UI in NHs indicate that approximately 41% to 55% of residents have some degree of UI (82,61,43). This probably underestimates the true prevalence for at least two reasons. First, the statistics were gathered before the full effects of the prospective payment system for acute hospitals on NH case mix were determined. Prospective hospital payment has resulted in the more rapid discharge to NHs of subacutely ill patients, among whom the prevalence of UI is probably high. Second, prevalence studies have determined continence status by the report of nursing staff, rather than by directly checking the wet/dry status of residents. In our experience, the latter method is more sensitive in detecting UI and has been used as the major outcome measure in the intervention trials that will be discussed later in the chapter.

One study examined the incidence and remission patterns of UI in the NH setting (66). Among a cohort of 430 residents of 8 NHs, UI developed in 27% within 2 months of admission and an additional 19% within 1 year. UI remitted in 23% within 2 months and an additional 22% within 1 year after admission. Although these data must be interpreted cautiously, they do suggest that continence status among NH residents is dynamic, similar to the phenomenon described among community-dwelling elderly (29). Further research is necessary to clearly identify factors associated with the development and remission of UI in the NH setting.

Several studies have identified factors associated with the presence of UI among NH residents. The strongest associations are with impaired functional status, especially immobility (64,67); impaired cognitive function and dementia (61,64,67,38,101); and stool incontinence, with 60%-80% of urinary incontinent residents also manifesting stool incontinence (90,61). These data strongly suggest the importance of functional disability in the pathogenesis of UI in the NH setting. Several studies have demonstrated an association between UI and bacteriuria (but not symptomatic urinary tract infection) (55).

The importance of this association is unclear, because no studies have documented that eradicating the bacteriuria either cures or changes the frequency of the UI (3,54,62). In contrast to studies of community-dwelling elderly, increasing age and female sex are not strongly associated with UI among NH residents (61,43,20). This finding again highlights the strong association between UI and functional disabilities in the NH setting.

CONSEQUENCES

UI has been purported to have adverse effects on physical health, psychosocial well-being, and the costs of care. Although UI in the NH has been associated with pressure sores and other skin problems, and with urinary tract infection (61), a cause-and-effect relationship has never been proven. Because the incidence of both pressure sores and symptomatic urinary tract infection is relatively low, it would take a large-scale clinical trial to demonstrate the impacts of improvements in UI on these conditions. A potentially hidden consequence of UI in the NH is falls. Many anecdotal reports suggest that incontinent NH residents frequently fall on the way to the bathroom (sometimes slipping in their own incontinent urine). Some studies have in fact suggested that the bathroom is a frequent site of falls among NH residents (76). No studies have, however, ever reported that an incontinence management program reduces the incidence of falls in the NH.

Among community-dwelling elderly, UI is associated with embarrassment, frustration, interference with social activities, and even depression (98,42,30,52). Such adverse psychosocial effects have been much more difficult to document among NH residents (64). This is probably in large part due to the difficulty in identifying these effects in residents with significant degrees of dementia. Improved measures of psychosocial functioning and quality of life will be necessary in order to document the effects of improved management for UI (as well as for interventions for other conditions) in the NH population. Among NH staff, UI is clearly seen as a difficult and onerous condition to manage (100,17). One study, however, failed to change the knowledge and attitudes of NH staff with an incontinence intervention program (15).

The economic costs of managing UI in NHs are staggering. Considering the costs of labor, supplies, and laundry necessary to manage UI and its complications, various assumptions have yielded estimates between \$0.5 and \$3 billion annually (in 1984 dollars) (60,35). Although no studies have documented that an effective incontinence management program will substantially reduce these costs (84,36), we believe that a well-designed and targeted program will reduce UI, reduce complications, and if not reduce cost, utilize resources more appropriately.

PATHOPHYSIOLOGY

Potentially reversible factors can cause or contribute to UI among NH residents. Such factors include delirium, mobility problems, acute urinary retention, acute urinary tract infection, atrophic vaginitis and urethritis in women, fecal impaction, a variety of drugs, and conditions that cause polyuria (e.g., poorly controlled diabetes) (65,37). The incidence of these factors among incontinent NH residents and the impact of treating them on continence status or the frequency of UI has not been well studied. These factors are likely to be much more common among residents admitted from acute hospitals and residents who develop the new onset of UI while in the NH, as opposed to those residents with chronic UI.

Several studies have demonstrated that the most common urodynamic abnormality among incontinent NH residents is detrusor hyperactivity (also referred to as detrusor instability or detrusor hyperreflexia) (41,75,73,68,63). This urodynamic finding has been demonstrated in 50%-75% of residents who have undergone a urodynamic evaluation. Advanced urodynamic investigations have shown that as many as one half of residents with detrusor hyperactivity also have impaired bladder contractility and empty less than one third of their bladder contents with the involuntary bladder contraction (detrusor hyperactivity with impaired contractility or DHIC) (75,73). The clinical importance of this finding is under investigation, but it may be very important in the pathogenesis of the frequent, small volume nature of incontinent episodes among NH residents. In contrast to elderly community-dwelling incontinent women, stress UI with sphincter weakness is less common among female residents. In part this may reflect the difficulty in documenting stress incontinence in cognitively and mobility-impaired residents who have relatively small bladder capacities due to concomitant detrusor hyperactivity. Overflow UI, due to an obstruction or an acontractile bladder, occurs in approximately 5%-10% of incontinent NH residents. Though less common than urge UI, stress and overflow UI are important to recognize because they may require different treatment and management approaches than urge UI.

A fundamental question remains about the pathophysiology of UI among NH residents. As most incontinent residents have *both* detrusor hyperactivity *and* functional impairments related to toileting skills, the relative importance of each remains unclear. In addition, detrusor hyperactivity has been found in some *continent* elderly individuals (20,7). Will eliminating the detrusor hyperactivity cure the UI without intervention for the functional impairments? Does managing the functional impairments by providing toileting assistance cure the UI without specific treatment for the detrusor hyperactivity? The answers to these questions have important implications for the treatment and management of UI in this population. Data presented later in this chapter suggest that at least for some incontinent NH residents the answer to the second question is yes.

MEDICAL AND NURSING ASSESSMENT

No studies have clearly defined the optimal medical and nursing assessment of incontinent NH residents. The NIH Consensus Conference (1989) statement, guidelines about to be promulgated by the Agency for Health Care Policy Research, and Resident Assessment Protocols (RAPs) published in conjunction with the new NH Minimum Data Set (MDS) (28) each offer recommendations for the diagnostic evaluation of incontinent patients. These recommendations are generally based on expert opinion, rather than on data that demonstrate specific aspects of the evaluation that improve outcome.

Studies have suggested that the vast majority of incontinent NH residents receive no formal diagnostic evaluation (90,61). On the other hand, recent research has shown that advanced urodynamic techniques are feasible and safe among incontinent residents (75). Given the costs of urological and/or gynecologic evaluations (including cystoscopy and radiologic studies) and of complex urodynamic evaluations (60,35) and the logistical difficulties of getting residents to centers with equipment and expert personnel (or vice versa), it is unlikely that these diagnostic techniques will achieve widespread use in the NH population. The critical issue is to identify which residents benefit from these relatively invasive and expensive procedures. Like any other diagnostic test, these techniques are appropriately used only when the information obtained alters the way a patient is treated and leads to a better patient outcome.

We believe that the medical and nursing assessment of an incontinent resident should have three goals:

1. Identifying reversible factors that may be causing or contributing to the UI
2. Identifying residents who should have a more extensive diagnostic evaluation, including urological or gynecological examination and/or complex urodynamic testing
3. Determining the most appropriate treatment or management plan

The identification of the potentially reversible factors noted earlier can be accomplished by a history, medical record review, and targeted physical examination (65,37,71,70). Although these factors may be more prevalent among newly admitted NH residents and those with the new onset of UI, they also contribute to chronic UI. Studies are lacking, however, to document the impacts of treating these reversible factors. It certainly makes clinical sense to diagnose and appropriately manage delirium, acute changes in mobility that interfere with toileting, fecal impaction, conditions that cause polyuria (e.g., diabetes, volume overload from venous insufficiency, or congestive heart failure), and side effects from a variety of drugs. Atrophic vaginitis and urinary tract infection (UTI) are also listed as potentially reversible causes of UI. No studies have systematically defined and treated atrophic vaginitis in residents. A study examining the impact of treating atrophic vaginitis on UI among residents is needed. UTI may be difficult to define in the NH population because of the relatively high prevalence of "asymptomatic" bacteriuria (approximately 20%-40%) (99,4). A question remains as to whether UI represents a symptom of bacteriuria in the population. Well-designed clinical trials have suggested that treating bacteriuria in residents does not significantly influence morbidity and mortality (47, 48). Studies among noninstitutionalized elderly with infrequent UI suggest that eradicating bacteriuria does not change the symptoms of UI (3,51). One small pilot study suggested the same findings (54). We are presently conducting a clinical trial with adequate statistical power to determine if eradicating bacteriuria reduces the frequency and/or volume of UI in the NH population.

Several studies have addressed the issue of the optimal extent of the diagnostic evaluation for geriatric UI (75,68,63,18,33,21,50,74); some of these have included NH residents (75,68,63,74). Because urologic and gynecologic evaluations and complex urodynamic testing are expensive and relatively invasive, yet capable of detecting conditions that require specific intervention, it is important to identify which incontinent residents will benefit from these evaluations. Table 5.1 lists what we believe to be appropriate indications for further evaluation of incontinent residents based on the limited data available (65,37,63,71,74,62). These recommendations presume that: (a) the resident has had a targeted history, physical examination, urinalysis, and postvoid residual determination; and (b) that conditions detected during the further evaluation would be acted upon (e.g., the resident is willing and able to undergo surgery if obstruction or severe stress incontinence is diagnosed).

The role of a simple urodynamic evaluation in the assessment of incontinent residents is not clear. Simple or "bedside" urodynamics can be helpful in differentiating stress, urge, mixed stress/urge, and overflow UI (62,63). A question remains as to whether it is helpful to define the exact type of UI in all NH residents. Recent studies of behavioral interventions, both among community-dwelling (25,8,24, 97,9,13,10,14) and NH populations (77,79,80,84-86,37,22,12,45,87,88,19), suggest that these interventions are helpful for stress, urge, and mixed UI. Thus an argument can be made that if behavioral intervention is to be the initial therapy, it can be implemented without knowing the exact type of UI. This is obviously not true if pharmacologic or surgical treatment is being considered. In addition, recent studies suggest that urodynamic classification is not helpful in identifying residents who respond well to the behavioral intervention of prompted voiding (77,79,81,86). We are currently conducting a clinical trial to determine if a "bedside" urodynamic evaluation adds information to the other components of the medical and nursing assessment that is helpful in efficiently targeting behavioral and/or pharmacologic interventions for UI among NH residents.

TREATMENT VERSUS MANAGEMENT OF URINARY INCONTINENCE

A distinction can be made between "treatment" and "management" interventions for UI in the NH setting. The goals of treatment are patient oriented and designed to change the function of the lower urinary tract. Surgery, pharmacological interventions, muscle retraining, and biofeedback procedures can be categorized as "treatment" procedures. The management approach is caregiver oriented and teaches caregivers new behaviors that can improve or even reverse incontinence symptoms. There is no direct effort to change urinary tract functioning. It has been documented that both institutional and

Table 5.1 Criteria for Referral of Elderly Incontinent Patients for Urologic, Gynecologic, or Urodynamic Evaluation

Criteria	Definition	Rationale
History		
Recent history of lower urinary tract or pelvic surgery or irradiation	Surgery or irradiation involving the pelvic area or lower urinary tract within the past 6-12 months	A structural abnormality relating to the recent procedure should be sought
Relapse or rapid recurrence of a symptomatic urinary tract infection	Onset of dysuria, new or worsened irritative voiding symptoms, fever, suprapubic or flank pain associated with significant growth of a urinary pathogen; symptoms and bacteriuria return within 4 weeks of treatment	A structural abnormality or pathologic condition in the urinary tract predisposing to infection should be excluded
Physical Examination		
Marked pelvic prolapse	Pronounced uterine descensus to or through the introitus or a prominent cystocele that descends the entire height of the vaginal vault with coughing during speculum examination	Anatomic abnormality may underlie the pathophysiology of the incontinence and may require surgical repair
Stress incontinence that has failed or cannot be managed by nonsurgical therapy or stress incontinence in a man	Stress incontinence demonstrated standing or supine; urine, generally drops or small volumes, leaks coincident with increasing abdominal pressure by vigorous coughing	Surgical procedures are generally well tolerated and successful in properly selected elderly women who have stress incontinence that responds poorly to more conservative measures; stress incontinence in a man suggests sphincter damage
Marked prostatic enlargement and/or suspicion of cancer	Gross enlargement of the prostate on digital exam; prominent induration or asymmetry of the lobes	An evaluation to exclude prostate cancer that requires curative or palliative therapy should be undertaken

Severe hesitancy, straining, and/or interrupted urinary stream	Straining to begin voiding and a dribbling or intermittent stream at a time the patient's bladder feels full	Signs suggestive of obstruction or poor bladder contractility are present
Postvoid Residual		
Difficulty passing a 12- or 14-French straight catheter	Catheter passage is impossible or requires considerable force or a larger, more rigid catheter	Anatomic blockage of the urethra or bladder neck may be present
Postvoid residual volume >200 ml	Volume of urine remaining in the bladder within 5-10 minutes after the patient voids spontaneously in as normal a fashion as possible	Anatomic or neurogenic obstruction or poor bladder contractility may be present
Urinalysis		
Hematuria (sterile)	Greater than 5 red blood cells per high-power field on microscopic exam in the absence of infection	A pathologic condition in the urinary tract should be excluded
Uncertain diagnosis	After the history, physical exam, simple tests of lower urinary tract function, and urinalysis, none of the other referral criteria are met and an appropriate treatment plan cannot be developed based on the findings	A complex urodynamic evaluation may help better define and reproduce the symptoms associated with the incontinence and target treatment

SOURCE: Ouslander et al. (1990b).

community-dwelling elderly can maintain continence with such management strategies even in the presence of lower urinary tract abnormalities (24,77,79,81,86,44). For example, many incontinent episodes reflect a failure to compensate for problems such as low bladder capacity that make accidents likely. Some elderly people may have to be taught to go to the bathroom more frequently and at times that they do not feel a strong urge to go. Such frequent toileting may reduce bladder pressure and decrease the number of accidents. Some elderly individuals may not be able to get to a toilet quickly enough, or in the case of NH residents, may not be able to toilet independently at all. Consistent toileting assistance is therefore essential to the success of any intervention for immobile incontinent residents.

Based on data that will be presented below, we believe that after an initial assessment rules out potentially reversible conditions and conditions requiring further evaluation, management approaches should be attempted before other more specific treatments with most residents for at least four reasons: (a) they are simple and noninvasive and will effectively reduce UI in many residents, even those who are very frail, (b) these approaches do not require expensive equipment or extensive professional involvement, (c) residents responsive to certain toileting programs can be identified in a 4- to 6-day assessment period, and (d) the assessment period provides information about the residents who do not respond to toileting that can be used to plan the next stage of intervention. For many residents, a treatment intervention designed to change urinary tract functioning will be the next option attempted.

MANAGEMENT APPROACHES

Overview

Several toileting management approaches to UI in the NH have been described. In general, they all involve some type of timed toileting program, either on a fixed schedule ("scheduled toileting" and "prompted voiding") or a variable schedule ("habit training") (Table 5.2). The logic of toileting management is that if residents are taught to void frequently in toileting receptacles they will not be incontinent between toileting opportunities. This logic holds true only if residents can do two things: (a) start the voiding process if given access to a toilet, and (b) hold urine during intervals between toiletings. Many residents have these abilities and will thus benefit

Table 5.2 Examples of Toileting Management for Urinary Incontinence in Nursing Homes

Approach	Description
Scheduled Toileting	Placing the resident on a commode or bedpan at fixed intervals regardless of whether the resident indicates a desire to go
Habit Training	Establishing a consistent individual pattern of voiding and toileting the resident according to individual pattern or habit
Prompted Voiding	Systematically contacting the resident to provide an opportunity to toilet but only toileting upon affirmative response to a prompt to void

from toileting management procedures. Several major problems must be resolved if toileting management programs are to work. For habit training, the resident's schedule of voiding must be established, and it must be predictable. Unfortunately, predictable voiding schedules cannot be identified for some residents. It may therefore be impossible to specify a critical time in which toileting assistance opportunities would be most successful. The second problem arises even if individualized resident voiding schedules can be identified: It is difficult for staff to remember a variety of individualized resident schedules. The nature of nurse's aides' work demands does not easily accommodate multiple, individualized resident-contact strategies (19).

Scheduled toileting programs are simpler to manage than habit training programs. Scheduled toileting involves contacting the resident on a fixed time schedule (usually 2 hours) and providing toileting assistance (87). There are no specific communication steps that are followed in simple scheduled-toileting protocols, and how the staff induces residents to toilet is left unspecified. In most cases, residents are toileted with minimal preparation or verbal interaction. Toileting becomes a habit or routine in which the resident plays a passive role.

Prompted voiding is a variation of scheduled toileting that includes a communication protocol (65,77). Aides are trained to talk to residents in a specific manner. These communication steps help reduce resident passivity and facilitate the toileting process. Efforts are made to encourage residents to take more responsibility and to request toileting assistance, and they are only toileted when they respond affirmatively to a prompt. Prompted voiding takes a little

Table 5.3   Evaluations of Toileting Management for Incontinence in
                Nursing Homes

Reference	N	Age	Sex	Percent Improvement in Wetness
55	126	86	M,F	50
37	11	—	M,F	42
62	65	85	M,F	26
63	62	76	M,F	28
52	86	—	M,F	33
65	92	81	M,F	38
66	4	78	M,F	34
68	10	78	F	21
69	20	—	M	85
71	14	77	M,F	44
11	21	82	M,F	49

NOTE: Toileting management interventions consisted of scheduled toileting, habit training, or prompted voiding; some interventions were combinations of these techniques (see text); wetness is generally measured by checks every 1 or 2 hours (see text).

more time than simple scheduled toileting, but we believe it involves a more mature and humane interaction with residents. At worst, aides will not verbally interact well with residents, and prompted voiding will be reduced to a simple scheduled-toilet protocol. At best, verbal interaction will produce a more responsible, dry, and energetic resident.

Table 5.3 summarizes the results of several clinical trials of toileting management approaches for UI. A recent panel convened by the Agency for Health Care Policy Research (AHCPR) reviewed these 13 articles (79-81,84-86,68,37,22,12,45,17,88). The articles report outcome data for 428 residents who ranged in age 76 to 86 years. Measurements of effectiveness reported in the studies reflect an increase in percent of checks dry or a decrease in percent of checks wet over a treatment period. The outcome measure, "percent checks wet," was expressed as percent of all physical checks done during the day in which resident were detected as wet. The number of physical checks completed in the studies ranges from 7 to 14 per day. Each of the studies reported an improvement with the management interventions. The average percent wet observed at the beginning of the treatment across all studies was 31.1% of checks wet. The average percent wet observed at the end of treatment was 19.2%. The impact of the improvement on wet rates for the cost of incontinence was estimated to be $90 million per year (AHCPR, unpublished data).

For reasons alluded to above, we have had the most experience with prompted voiding. The remainder of this section discusses issues we believe to be critical in making prompted voiding a cost-effective, practical, and accepted part of NH practice.

Who Responds to Toileting Management?

Despite the overall success of toileting management interventions, it is clear that not all NH residents are responsive. Many residents cannot either initiate the voiding process when placed on the toilet or store urine between the scheduled toileting opportunities. In one controlled study of every 2 hours prompted voiding among 126 NH residents, one of us reported that 33% of the residents reduced incontinence frequency to fewer than one episode per day (77). Another 35% reduced incontinence frequency by two episodes per 12-hour period, but continued to be wet more than one time per day. Subjects who were most responsive had larger bladder capacities (as measured by maximum voiding volume) and lower frequencies of voiding during baseline assessment periods. For example, the maximum voided volume of a responsive subject (calculated as the largest void over a 1-day period) averaged 223, whereas a maximum voided volume of an unresponsive subject averaged 159. Mental status scores were not predictive of a subject's responsiveness. The behavioral variable that was most predictive of how well a subject would respond to the intervention was the subject's ability to initiate toileting as measured by the statistic, "appropriate toileting percentage." To calculate this statistic, the subject is prompted to toilet every 2 hours from 7 a.m. to 7 p.m. for a period of 1 to 3 days. The number of times that a subject successfully toilets is divided by the total number of voids (toileting plus incontinence episodes). For example, assume the number of times a subject toilets is 3 and the number of incontinence episodes is 3. The appropriate toileting percentage would be 3 divided by 3 + 3 = 50%. Subjects' appropriate toileting percentages on the first assessment day was a highly significant predictor of their responsiveness to the prompted voiding intervention. The higher the appropriate toileting percentage, the more likely they would be responsive. The fact that subjects' responsiveness can be assessed by their appropriate toileting ability over a brief assessment period suggests that NH caregivers can efficiently identify residents who might benefit from prompted voiding. The procedures to organize such an assessment over a 6-day assessment period are described in a recent book (78). As noted earlier, we are currently involved in a clinical trial to validate these assessment procedures, so that the simplest and least invasive assessment protocol can be designed to identify residents likely to respond well to the prompted voiding.

Continence Maintenance Issues

As described above, numerous studies have shown that a large percentage of NH residents will improve if staff prompt the residents and consistently provide toileting assistance. This consistent prompting is a management technique that compensates for the cognitive and physical impairments that prevent the incontinent resident from independent toileting. As the residents remain physically and cognitively impaired, the prompted voiding procedure must be continuously implemented if continence is to be maintained. Unfortunately, there is clear evidence that staff have difficulty maintaining continence programs (19,82).

One primary reason for the failure of nursing staff to maintain toileting programs may be the fact that toileting residents is more time consuming than changing the residents. The average time involved in a toileting episode is 7.5 minutes, whereas the average time in a cleaning episode is 4.5 minutes (84). Exaggerating this time differential even further is the fact that NH staff do not change residents after every incontinence episode. This was demonstrated in a study in which the average wet frequency of a group of residents at two NHs was 3.8 times per day, and staff changed these residents only 2.1 times per day (84). In one study of prompted voiding the average amount of time research staff spent in toileting residents who were responsive to the program over a 5-day period was 19.2 minutes per 8-hour shift. The average amount of time indigenous NH staff spent changing and toileting these same residents during another 5-day period was 6.2 minutes. Thus, an increase of 14 minutes per resident per shift would have been required if staff were to toilet residents at sufficient frequencies to maintain continence (84).

Given the fact that prompted voiding requires increased nursing aide work activity, it is no surprise that simply training staff about why or how to implement prompted voiding is not sufficient to maintain continence (15). The failure of a formalized training program to produce continence maintenance in over 100 residents in 6 NHs was described in a recent study (82). In this study, research staff worked directly with nursing aides to demonstrate the prompted voiding procedures. Aides first observed the prompted voiding routines and were then asked to perform the prompted voiding while observed by research staff. A 1-page protocol for residents who proved responsive to prompted voiding programs was formulated and given to supervisors and nursing aides with a description of how well the resident responded, as well as a recommended toileting schedule. Toileting forms were placed on the door of each resident's room and aides were encouraged to prompt residents according to the prescribed schedule and to record toileting activities. Group in-service activities were held with NH staff on each floor to describe the protocols and to start the program. Measures of resident wetness were collected by research staff 2 weeks and 6 weeks after the program was turned over to the indigenous NH nursing staff. Wetness frequencies during a 2-week follow-up check had returned to the high levels observed during pretreatment periods. It is clear from this study that training alone is not sufficient to motivate staff to maintain toileting programs. Follow-up staff management procedures in addition to this training would appear necessary to maintain continence over longer time periods.

Continence Maintenance Interventions

One approach to maintaining the intervention is to give ongoing feedback to the staff responsible for the prompted voiding. Four residents in one NH were subjects of a group feedback continence maintenance intervention (12). Each resident was assigned a toileting schedule and feedback was given in biweekly meetings with nursing staff about the percentage of scheduled resident toiletings that staff recorded as occurring. The feedback provided averaged data and hence the individual performance of aides were not displayed. Such biweekly group feedback maintained the percentage of assigned toiletings and improved dryness rates for 4 to 5 months. After this time period, there was some evidence of deterioration in staff compliance to the toileting regimen. An individual feedback system was then added in which each aide was provided bar graph information about the percentage of assigned toiletings that the individual aide had recorded as occurring. This individualized feedback system increased compliance to the toileting schedule back to the level observed during the early phases of the group feedback.

A second study evaluated the effects of an incontinence management program based on the quality control techniques utilized in business and industry to maintain consistent levels of employee performance (84). This quality control technology has three major components: (a) standards of job performance are defined, (b) job performance is monitored and compared to these standards, and (c) methods to improve performance are investigated when job standards are not met. Job standards were set based on a 4-day assessment in which all residents were prompted on a 2-hour schedule by research staff. All residents who responded to prompted voiding with a wetness rate of approximately one time per day or less during the 4-day assessment period were selected from the continence maintenance program. Job performance criteria were set by calculating the average number of checks in which the responsive residents were found wet during the assessment period. The variability of expected resident wetness was calculated by the standard deviation across the 24 checks completed during the 4 days (6 checks per day for 4 days).

Once the average number of residents expected to be wet and the standard deviation is calculated from the assessment data, the nurse manager knew how many residents should be wet if they were prompted on a 2-hour schedule. In general, the percentage of residents wet at any given hour should be within the average or within two standard deviations from the average. If the number found wet is more than two standard deviations from the average, intervention is not doing well. For example, the average number of residents found wet on any check during the assessment period for NH 1 was 10% with a standard deviation of 9%. These 10 residents were turned over to the nursing staff for continence maintenance. Supervisory nurses could now implement job monitoring by making rounds and noting the number of residents wet. If zero to three residents were found wet (between the average and two standard deviations from average), then supervisors could conclude that the toileting program was as effective as it was during the initial assessment period. If four or more residents were found wet (more than two standard deviations from the average expected wetness), one could assume that the program is not working well. Individual feedback can be given to the aides and efforts made to identify the work measures that contribute to the unusually high work samples.

This system was implemented in seven NHs with 76 residents, and nursing staff was able to maintain the improved levels of wetness observed during the assessment period for a 6-month interval (83). These studies document that it is possible with training and follow-up management to maintain improved continence status in NH residents. We believe this management intervention is capable of significantly improving incontinence and maintaining improvement in a large number of residents.

Residents Unresponsive to Prompted Voiding

Three major groups of residents can be identified during the brief prompted voiding assessment period based on their toileting and voiding behavior: (a) some residents will reduce incontinence frequencies to less than one per day and will appropriately toilet more than 50% of the time, (b) some residents will significantly reduce the frequency of their incontinence episodes but continue to be wet two or more times per day and appropriately toilet less than 50% of the time, and (c) some residents will not change their wetness frequency or increase their appropriate toileting rates. The second group of residents appear to be capable of some bladder control by changing their incontinence frequency and by increasing their appropriate toileting rates. In addition, they appear adequately motivated and cognitively capable of responding to verbal prompts for toileting assistance. These residents are thus the most logical candidates for a treatment intervention designed to improve bladder function to the point that they would be more responsive to a toileting management program. Treatment approaches that could be attempted with these residents are described in the next section of this chapter. Residents who fail to respond to the treatment interventions and most of the unresponsive residents in the third group are candidates for conservative management with absorbent garments and regular checking and changing.

TREATMENT APPROACHES

Behavioral Treatments

Behavioral treatments have been used successfully for UI in several studies of community-dwelling elderly (25,8,24,87,9,13,10,14). These treatments include bladder training, pelvic muscle exercises, and biofeedback. All of these treatments require cooperation, motivation, and learning by the incontinent person. They thus may not be viable approaches to many of the more severely impaired incontinent residents who do not respond to a simple prompted voiding program.

Bladder training involves three primary components: (a) an educational program, (b) scheduled voidings, and (c) positive reinforcement. The education program usually combines written material and a visual and verbal instructional package addressing the mechanics of the lower urinary tract. The voiding schedule incorporates a plan for progressively longer intervals between mandatory voidings and can employ distraction or relaxation techniques to help inhibit voiding in between scheduled voiding opportunities. By gradually increasing the intervals between voidings, this procedures corrects the maladaptive behavior of frequent voiding, improves the ability to suppress bladder instability, and may eventually diminish urgency. Bladder training has been shown to be effective for urge, stress, and mixed UI among outpatient older women (24,14). Its applicability to most NH residents is uncertain because of the learning required. A bladder training program would be helpful among residents admitted from an acute hospital with an indwelling catheter in whom the catheter is removed (65). No studies have, however, reported on the effectiveness of bladder training in the NH setting.

Pelvic muscle ("Kegel") exercises can improve urinary control by strengthening the pupococcygus muscle (97,13). The first step in pelvic muscle exercises is to establish better discrimination of muscle function. Biofeedback is often used to assist individuals in gaining such pelvic muscle awareness (97,13,10). The exercises are performed by drawing in the vaginal muscles and anal sphincters as if to control urination or defecation without contracting abdominal, buttock, or thigh muscles. Many studies have documented improvements in UI with pelvic muscle exercises, even among individuals who have had multiple surgical repairs (97). As is the case for bladder training, there is no evidence to suggest how many NH residents will be capable of responding on interventions that require active learning and practice.

Biofeedback describes a group of procedures that use electronic or mechanical instruments to display information about neuromuscular activity. This information is turned into the form of audible signals or visual displays and can be used to shape responses that tend to lead to improved physiological functioning. Biofeedback is generally used in combination with pelvic muscle exercises and other techniques such as bladder training and fluid and diet manipulation (8,13,10). It aims to alter bladder and sphincter dysfunction by teaching individuals to change physiological responses that moderate bladder control. Biofeedback has been shown to be highly effective in reducing incontinence in several studies (13,10,14). There is no evidence concerning the number of residents who may prove responsive to such a procedure. Studies performed in France (2) and in male residents in a Veterans Administration NH (49) suggest that some incontinent residents may improve after biofeedback therapy.

Further research is needed to determine if biofeedback will be useful in large numbers of residents.

Electrical stimulation is a technique sometimes used in conjunction with other behavioral treatments. Different stimulation frequencies are used to treat stress and urge UI (23). One small study found no effect of electrical stimulation on the frequency of UI in NH residents (39). Several methodologic issues (such as sample size, duration of stimulation, lack of an adjunctive toileting program) limit the conclusions that can be drawn from this study. Because of the high prevalence of detrusor instability and detrusor hyperreflexia among incontinent residents, and the potential ability of electrical stimulation to inhibit involuntary bladder contractions, further study of electrical stimulation for UI in the NH is warranted.

Pharmacologic Treatment

Several studies have suggested that pharmacologic treatment with anticholinergic agents (e.g., propantheline, oxybutynin) directed at urge incontinence and detrusor hyperactivity is not effective among incontinent individuals with significant impairments of cognitive and physical functioning in both community and institutional settings (54,16,100,101,92). Small sample sizes, difficulties with the definition and measurement of outcomes, and lack of adjunctive toileting management may have masked some treatment effect. No studies have addressed the pharmacologic treatment of stress UI in the NH population. We believe that drug therapy *alone* will not be effective for the large number of incontinent residents with predominantly urge type UI, largely because inhibiting the involuntary bladder contractions will not make them continent if cognitive and physical impairments continue to prevent appropriate toileting behavior. We have therefore initiated a clinical trial, along the lines of a previously reported pilot study (54), to determine if a bladder relaxant drug is effective when *combined* with prompted voiding among residents with urge UI who fail to respond to prompted voiding alone.

Surgical Treatment

Surgical intervention is necessary if a pathologic lesion (tumor, stone) is identified or if obstruction is causing urinary retention, infection, and potential upper urinary tract damage. Surgery is also performed for stress UI that is not responsive to behavioral and/or pharmacologic treatments. Although several studies have suggested that surgery for stress UI is highly effective (short-term cure rates over 80% for first surgery), even in the elderly (69,89), no studies have examined the efficacy of surgery in frail elderly NH residents. Concomitant medical and psychiatric conditions, previous genito-urinary surgery, and the common occurrence of detrusor hyperactivity (in association with stress UI) among residents may all reduce the chances of surgical success. Lacking data from clinical trials, the decision to consider surgery for stress UI in a resident must be made on an individualized basis, considering the factors noted above as well as the resident's perceptions of the potential risks and benefits of the procedure.

PADS AND UNDERGARMENTS

Highly absorbent launderable or disposable pads and incontinence undergarments are the most common method of managing UI in the NH. Several types of garments and padding are available that are effective in absorbing large amounts of urine (5). Disposable products appear to be at least as, if not more cost-effective than launderable products (35), although the potential environmental hazards of large-scale disposable product use must also be considered. This method of management is certainly appropriate for the subgroup of incontinent residents who are identified for palliative incontinence care. Pads and garments may also be very helpful at night for residents who are managed by prompted voiding and/or other interventions during the day and evening.

These containment devices should not, however, be used as the sole solution to UI in the NH, or in a manner that fosters further dependency. When pads or garments are used, residents should still be regularly checked, toileted, and/or changed if necessary in order to avoid skin irritation and breakdown. Environmental considerations, such as bathroom and commode design, and the appropriate use of toilet substitutes are also relevant to managing UI in NHs (6).

CATHETERS AND CATHETER CARE

Three basic types of catheters and catheterization procedures are used for the management of urinary incontinence in NHs: external catheters, intermittent straight catheterization, and chronic indwelling catheterization. External catheters are the most common method of managing UI in Veterans Administration NHs (56). Studies of complications associated with the use of these devices have been limited, but existing data suggest that male residents with external catheters are at increased risk of developing symptomatic UTIs (58). External catheters should therefore only be used to manage intractable incontinence in male residents who do not have urinary retention and who are extremely physically dependent. As with incontinence undergarments and padding, these devices should not be used as a matter of convenience, as they may foster dependency. Contrary to popular belief, by simply cleaning the penis with betadine, applying a new catheter, and collecting the first voided urine, one can use the external catheter to collect urine specimens that accurately reflect bladder urine (59). Use of this simple technique will avoid false-positive cultures and the discomfort of straight catheterization in residents suspected of having an infection. An external catheter for use in females is now commercially available, but its safety and effectiveness have not been well documented in the NH.

Intermittent catheterization is used in the management of urinary retention and overflow UI. Overflow UI accounts for less than 10% of UI in NHs. The procedure involves straight catheterization two to four times daily, depending on residual urine volumes. Studies conducted largely among younger paraplegics have shown that this technique is practical, and as compared with chronic catheterization, reduces the risk of symptomatic infection (40). Intermittent self-catheterization has also been shown to be feasible for elderly female outpatients who are functional and both willing and able to catheterize themselves (1). However, studies carried out in young paraplegics and elderly female outpatients cannot automatically be extrapolated to the NH population. The technique may be useful for certain residents, such as women who have undergone bladder neck suspension, or following removal of an indwelling catheter in a bladder retraining protocol. One small study has suggested that this technique may be practical in male residents (91). Elderly residents, however, may be difficult to catheterize, and the anatomic abnormalities commonly found in the lower urinary tract of residents may increase the risk of infection due to repeated straight catheterizations. In addition, using this technique in an institutional setting (which may have an abundance of organisms relatively resistant to many commonly used antimicrobial agents) may pose an unacceptable risk of nosocomial infections. Using sterile catheter trays for these procedures would be very expensive. Thus, it may be extremely difficult to implement such a program in a typical NH.

Table 5.4 Indications for Use of a Chronic Indwelling Catheter

1. Urinary retention that:
   a. Is causing persistent overflow incontinence, symptomatic infections, or renal dysfunction
   b. Cannot be corrected surgically or medically
   c. Cannot be managed practically with intermittent catheterization
2. Skin wounds, pressure sores, or irritations that are being contaminated by incontinent urine
3. Care of the terminally ill or severely impaired for whom bed and clothing changes are uncomfortable or disruptive
4. Preference of resident when he/she has failed to respond to more specific treatments

SOURCE: Ouslander et al. (1990b).

Chronic indwelling catheterization is probably overused in the NH and has been shown to increase the incidence of a number of other complications, including chronic bacteriuria, symptomatic UTI, bladder stones, periurethral abscesses, and even bladder cancer (93-95,57). The prevalence of indwelling catheter use varies considerably, but one recent study in Maryland NHs showed a prevalence of about 10% (or about 20% of incontinent residents) (96). Elderly residents, especially men, managed by this technique are at relatively high risk of developing symptomatic UTI. In one study of 54 male NH residents with indwelling catheters followed prospectively for a mean of 9 months, only 20% did not get at least one symptomatic UTI. The incidence of UTI was much higher than in residents without indwelling catheters (57). The incidence of symptomatic UTI among female NH residents with indwelling catheters is higher than in those without catheters, but not as high as in male catheterized residents (93). Given these risks, it seems appropriate to recommend that the use of chronic indwelling catheters be limited to certain specific situations. Table 5.4 lists what we believe to be appropriate indications for the use of chronic indwelling catheters in NH residents. Although these indications have been used in federal guidelines to surveyors, they are based on opinion and not data. We have planned a study to use the expert consensus methodology developed at the RAND Corporation to identify more objectively and more specifically appropriate indications for chronic indwelling catheter use in NHs. When indwelling catheterization is used, certain principles of catheter care should be observed to attempt to minimize complications (Table 5.5). Some, but not all of these principles are supported by data in the literature (65).

Table 5.5 Key Principles of Chronic Indwelling Catheter Care

1. Maintain sterile, closed, gravity drainage system
2. Avoid breaking the closed system
3. Use clean techniques in emptying and changing the drainage system; wash hands between patients in institutionalized setting
4. Secure the catheter to the upper thigh or lower abdomen to avoid perineal contamination and urethral irritation due to movement of the catheter
5. Avoid frequent and vigorous cleaning of the catheter entry site; washing with soapy water once per day is sufficient
6. Do not routinely irrigate
7. If bypassing occurs in the absence of obstruction, consider the possibility of a bladder spasm which can be treated with a bladder relaxant
8. If catheter obstruction occurs frequently, increase the patient's fluid intake and acidify the urine if possible
9. Do not routinely use prophylactic or suppressive urinary antiseptics or antimicrobials
10. Do not do routine surveillance cultures to guide management of individual patients as all chronically catheterized patients have bacteriuria (which is often polymicrobial) and the organisms change frequently
11. Do not treat infection unless the patient develops symptoms; symptoms may be nonspecific and other possible sources of infection should be carefully excluded before attributing symptoms to the urinary tract
12. If a patient develops frequent symptomatic urinary tract infections, a genitourinary evaluation should be considered to rule out pathology such as stones, periurethral or prostatic abscesses, chronic pyelonephritis

SOURCE: Ouslander et al. (1990b).

CONCLUSIONS AND FUTURE DIRECTIONS

Much has been learned about the epidemiology, correlates, consequences, pathophysiology, and management of UI in NHs over the last several years. In this chapter we have synthesized the results of a large number of studies and attempted to present what we believe to be their implications for clinical care based on current knowledge.

Several directions for future research have been suggested. The optimal extent of the diagnostic evaluation of incontinent residents remains unclear. More research is needed to better define what assessment procedures and diagnostic tests are useful in targeting various management and treatment options to those most likely to respond. The contributions of bacteriuria and atrophic vaginitis to the development and severity of UI in the NH population need to be clarified. The clinical significance of detrusor hyperactivity with impaired contractility (DHIC) and the implications of this urodynamic finding for therapeutic interventions need to be determined.

Although prompted voiding is effective in selected NH residents, strategies need to be further developed and tested in order to motivate indigenous NH staff to maintain an effective management intervention. Improved pharmacologic treatments and incontinence garments will make important contributions to the care of incontinent residents. Appropriate indications for chronic indwelling catheters are needed, as are better methods to prevent symptomatic infections among those NH residents who are managed with these devices. Finally, we believe that the effects of interventions for UI among residents beyond improvements in dry (or wet) rates need to be documented. Whether improved incontinence care leads to a better quality of life for residents remains to be determined. We have recently begun a series of studies that examine the effects of interventions for UI on agitation, sleep/wake patterns, responsiveness, and social engagement in order to answer this critical question.

REFERENCES

1. Bennett, C. J., & Diokno, A. C. (1874). Clean intermittent self-catheterization in the elderly. *Urology, 24,* 43-45.
2. Bizien, J. (1987). Paper presented at the Gerontology Research Center, Baltimore, MD.
3. Boscia, J. A., Kobasa, W. D., Abrutyn, E., et al. (1986a). Lack of association between bacteriuria and symptoms in the elderly. *American Journal of Medicine, 81,* 979-982.
4. Boscia, J. A., Kobasa, W. D., Knight, R. A., et al. (1986b). Epidemiology of bacteriuria in an elderly ambulatory population. *American Journal of Medicine, 80,* 208-214.
5. Brink, C. A. (1990). Absorbent pads, garments, and management strategies. *Journal of the American Geriatrics Society, 38,* 368-373.
6. Brink, C. A., & Wells, T. J. (1986). Environmental support for geriatric incontinence: Toilets, toilet supplements and external equipment. *Clinics in Geriatric Medicine, 2,* 829-840.
7. Brocklehurst, J. C., & Dillane, J. B. (1966). Studies of the female bladder in old age: 2. Cystometrograms in 100 incontinent women. *Gerontology Clinics, 8,* 306-319.
8. Burgio, K. L., & Burgio, L. D. (1986). Behavior therapies for urinary incontinence in the elderly. *Clinics in Geriatric Medicine, 2,* 809-827.
9. Burgio, K. L., & Engel, B. T. (1990). Biofeedback-assisted behavioral training for elderly men and women. *Journal of the American Geriatrics Society, 38,* 338-340.
10. Burgio, K. L., Whitehead, W. E., & Engel, B. T. (1985). Urinary incontinence in elderly—bladder-sphincter biofeedback and toilet skills training. *Annals of Internal Medicine, 104,* 507-515.
11. Burgio, L. D. (1990). A staff management system for maintaining improvements in continence with elderly nursing home residents. *Journal of Applied Behavior Analysis, 23,* 111-118.

12. Burns, P. A., Marecki, M., Dittmar, S. (1985). Kegel's exercises with biofeedback therapy for treatment of stress incontinence. *The Nurse Practitioner, 10,* 34.
13. Burns, P. A., Pranikoff, K., Nochajski, T., et al. (1990). Treatment of stress incontinence with pelvic floor exercises and biofeedback. *Journal of the American Geriatrics Society, 38,* 341-344.
14. Burton, J. R., Pearce, K. L., Burgio, K. L., et al. (1988). Behavioral training for urinary incontinence in elderly patients. *Journal of the American Geriatrics Society, 36,* 693-698.
15. Campbell, E. B., Knight, H., Benson, M., et al. (1991). Effect of an incontinence training program on nursing home staff's knowledge, attitudes and behavior. *Gerontologist, 31*(6), 788-794.
16. Castleden, C. M., Duffin, H. M., Asher, M. J., et al. (1985). Factors influencing outcome in elderly patients with urinary incontinence and detrusor instability. *Age and Ageing, 14,* 303-307.
17. Colling, J. (1988). Educating nurses to care for the incontinent patient. *Nursing Clinics of North America, 23*(1), 279-289.
18. Colling, J., Ouslander, J., Hadley, B., et al. (in press). The effects of patterned urge response toileting (PURT) on urinary incontinence in nursing home residents. *Journal of the American Geriatrics Society.*
19. Diokno, A., Wells, T., & Brink, C. (1987). Urinary incontinence in elderly women: Urodynamic evaluation. *Journal of the American Geriatrics Society, 35,* 940-946.
20. Diokno, A. C., Brown, M. B., Brock, B. M., et al. (1988). Clinical and cystometric characteristics of continent and incontinent noninstitutionalized elderly. *Journal of Urology, 140,* 567-571.
21. Eastwood, H. D. H., & Warrell, R. (1984). Urinary incontinence in the elderly female: Prediction in diagnosis and outcome of management. *Age and Ageing, 13,* 230-234.
22. Engel, B. T., Burgio, L., McCormick, K., et al. (1990). Behavioral treatment of incontinence in the long term care setting. *Journal of the American Geriatrics Society, 38,* 361-363.
23. Fall, M., Ahlstrom, K., Carlsson, C. A., et al. (1986). Contelle: Pelvic floor stimulator for female stress-urge incontinence. *Journal of Urology, 26*(3), 282-287.
24. Fantl, J. A., Wyman, J. F., McClish, D. K., et al. (1991). Efficacy of bladder training in older women with urinary incontinence. *Journal of the American Medical Association, 265,* 609-613.
25. Hadley, E. (1986). Bladder training and related therapies for urinary incontinence in older people. *Journal of the American Medical Association, 256*(3), 372-379.
26. Health Care Financing Administration. (1989a). *Interpretive guidelines for skilled nursing facilities and intermediate care facilities.* Washington, DC.
27. Health Care Financing Administration. (1989b, February 2). Medicare and Medicaid requirements for long term care facilities. *Federal Register, 54*(21).
28. Health Care Financing Administration. (1990). *Resident assessment system for long term care facilities.* Washington, DC.
29. Herzog, A. R., & Fultz, N. H. (1990). Prevalence and incidence of urinary incontinence in community-dwelling populations. *Journal of the American Geriatrics Society, 38,* 273-281.
30. Herzog, A. R., Fultz, N. H., Brock, B. M., et al. (1988). Urinary incontinence and psychological distress among older adults. *Psychology and Aging, 3,* 155-161.
31. Hilton, P., & Stanton, S. L. (1981). Algorithmic method for assessing urinary incontinence in elderly women. *British Medical Journal, 282,* 940-942.

32. Hu, T.-W. (1986). The economic impact of urinary incontinence. *Clinics in Geriatric Medicine, 2,* 673-687.
33. Hu, T.-W. (1990). Impact of urinary incontinence on health-care costs. *Journal of the American Geriatrics Society, 38,* 292-295.
34. Hu, T.-W., Igou, J., Kaltreider, L., et al. (1989b). A clinical trial of a behavioral therapy to reduce urinary incontinence in nursing homes. *Journal of the American Medical Association, 261,* 2652-2656.
35. Hu, T.-W., Kaltreider, L. D., Igou, J. (1990). Disposable versus reusable diapers: A controlled experiment in a nursing home. *Journal of Gerontological Nursing, 16,* 19-24.
36. Hu, T.-W., Kaltreider, L. D., Igou, J. F., et al. (1989a). Cost effectiveness of training incontinent elderly in nursing homes: A randomized clinical trial. *Health Services Research, 25,* 3.
37. Kane, R. L., Ouslander, J. G., & Abrass, I. B. (1984). *Essentials of clinical geriatrics.* New York: McGraw-Hill. Chapter 6.
38. Jewett, M.A.S., Fernie, G. R., Holliday, P. J., et al. (1981). Urinary dysfunction in a geriatric long-term care population: Prevalence and patterns. *Journal of the American Geriatrics Society, 29,* 211-214.
39. Lamhut, P., Jackson, T. W., Wall, L. L. (1986). The treatment of urinary incontinence with electrical stimulation in nursing home patients. *Journal of the American Geriatrics Society.*
40. Lapides, J., & Diokno, A. C. (1983). Clean, intermittent self-catheterization. In S. Raz (Ed.), *Female urology.* Philadelphia: Saunders.
41. Leach, G. E., & Yip, C.-M. (1986). Urologic and urodynamic evaluation of the elderly population. *Clinics in Geriatric Medicine, 2,* 731-755.
42. Mitteness, L. S. (1990). Knowledge and beliefs about urinary incontinence in adulthood and old age. *Journal of the American Geriatrics Society, 38,* 374-378.
43. Mohide, E. A. (1986). The prevalence and scope of urinary incontinence. *Clinics in Geriatric Medicine, 2,* 639-655.
44. McClish, D. K., Fantl, A. J., Wyman, J. F., et al. (1991). Bladder training in older women with urinary incontinence: Relationship between outcome and changes in urodynamic observations. *Obstetrics and Gynecology, 77,* 281-286.
45. McCormick, K. A., Cella, M., Scheve, A., et al. (1990, December). The cost-effectiveness of treating incontinence in the severely mobility-impaired long-term care residents. *Quality Review Bulletin,* pp. 439-443.
46. National Institutes of Health Consensus Conference. (1989). Urinary incontinence in adults. *Journal of the American Medical Association, 261,* 2685-2690.
47. Nicolle, L. E., Bjornson, J., Harding, G. M. K., et al. (1983). Bacteriuria in elderly institutionalized men. *New England Journal of Medicine, 309,* 1420-1425.
48. Nicolle, L. E., Mayhew, J. W., & Bryan, L. (1987). Prospective randomized comparison of therapy and no therapy for asymptomatic bacteriuria in institutionalized women. *American Journal of Medicine, 83,* 27-33.
49. O'Donnell, P. (1986). Personal communication.
50. Ouslander, J. G. (1986). Diagnostic evaluation of geriatric urinary incontinence. *Clinics in Geriatric Medicine, 2,* 715-730.
51. Ouslander, J. G. (1989a). Asymptomatic bacteriuria and incontinence. *Journal of the American Geriatrics Society, 37,* 197-198.
52. Ouslander, J. G. (1989b). Urinary incontinence: Out of the closet. *Journal of the American Medical Association, 261,* 2695-2696.
53. Ouslander, J. G., & Abelson, S. (1990a). Perceptions of urinary incontinence among elderly outpatients. *Gerontologist, 30,* 369-372.

54. Ouslander, J. G., Blaustein, J., Connor, A., et al. (1988). Habit training and oxybutynin for incontinence in nursing home patients: A placebo-controlled trial. *Journal of the American Geriatrics Society, 36,* 40-46.

55. Ouslander, J. G., & Bruskewitz, R. (1989a). Disorders of micturition in the aging patient. *Advances in Internal Medicine, 34,* 165-190.

56. Ouslander, J. G., & Fowler, E. (1985). Incontinence in VA nursing home units. *Journal of the American Geriatrics Society, 33,* 33-40.

57. Ouslander, J. G., Greengold, B. A., & Chen, S. (1987a). Complications of chronic indwelling urinary catheters among male nursing home patients: A prospective study. *Journal of Urology, 138,* 1191-1195.

58. Ouslander, J. G., Greengold, B. A., & Chen, S. (1987b). External catheter use and urinary tract infections among incontinent male nursing home patients. *Journal of the American Geriatrics Society, 35,* 1063-1070.

59. Ouslander, J. G., Greengold, B. A., Silverblatt, F. J., et al. (1987c). An accurate method to obtain urine for culture in men with external catheters. *Archives of Internal Medicine, 147,* 286-288.

60. Ouslander, J. G., & Kane, R. L. (1984). The costs of urinary incontinence in nursing homes. *Medical Care, 22,* 69-79.

61. Ouslander, J. G., Kane, R. L., & Abrass, I. B. (1982). Urinary incontinence in elderly nursing home patients. *Journal of the American Medical Association, 248,* 1194-1198.

62. Ouslander, J. G., Leach, G. E., Staskin, D. R. (1989b). Simplified tests of lower urinary tract function in the evaluation of geriatric urinary incontinence. *Journal of the American Geriatrics Society, 37,* 706-714.

63. Ouslander, J. G., Leach, G., Staskin, D., et al. (1989c). Prospective evaluation of an assessment strategy for geriatric urinary incontinence. *Journal of the American Geriatrics Society, 37,* 715-714.

64. Ouslander, J. G., Morishita, L., Blaustein, J., et al. (1987d). Clinical, functional, and psychosocial characteristics of an incontinent nursing home population. *Journal of Gerontology, 42(6),* 631-637.

65. Ouslander, J. G., Osterweil, D., & Morley, J. (1990b). *Medical care in the nursing home.* New York: McGraw-Hill.

66. Ouslander, J., Palmer, M., Brant, L., et al. (1990c). Urinary incontinence in nursing homes: Incidence, remission and associated factors. *Journal of the American Geriatrics Society, 38,* A24.

67. Ouslander, J. G., Uman, G. C., Urman, H. N., et al. (1987e). Incontinence among nursing home patients: Clinical and functional correlates. *Journal of the American Geriatrics Society, 35,* 324-330.

68. Pannill, F. C., III, Williams, T. F., & Davis, R. (1988). Evaluation and treatment of urinary incontinence in long term care. *Journal of the American Geriatrics Society, 36,* 902-910.

69. Raz, S. (1990). Vaginal surgery for stress incontinence. *Journal of the American Geriatrics Society, 38,* 345-347.

70. Resnick, N. M. (1990a). Initial evaluation of the incontinent patient. *Journal of the American Geriatrics Society, 38,* 311-316.

71. Resnick, N. M. (1990b). Noninvasive diagnosis of the patient with complex incontinence. *Gerontology, 36(Suppl 2),* 8-18.

72. Resnick, N. M., & Ouslander, J. G. (Eds.). (1990). NIH consensus conference on urinary incontinence. *Journal of the American Geriatrics Society, 38,* 263.

73. Resnick, N., & Yalla, S. V. (1987). Detrusor hyperactivity with impaired contractile function: An unrecognized but common cause of incontinence in elderly patients. *Journal of the American Medical Association, 257,* 3076-3087.

74. Resnick, N. M., Yalla, S. V., & Laurino, E. (1986). An algorithmic approach to urinary incontinence in the elderly. *Clinical Research, 34,* 832A.

75. Resnick, N. M., Yalla, S. V., & Laurino, E. (1989). The pathophysiology of urinary incontinence among institutionalized elderly persons. *New England Journal of Medicine, 320,* 1-7.

76. Robbins, A., Rubenstein, L., Josephson, K., et al. (1989). Predictors of falls among elderly people. *Archives of Internal Medicine, 149,* 1628-1633.

77. Schnelle, J. F. (1990). Treatment of urinary incontinence in nursing home patients by prompted voiding. *Journal of the American Geriatrics Society, 38,* 356-360.

78. Schnelle, J. F. (1991). *Managing urinary incontinence in the elderly.* New York: Springer.

79. Schnelle, J. F., Newman, D. R., Abbey, J. C., et al. (1990c). Urodynamic and behavioral analysis of incontinence in nursing home patients. *Behavior Health and Aging, 1,* 41-49.

80. Schnelle, J. F., Newman, D. R., & Fogarty, T. (1990a). Statistical quality-control in nursing homes: Assessment and management of chronic urinary incontinence. *Health Services Research, 25*(4), 627-637.

81. Schnelle, J. F., Newman, D. R., Fogarty, T., et al. (1990b). Management of patient continence in long-term care nursing facilities. *Gerontologist, 30,* 373-376.

82. Schnelle, J. F., Newman, D. R., Fogarty, T. E., et al. (1991). Assessment and quality control of incontinence care in long-term nursing facilities. *Journal of the American Geriatrics Society, 39,* 165-171.

83. Schnelle, J. F., Newman, D. K., White, M., et al. (1991). *Maintaining continence in nursing home residents through the application of industrial quality control.* Manuscript in preparation.

84. Schnelle, J. F., Sowell, V. A., Hu, T. W., et al. (1988). Reduction of urinary incontinence in nursing homes: Does it reduce or increase costs? *Journal of the American Geriatrics Society, 36,* 34-39.

85. Schnelle, J. F., Traughber, B., Morgan, D. B., et al. (1983). Management of geriatric incontinence in nursing homes. *Journal of Applied Behavior Analysis, 16,* 235-241.

86. Schnelle, J. F., Traughber, B., Sowell, V. A., et al. (1989). Prompted voiding treatment of urinary incontinence in nursing home patients. *Journal of the American Geriatrics Society, 37,* 1051-1057.

87. Sogbein, S. K., et al. (1982). Behavioral treatment of urinary incontinence in geriatric patients. *Canadian Medical Association Journal, 127,* 863-864.

88. Spangler, P. F., et al. (1984). The management of dehydration and incontinence in nonambulatory geriatric patients. *Journal of Applied Behavior Analysis, 17,* 397-401.

89. Stanton, S. L. (1990). Suprapubic approaches for stress incontinence in women. *Journal of the American Geriatrics Society, 38,* 348-351.

90. Starer, P., & Libow, L. S. (1985). Obscuring urinary incontinence: Diapering the elderly. *Journal of the American Geriatrics Society, 12,* 842-846.

91. Terpenning, M. S., Allada, R., & Kauffman, C. A. (1989). Intermittent urethral catheterization in the elderly. *Journal of the American Geriatrics Society, 37,* 411-416.

92. Tobin, G. W., & Brocklehurst, J. C. (1986). The management of urinary incontinence in local authority residential homes for the elderly. *Age and Ageing, 15,* 292-298.

93. Warren, J. W., Damron, D., Tenney, J. H., et al. (1987). Fever, bacteremia and death as complications of bacteriuria in women with long-term urethral catheters. *Journal of Infectious Diseases, 155,* 1151-1158.

94. Warren, J. W., Muncie, H. L., Jr., Berquist, E. J., et al. (1981). Sequelae and management of urinary infection in the patient requiring chronic catheterization. *Journal of Urology, 125,* 1-7.

95. Warren, J. W., Muncie, H. L., Jr., & Craggs-Hall, M. (1988). Acute pyelonephritis associated with bacteriuria during long-term catheterization: A prospective clinicopathological study. *Journal of Infectious Diseases, 158*(6), 1341-1346.

96. Warren, J. W., Steinbert, L., Hebel, R. J., et al. (1989). The prevalence of urethral catheterization in Maryland nursing homes. *Archives of Internal Medicine, 149,* 1535-1537.

97. Wells, T. J. (1990). Pelvic (floor) muscle exercises. *Journal of the American Geriatrics Society, 38,* 333-337.

98. Wyman, J. F., Harkins, S. W., & Fantl, J. A. (1990). Psychosocial impact of urinary incontinence in the community-dwelling population. *Journal of the American Geriatrics Society, 38,* 282-288.

99. Yoshikawa, T. T., & Norman, D. C. (1987). *Aging and clinical practice: Infectious diseases.* New York: Igaku-Shoin.

100. Yu, L. C., & Kaltreider, D. L. (1987). Stressed nurses dealing with incontinent patients. *Journal of Gerontological Nursing, 13,* 27-30.

101. Yu, L. C., Rohner, T. J., Kaltreider, L. D., et al. (1990). Profile of urinary incontinent elderly in long-term care institutions. *Journal of the American Geriatrics Society, 38,* 433-439.

102. Zorzitto, M. L., Holliday, P. J., Jewett, M. A. S., et al. (1989). Oxybutynin chloride for geriatric urinary dysfunction: A double-blind placebo-controlled study. *Age and Ageing, 18,* 195-200.

103. Zorzitto, M. L., Jewett, M. A. S., Fernie, G. R., et al. (1986). Effectiveness of propantheline bromide in the treatment of geriatric patients with detrusor instability. *Neurourology and Urodynamics, 5,* 133-140.

6

A Review of Research on Common Bowel Problems in the Nursing Home

CATHY A. ALESSI, M.D.
CYNTHIA T. HENDERSON, M.D., M.P.H.,
F.A.C.N.
KAREN M. LINDERBORN, M.S., R.N.-C.

Problems with bowel function are common among nursing home (NH) residents, whether they are elderly or disabled younger persons. Constipation, fecal impaction, diarrhea, fecal incontinence, and bowel complications of enteral tube feedings may all have a major effect on resident comfort and health. Frequent contributors include drug therapy, immobility, a diet deficient in fiber and/or fluid, gastrointestinal (GI) disease, acute and chronic conditions that affect bowel function, functional impairment, cognitive impairment, chronic laxative use, and characteristics of tube feeding formulas. Until recently there has been little research to guide treatment, but as interest in NH research in general has grown, there has also been an increase in investigations of bowel problems in this setting.

Most research on bowel problems in the NH has addressed constipation. Complications of tube feedings, though primarily studied in non-NH settings, are nonetheless important in NH residents. Constipation and GI complications of tube feeding will be the major focus of this review. There will be briefer discussions of fecal impaction, diarrhea, and fecal incontinence as there is less information available these topics, particularly in long-term care settings. The appropriate use of diagnostic procedures to evaluate these problems in NH residents has not been well studied but will be reviewed here.

The authors gratefully acknowledge the secretarial assistance of Wendy Barnett.

Finally, the agenda for future research on bowel problems in the NH will be addressed, drawing on the experiences and results of research to date.

CONSTIPATION

Definition of Constipation

Two aspects of bowel function are included in the definition of constipation: difficulty passing stools and infrequent stools. As people who have difficulty passing stools describe straining with bowel movements, difficulty passing stools is usually evaluated in research by subject questionnaires, descriptions of stool consistency, or measurement of stool water content (65). The other aspect of constipation, infrequent bowel movements, is usually evaluated in research with counts of bowel movements, days without bowel movements, or measures of intestinal transit time with radio-opaque or radioisotope markers.

Epidemiology of Constipation

Community-Living Persons

Much of the earlier epidemiological work on constipation in older persons has focused on those living at home. These community-based surveys show that bowel function varies widely among normal individuals and ranges from three bowel movements per day to three per week (22). From 78% to 96% of older people at home have bowel frequency within this normal range, with 55% having a daily bowel movement. Even though this suggests the majority of older people in the community have normal bowel frequency, studies show that the elderly commonly complain about infrequent bowel movements and over half use laxatives (22,24,73,112).

Sonnenberg and Koch (1989) reviewed the epidemiology of constipation in the United States based on four national surveys. This review pointed out that more than 4 million persons complain of frequent constipation, making it the most common chronic digestive condition in the United States. The prevalence of complaints of constipation increases with age, ranging from 4.5% in the age group 65-74 to 10.2% in those over 75 years. Constipation was three times more common in women than in men, and 1.3 times more frequent in nonwhites than whites. The National Ambulatory Medical Care Survey (1980-1981) revealed that 2-3 million patients are annually prescribed cathartics and/or laxatives by practitioners. Use of over-the-counter drugs, which is probably enormous, is not included in this figure (105).

More recently, Sandler et al. (1990) reported that in the first National Health and Nutrition Examination Survey (NHANES-I) 12.8% of all respondents reported constipation, whereas 23.3% of those over age 60 reported constipation. A dietary role was suggested as constipated subjects reported lower consumption of several foodstuffs including dry beans and peas, milk, beverages, and fruits and vegetables.

Long-Term Care Residents

NH residents have an increased frequency of constipation and laxative use compared to community-based surveys. Wigzell (1969) found that among elderly institutionalized patients only 41% had normal bowel habits. Primrose and associates (1987) have reported that 58% of residents in registered NHs and 73% of residents on long-stay geriatric wards use laxatives. Similarly, Lamy and Krug (1978) found that 58% of residents in one NH were on laxatives, primarily saline laxatives, stimulants, and stool softeners. Of these subjects, none was managed with dietary intervention for treatment of constipation, such as by dietary fiber.

People with spinal cord injury, a group at high risk of requiring NH care, have received little attention as a group with chronic GI problems. Stone and colleagues (1990) demonstrated the frequency of these problems in their survey of 127 institutionalized spinal cord injury patients. Twenty-seven percent had significant symptoms, including difficulty with evacuation, chronic abdominal pain, gastroesophageal reflux, abdominal distention, and hemorrhoids. Twenty-three percent of these individuals had required hospitalization for GI complaints.

Causes of Constipation in the NH

Factors that may lead to constipation among residents are summarized in Table 6.1 (65,13,1). Most bowel intervention studies in NHs have focused on secondary and tertiary prevention rather than on primary prevention. The effect of potential primary interventions such as increasing mobility, correcting dentition, and improving access to toileting has not been studied. The only primary prevention

Table 6.1   Causes of Constipation in the Nursing Home

Primary causes
  Deficient fiber intake
  Deficient fluid intake
  Immobility
  Poor mastication, poor dentition
  Poor abdominal musculature
  Failure to respond to the urge to defecate (e.g., due to functional impairment)
Secondary causes
  Intrinsic bowel lesion (e.g., colon cancer or anorectal disease)
  Drugs (e.g., analgesics, antacids, anticholinergics)
  Neurologic disorders (e.g., dementia, stroke, spinal cord injury)
  Psychiatric disorders (e.g., depression)
  Endocrine/metabolic disorders (e.g., hypothyroidism)

SOURCE: Adapted from Alessi and Henderson (1988).

studies reviewed in this chapter involve increased dietary fiber and fluid intake. The other studies reviewed involve treatment of existing constipation.

Studies of the NH Diet

Most clinicians would agree that dietary intervention is the first step in the prevention and management of constipation (76). However, the NH diet may be inadequate to maintain normal bowel function. Studies demonstrate that many residents fail to meet recommended daily allowances (RDA) for essential nutrients. Although there is no RDA for fiber, fiber intake is often inadequate (see Chapter 7). In a survey of 14 NHs in Wisconsin, Sempos et al. (1982) found that no NH menu met the recommended daily allowances for all nutrients for both sexes, and the average crude fiber intake per day was low at 2.6 grams. One dietary survey in a private NH found that some residents had inadequate nutrient intake despite being served meal trays with a diet equaling or exceeding recommended allowances, due to failure of residents to eat enough (52). In comparing food choices of institutionalized versus independently living elderly, Clarke and Wakefield (1975) found that more NH residents had changed their traditional eating habits, which seemed to contribute to lower nutritional scores and decreased food intake. These studies suggest that although adequate nutrition may be present on the meal trays, menus were planned around an expected intake that was higher than residents actually consumed.

These epidemiologic and descriptive studies show that constipation is a significant problem in NHs, laxative use is common, and dietary interventions are not frequently practiced.

Intervention Studies on the Treatment of Constipation

Intervention trials of the management of constipation among the elderly and in the NH setting are reviewed below in three major categories: dietary fiber, laxatives, and nondrug therapies. This review includes studies carried out in long-term care and relevant studies carried out in other settings.

Dietary fiber is an important means of treatment of constipation (101). Trials of increased dietary fiber in outpatients (110,80,103) have demonstrated increased frequency of bowel movements, decreased intestinal transit time, improved stool consistency, and decreased laxative use. Similar results have been reported in most of the studies of dietary fiber conducted in the NH setting. A number of these studies are presented in Table 6.2. Variability in the study setting, duration, subjects, and type and amount of fiber used makes comparison across studies difficult.

Most of the studies reviewed in Table 6.2 were performed on geriatric or psychiatric long-stay wards or in NHs. A hospital geriatric evaluation unit and a general medical ward were the locations for the others. Study designs included pre- and posttreatment comparisons. There was limited use of controls and randomization, and infrequent use of placebo. As improvement in constipation can be a subjective outcome to measure, these problems in study design are significant. However, most of the studies have in common the use of bran or other fiber supplementation in breads, biscuits, cereal, or other foodstuffs. Some articles even provide recipes for bran-supplemented food items (50,48).

The majority of the studies in Table 6.2 showed benefit from the treatment of constipation with fiber. However, three randomized controlled studies (59,30,104) showed no increase in frequency of bowel movements with fiber supplementation. However, two of these studies were of short duration and involved acute care hospital patients observed for about 5 days (59) or in a geriatric unit for 1-3 weeks (104). It is unlikely that significant benefits from fiber supplementation would be detected in these short periods of observation. In the third trial (30), although the setting was a long-stay geriatric ward, the control group received a high-fiber diet without the addition of the bran supplement under study. The use of a high-fiber diet in controls may have made it difficult for the intervention group to show a significant difference. Fiber supplementation in tube-fed patients will be discussed later in this chapter.

Complications of fiber supplementation have been reported. Patients may complain of flatulence and mild abdominal discomfort early in fiber therapy, but these symptoms usually resolve over time. There is also some concern that fiber therapy may decrease food intake and decrease absorption of minerals. However, at least three studies have not shown deleterious effects of fiber supplementation on serum chemistries or minerals in an older population (5,98,49). Of some concern is a published letter that reported that although wheat bran supplementation among geriatric unit patients improved bowel frequency, half of treated subjects suffered "frequent and distressing fecal incontinence" while on bran (4).

With the above limitations in mind, the weight of current evidence suggests that dietary fiber supplementation can be a successful, safe method of treatment for constipation in selected NH and elderly patients. Features mentioned by several of the authors that may increase the likelihood of success include: titrating fiber dose to individual response, allowing longer periods of treatment, and using palatable forms of fiber to improve compliance.

Many drugs are available for the treatment of constipation. The major classes of these drugs and examples of brand names are listed in Table 6.3. Only a few of these drugs have been carefully studied in the NH setting and in the elderly; new drugs in particular have not been studied in these populations (62,75). Table 6.4 presents some intervention studies for the treatment of constipation with laxatives in NHs or long-stay wards. In general, these trials were of more rigorous design than the studies of dietary fiber listed in Table 6.2. The majority of these involved randomization and use of placebo controls. Some randomized trials compared two or more treatments, often with crossover of treatment.

The studies listed in Table 6.4 involve various durations of therapy with a wide range of laxatives. Several laxatives have been shown to be successful in the treatment of constipation in the NH. Although some authors claim their agent of choice to be the most beneficial, clinical decisions on the choice of agent for a particular individual should focus on reducing the risk of known side effects of these agents.

Some *nondrug and nonfiber* treatments of constipation have been suggested, particularly for the treatment of fecal impaction. Examples of these treatments are whole-gut irrigation and electrohydraulic lithotripsy, which are mentioned below in the discussion of fecal impaction. In addition, surgery has been used in the treatment of severe chronic constipation or anal outlet obstruction. The surgical

Table 6.3   Laxatives

Class	Agents	Example Brand Names
Bulk forming	Methylcellulose	Collogel, Hydrolose
	Psyllium	Konsyl, Metamucil
Emollient laxatives	Docusate sodium	Colace, Kasof
	Docusate calcium	Surfak
	Docusate potassium	Dialose
Lubricants	Mineral oil (oral)	
	Lubricant enemas	Fleets oil retention enema
		Saf-Tip
Saline laxatives	Magnesium salts	Citrate of Magnesia, Milk of
	(citrate, hydroxide, sulfate)	Magnesia, Epsom salts
	Sodium salts (phosphate, sulfate)	Fleets enema, Phosphosoda
Stimulant laxatives	Anthraquinones	
	Cascara	Nature's Remedy
	Senna	Senekot, Nytilaz, Perdiem
	Danthron	Dorbane
	Diphenylmethanes	
	Phenolphthalein	Ex-Lax, Feen-a-mint, Correctol
	Bisacodyl	Dulcolax, Carter's Pills
	Castor oil	Neoloid
Hyperosmotic laxatives	Glycerin suppositories	
	Lactulose	Chronulac, Cephulac
	Polyethylene glycol-saline solution	Golytely, Colyte

SOURCE: Adapted from Alessi and Henderson (1988).

procedures performed include colectomy with ileoanal anastomosis or anorectal myectomy (53,87,114). Most of the recent literature on surgical treatment of constipation comes from Great Britain and involves young, community-dwelling women with chronic constipation. Although some elderly subjects are included, none of these studies primarily involved NH residents.

FECAL IMPACTION

The causes of fecal impaction in the NH resident are the same as the causes of constipation (see Table 6.1). Read and colleagues (93) reported the presence of fecal impaction in 42% of patients admitted to geriatric units in Great Britain. The diagnosis of fecal impaction is usually made on rectal examination with the palpation of a fecal mass in the rectum. If the fecal mass is located in more proximal regions of the colon, abdominal x-ray may be needed to make the diagnosis. Complications of fecal impaction include fecal incontinence, rectal bleeding, stercoral ulcers, urinary retention, urinary tract infection, and bowel obstruction (1).

The traditional treatment of fecal impaction located in the rectum is manual disimpaction (1). However, some clinicians and authors consider manual disimpaction unnecessary and inhumane, and other methods have been suggested. For example, Smith and associates (1978) found whole-gut irrigation with saline solution via nasogastric tube to be a more successful and less humiliating method for the treatment of fecal impaction. The use of polyethylene glycol-saline solution (Golytely) has also been shown to be effective for the treatment of fecal impaction in older patients (91). Andorsky and Goldner (1990) reported successful treatment of younger community-living individuals with chronic constipation using daily, small-volume (8 ounces BID) administration of polyethylene glycol-saline solution. This regimen may prove useful in NH residents because of the lack of effect on electrolyte and fluid balance. Recently, Morgentaler and Koufman (1990) described the successful treatment of a large impacted calcified fecalith with electrohydraulic lithotripsy in a 76-year-old woman.

FECAL INCONTINENCE

Fecal incontinence is a very distressing problem in any setting, including the NH. Urinary and fecal incontinence have been well established to be a substantial source of caregiver stress (78). Prevalence rates of fecal incontinence range from 10% to 23% of residents in long-stay wards and residential homes in Great Britain and over half of long-term care patients (36). Fecal incontinence usually occurs together with urinary incontinence. In 1988, Burgio and co-workers reported that 82% of residents of a NH were incontinent of either bowel or bladder at least once per week. Of these incontinent residents, 75% were incontinent of both bowel and bladder, 22% had only urinary incontinence, and 3% had only bowel incontinence.

The major causes of fecal soiling and fecal incontinence include: fecal impaction, loss of the normal continence mechanism from neurologic disorder or trauma, problems that overwhelm a normal continence mechanism such as diarrhea or poor access to toileting, and psychological or behavioral problems (36,67). The treatment of fecal impaction is described above. Suggested measures for the treatment of the other etiologies of fecal incontinence include use of a bowel program, biofeedback, and cues to encourage appropriate bathroom use in demented patients (36). The appropriate bowel program depends on the cause of the fecal incontinence, but typically involves scheduled toileting to coincide with the gastrocolic reflex and/or administration of a suppository (23).

DIARRHEA IN THE NH

It is estimated that one third of residents in chronic care facilities have a significant episode of diarrhea each year, which is commonly overlooked and may be a serious, life-threatening problem (28,77,6). Diarrhea may be acute or chronic. In the NH, acute diarrhea is commonly infectious in origin, particularly due to cytotoxigenic *Clostridium difficile*. Cytotoxigenic *C. difficile* is found in a significant number of residents on admission to the NH and may be acquired after admission in others (38). Other organisms are common, however, and outbreaks of diarrhea secondary to food poisoning and *Clostridium perfringens* may occur. Infectious agents may be spread by person-to-person contact or contaminated food, such as *Shigella* species, *Salmonella* species, rotavirus, and Norwalk agent (79).

Thomas and co-workers (1990) studied postantibiotic colonization with *C. difficile* in a 233-bed long-term care facility. During a 6-month period, they found that one third of stool specimens collected from residents after a course of antibiotics were infected with *C. difficile*. Risk factors for *C. difficile* infection included ward location and stool incontinence, with 1-year mortality being significantly higher in infected residents.

Several authors have reported outbreaks of infectious diarrhea in the NH setting. In 1986, Ryan and colleagues reported an outbreak of diarrhea due to *Escherichia coli* that affected 34 of 101 residents in a NH. This investigation implicated hamburger as the vehicle of transmission, and outcomes ranged from mild illness to severe hemorrhagic colitis and death. Choi and coworkers (1990) reported an outbreak of salmonella gastroenteritis among 44 of 199 residents in a NH. No common source of infection was identified, and in this study, outcome ranged from mild diarrhea to severe diarrheal illness requiring acute hospitalization, but no deaths. An outbreak of acute, painless diarrhea due to *Aeromonas hydrophila* was reported by Bloom and Bottone (1990) among 17 residents on two contiguous floors of a 784-bed long-term care facility. The illness was self-limited in all but one resident, who died after one day of severe, fulminant diarrheal illness.

Research on the prevention of diarrhea in the NH is minimal, and therefore information must be gathered from studies done in other settings. For example, in 1989, Surawicz and co-workers described a double-blind, randomized, placebo-controlled trial in hospitalized patients to study the effect of a living yeast (*Saccharomyces boulardii*) to prevent antibiotic-associated diarrhea. There was a significant decrease in the incidence of diarrhea in patients who received the yeast, and there were no recognized side effects of the therapy. Risk factors found to be associated with the development of antibiotic-associated diarrhea were multiple antibiotic combinations and the administration of tube feeding.

Little information is available on interventions in the NH for the treatment of chronic diarrhea. In a randomized trial with crossover, Qvitzau et al. (1988) studied the effectiveness of a combination ispaghula husk and calcium compared to loperamide for the treatment of chronic diarrhea. The combination therapy was as effective as, and less expensive than loperamide.

BOWEL COMPLICATIONS OF ENTERAL TUBE FEEDINGS

Epidemiology of Tube Feeding in the NH

Tube feeding is relatively common in the NH setting. A cross-sectional study of a NH with 461 skilled nursing beds revealed 52 tube-fed residents (11.3%) (83). The duration of intubation ranged from 1 month to 6.4 years; half of tubes had been in place for over 1 year. The mean age of the tube-fed resident was 87 years, 86% were female, all were demented, and the average period of time the tube-fed residents had been in the NH was 5.5 years. Ciocon et al. (1988) reported similar findings in an 11-month prospective study of 70 tube-fed residents in a 527-bed skilled nursing facility. The mean age of the tube-fed subjects was 82 years, 86% were women, and mean duration of tube feeding was 6 months, with a range of 1 month to over 8 years.

Enteral tube feeding is typically used in NH residents who have adequate GI motility and absorption, but who for various reasons cannot meet their nutritional needs by oral intake (26). Common reasons for inadequate oral intake are refusal or inability to eat or swallow, or dysphagia (43,18). Among tube-fed residents, Peck et al. (1990) reported that weight loss was the most common indication for tube feeding followed by refusal to eat, dysphagia, and stroke.

Once the decision to initiate tube feeding has been made, a wide range of tubes and formulas, and several routes of delivery are available. Possible routes of delivery for tube feeding are nasogastric, nasoduodenal, gastrostomy, or jejunostomy (43). The multitude of tubes available are generally defined by their external diameter, composition, length, and presence or absence of a weighted tip. Many types of feeding formulas are commercially available. Put simply, these formulas differ with respect to the relative proportion of protein, carbohydrate, and fat and the degree of absorptive and digestive capacity that is required by the patient to utilize the formula (26). Standard formulas provide about 1 kcal/ml, nutrient dense formulas provide 1.5-2 kcal/ml.

Complications of Tube Feeding

Various GI and non-GI complications of tube feeding have been described. Common non-GI complications include aspiration with subsequent pneumonia, hyponatremia, and increased use of restraints (83,18,43). In some patients, aspiration pneumonia may result from GI causes such as delayed gastric emptying due to medications or partial gastric outlet obstruction from gastrostomy tube migration. Tube-related problems include self-extubation, tube misplacement, leakage at the insertion site, infection at the insertion site, clogged or kinked tubes, and difficulty with insertion (18).

GI complications associated with tube feeding include constipation, abdominal discomfort, nausea and vomiting, GI bleeding and diarrhea. Constipation is common and so are the primary causes of constipation listed in Table 6.1. Among tube-fed patients, the likelihood of significant immobility is high. Of 40 tube-fed patients studied by Henderson and colleagues (1992) in a chronic disease hospital, none were ambulatory. In addition, the lean body mass of these individuals was below the 50th age-appropriate body mass index percentile. This loss of skeletal muscle diminished abdominal muscle mass and tone, impairing the generation of intraabdominal pressure for defecation.

The incidence of abdominal discomfort (e.g., gas, distention) and vomiting related to tube feeding in long-term care is unknown. Vomiting and gastroesophageal reflux in chronic tube feeding may be due to gastrostomy tube migration and partial pyloric outlet obstruction, delayed gastric emptying due to medications, or the rate of formula infusion. The schedule used in tube feeding has been associated with gastroesophageal reflux and aspiration. In a summary of five case reports, Podell describes that symptoms of gastroesophageal reflux and aspiration resolved when tube feeding infusion was changed from continuous administration to intermittent infusion (250 to 500 ml four to five times per day) with the patient in an upright position (88). Patients with acute head injury frequently have gut dysmotility and intolerance of enteral feeding during the first 2 weeks (81). There is little information on the incidence and etiology of GI bleeding among tube-fed residents associated with tube feeding.

Diarrhea in Tube-Fed Patients

Hospital-based studies indicate that such diarrhea is common. Benya et al. (1991) point out that the published incidence of diarrhea associated with tube feeding varies widely—between 2.3% and 68%. In a study of 123 hospitalized patients who received tube feedings, 32 (26%) had documented diarrhea of greater than 500 ml per day for at least 2 consecutive days (25). Formula factors such as fiber content and osmolality have been implicated as causing diarrhea with tube feedings and are the subject of several intervention studies. However, other factors such as medications, hypoalbuminemia, infectious agents, bacterial contamination of formula, and infusion rate have also been implicated as contributing to diarrhea (61,43,60,44).

Formula Factors

A number of authors have reported clinical evidence that formula composition affects bowel complications of tube feeding. Table 6.5 summarizes some of these studies. Only two of these studies were carried out in a long-term care population (31,29).

Fiber supplementation is commonly used to manage patients who develop constipation or diarrhea with tube feedings (34). Much of the evidence for fiber supplementation comes from non-NH populations in healthy, young volunteers.

Fiber supplementation of enteral feedings decreases liquid stools compared to nonsupplemented feedings (100,115). In critically ill patients, fiber supplementation of tube feedings has had mixed results (32,33,37,41,42). The results of these studies suggest that fiber supplementation leads to firmer stools. However, other factors such as antibiotics, hypoalbuminemia, and infection seem to play a more important role in diarrhea in acutely ill patients. In hospitalized patients who are not critically ill, fiber supplementation has been associated with increased stool weight and firmer stools (46,72).

There is less information available on fiber supplementation of tube feedings in the NH setting. Fischer et al. (1985) conducted a randomized crossover trial of a soy polysaccharide supplemented formula to evaluate the effect on bowel function in nonambulatory, tube-fed NH residents. They found no increase in stool frequency or GI transit time although they did demonstrate an increase in stool weight. Unfortunately, the subjects received the fiber-containing diet for only 2 weeks, probably an insufficient time of observation. Caloric intakes in study patients (mean 1073 kcal ± 188) were significantly lower than the 1560 kcal recommended by the formula manufacturer to provide adequate fiber intake.

There is considerable variability in the composition and amount of fiber supplied by individual formulas that may make results of long-term use difficult to evaluate, especially if patients are not maintained on the same formula for prolonged periods (35). One physiologic difference between various fiber sources is in stimulation of colonic fermentation and short-chain fatty acid absorption, which has been implicated in various colonic abnormalities and metabolic processes. For example, McBurney and Thompson (1991) reported differences in fermentability among five commercially available dietary fruit fiber supplements. Most commercial enteral nutrition formulas contain soy polysaccharide as the fiber source.

Nonfiber containing formulas have been studied for their role in diarrhea as well. McCamman et al. (1977) compared three low-residue defined formula diets (Vivonex, Flexical, and Precision LR) in normal volunteers in a randomized crossover design. There were no significant differences in stool frequency between the formulas, and with all three, stool weight and frequency of defecation decreased over time. In critically ill patients, Brinson and Kolts (1988) found no difference in stool frequency or fecal weight in intensive care unit patients on an isotonic nonfiber-containing formula versus a peptide-based formula. However, subjects' stools on the isotonic formula were more watery. Jones et al. (1983) reported a comparison of an isotonic formula with a more hypertonic, elemental formula and found no difference in the incidence of diarrhea in hospitalized patients. The diarrhea that did occur was attributable to antibiotics in most cases. Keohane et al. (1984) found that GI side effects were similar in subjects randomized to either a hypertonic solution with or without a starter regimen of diluted formula, or an isotonic solution. In this study of hospitalized noncritically ill patients, diarrhea was significantly associated with concurrent treatment with antibiotics. In 1990, Viall and colleagues described a study of two enteral feeding formulas, a soy hydrolysate and a casein formula. Both formulas were isotonic, low in residue, lactose free, and isocaloric, but differed in the type and concentration of protein and medium-chain triglycerides. There was no difference in incidence of diarrhea, but the soy hydrolysate formula group had less frequent bowel movements and less vomiting. These differences were less significant after controlling for antibiotic use as a covariate.

As in the case of the studies of fiber-containing products, there is a need to replicate the above studies in the NH. Feller et al. (1990) undertook the study of three nonfiber-containing formulas to evaluate serum proteins in a small sample of demented, bedridden residents. The formulas used were a whole protein, a peptide-based, and an amino-acid-based formula. Although they found no GI side effects with any of the different formulas, the evaluation of GI problems was not a primary study endpoint, limiting interpretation of the data in this regard.

Nonformula Factors

Various nonformula factors have been associated with diarrhea in tube feeding including: patient characteristics, medications, infection and contamination, malnutrition and hypoalbuminemia, and rapid infusion rate. Patient characteristics associated with diarrhea in tube feeding include preexisting loose stools and severity of illness. For example, in a small sample of hospitalized surgical patients, Hoffmeister and Dobbie (1977) found that tube feeding with an isotonic, lactose-free formula (Isocal) only produced diarrhea and increased stool weight in those patients who had loose stools at baseline prior to starting tube feedings. Evidence of the frequent occurrence of diarrhea in critically ill patients was noted by Hart and Dobb (1988), who found that over half of tube-fed intensive care unit patients developed diarrhea. Pesola et al. (1989) found that an isotonic, low-residue formula (Isocal) did not cause diarrhea in hospitalized nonintensive care unit patients or nonhospitalized volunteers. The same formula did cause diarrhea in 36% of a sample of intensive care unit patients (86). In a subsequent study, Pesola et al. (1990) found that a hypertonic, low-residue formula (Ensure Plus) did not cause diarrhea in nonintensive care unit patients and normal volunteers. From these investigations, it appears that severity of illness is a significant correlate of diarrhea in tube-fed patients.

Medications, especially antibiotics, are also associated with diarrhea in the tube-fed population. Antimicrobial agents alter the normal intestinal flora, leading to bacterial overgrowth and diarrhea. In a study of diarrhea associated with tube feeding in the acute hospital setting, Edes et al. (1990) found medications directly responsible for diarrhea in 61% of cases. Of the intervention studies reviewed in Table 6.5, three found the use of antibiotics to be an important factor in the development of diarrhea (51,41,37). One study of diarrhea in intensive care unit patients (54) found a significant increase in the incidence of diarrhea in patients on nasogastric feeding and in those on cimetidine, but no increased incidence in those receiving antibiotic therapy. It is possible that hypochlorhydria in these individuals may have contributed to small bowel bacterial overgrowth and diarrhea. This concept has significant implications for the NH population due to the frequent and often prolonged use of H_2 blocker therapy.

Infectious diarrhea is an important problem in the NH, as described in an earlier section of this chapter. Infectious diarrhea can occur in the tube-fed patient and complicate the differential diagnosis of diarrhea. In addition, bacterial contamination of formula can lead to diarrhea. Contamination can occur when inappropriate handling techniques are used during the preparation or administration of tube feedings, or when the feedings are hung for too long at room temperature (60). Fagerman (1992) reported reduced contamination of enteral formula in two hospitals following changes in nursing procedures. Changes included use of sterile water for dilution, a new formula administration bag every 24 hours, alcohol swabs to clean can lids before opening, rinsing and air drying formula bags between intermittent feedings, and limiting formula hang time to 4 hours. The type of infusion pump used may also influence bacterial contamination risk. Payne-James et al. (1992) demonstrated in the hospital setting that bacterial contamination of formula can occur during continuous formula infusion when the pump lacks a drip chamber. These findings, though not reported in the NH setting, are potentially very applicable to tube feeding practices in NHs.

Malnutrition and hypoalbuminemia have also been implicated as contributing to diarrhea in tube-fed patients. Malnutrition can lead to a loss of intestinal villi and enzymes and a subsequent loss in intestinal absorptive capacity leading to diarrhea (21,60). Hypoalbuminemia alters intravascular osmotic forces, which can also impair intestinal absorptive capacity and is thought by some to lead to diarrhea, particularly in critically ill patients (10). Intervention studies listed in Table 6.5 that implicate malnutrition and/or hypoalbuminemia in diarrhea in tube-fed patients include the studies by Guenter et al. (1991) and Brinson and Kolts (1988), both involving critically ill hospitalized patients. However, in the two studies by Pesola and colleagues (1989, 1990), intensive care unit patients who developed diarrhea with tube feedings actually had higher albumin levels than those who did not develop diarrhea, and serum albumin level was not correlated with diarrhea. Because a substantial proportion of tube-fed NH patients are hypoalbuminemic and malnourished, it would be useful to have studies that evaluate the relationship of these factors to diarrhea (45,18).

Finally, rapid infusion rate has been described as a cause of diarrhea with tube feedings. This issue has been addressed primarily by reports of clinical experience and case reports. It has been suggested that continuous pump-assisted feeding at a slow rate in addition to isotonic feeding formula will relieve diarrhea in some jejunostomy-fed patients (44).

DIAGNOSTIC STUDIES FOR EVALUATION OF GASTROINTESTINAL PROBLEMS

Fecal occult blood testing has been widely advocated for colorectal cancer screening in ambulatory populations. It is also frequently used in the evaluation of hospitalized patients. However, the role of fecal occult blood testing in the NH setting remains to be defined. Klos et al. (1991) evaluated the pattern of fecal occult blood test use in a large nursing facility. Thirty-seven percent of the residents had been tested. The majority of tests (61%) were performed for routine screening, of which 8.5% had positive results. The remaining tests were indicated for evaluation of diagnostic findings or to look for complications of medication use (e.g., NSAIDS). Of these patients, 24% had positive results. In over half the cases where occult blood testing was done as a screening measure, no additional diagnostic testing was performed. In most cases, the patient refused further workup. When there was a follow-up evaluation, no diagnosis was made in 68% of the cases. The use of procedures to further investigate positive fecal occult blood was more common when the fecal testing was done because of a diagnostic finding. However, no diagnosis explaining the positive fecal test was found in 46% of these individuals.

For the evaluation of lower GI tract disorders the barium enema is commonly used although its efficacy is questionable due to the high incidence of inadequate preparation. Tinetti et al. (1989) retrospectively reviewed the charts of 140 hospitalized patients over age 65 who underwent barium enema. In 31%, results were uninterpretable due to retention of fecal material or patients' inability to retain the barium. Patients with confusion, cachexia, fecal incontinence, or diarrhea were more likely to have an incomplete examination. Of the adequate exams, 25% were abnormal with obstruction, narrowing, mass lesions, malignancy, and polyps most commonly seen. A study of similar design was conducted by Gurwitz et al. (1992), who reviewed charts of 171 elderly long-term care patients and found that 52% of the barium enemas were inadequate, usually due to poor bowel preparation. Gurwitz et al. found that of the patients with an interpretable study, 64% had a diagnostic finding, and that of the 18 patients with a colonic polyp or cancer, more than 40% underwent no further evaluation or treatment. Follow-up barium or colonoscopy in the 88 patients with inadequate exams was undertaken in only 14%. Tinetti et al. reported that colonoscopy was performed in 9 of the 43 patients with inadequate barium enemas, and 8 patients had upper gastrointestinal series.

FUTURE RESEARCH

Many questions remain on the prevention and treatment of bowel problems in the NH. Constipation among residents able to eat by mouth is probably the most thoroughly studied bowel problem in this setting. An important area of future research is to clarify the factors that should guide the choice of particular therapies. A crucial first step in this regard is the identification and assessment of preexisting GI disorders in NH patients. It is likely that a successful institutional program would involve institution-wide supplementation of the NH diet with fiber after a careful screening for those residents who are likely to have complications from fiber. This could be done in conjunction with measures to affect the other primary causes of constipation that are common in the NH, such as improving dentition, fluid intake, and access to toileting. Other drug therapies in residents would then be instituted in those residents who do not respond to these measures.

Research on the prevention and management of diarrhea and fecal incontinence in the NH is minimal and is an area open for future research. Even epidemiologic data is lacking for these common bowel problems.

There is room for additional investigation of enteral tube feedings. Much of the research reviewed here focused on the choice of feeding formula. The type of fiber supplement in enteral formula may have significant clinical effects, and fiber from a variety of sources needs to be evaluated in long-term studies that last beyond a few months. The extent to which diarrhea is associated with enteral feeding or other factors needs to be established in long-term care residents, so the results of existing studies from hospital settings can be properly interpreted. In addition, the increasing evidence that other nonformula factors such as antibiotic use and hypoalbuminemia may be as important or more important than the choice of formula warrants newer interventions aimed at these factors. It is also important to point out that large-scale, randomized, controlled trials comparing the GI effects of pump-assisted versus gravity drip tube feedings have yet to be performed. A technology assessment approach is urgently needed in the evaluation of this nutrition support modality.

Once bowel problems are identified, the most effective and clinically appropriate diagnostic approach should be employed. However, there is insufficient research to guide clinicians' choices. Significant ethical dilemmas and ageist biases may surface in the decision-making process when diagnostic interventions are to be used in frail NH residents. Without doubt, future research should evaluate the efficacy of upper and lower GI endoscopy and radiography, as well as other diagnostic modalities in this population.

In summary, bowel problems in the NH are a common concern for residents and staff. Current research, when available, has focused on constipation and tube feedings, with only minimal work done on other important bowel problems. Further studies are essential to help clinicians prevent and treat bowel problems in the NH.

REFERENCES

1. Alessi, C. A., & Henderson, C. T. (1988). Constipation and fecal impaction in the long-term care patient. *Clinics in Geriatric Medicine, 4*, 571-588.
2. Andersson, H., Bosaeus, I., Falkheden, T., et al. (1979). Transit time in constipated geriatric patients during treatment with a bulk laxative and bran: A comparison. *Scandinavian Journal of Gastroenterology, 14*, 821-826.

3. Andorsky, R. I., & Goldner, F. (1990). Colonic lavage solution (polyethylene glycol electrolyte lavage solution) as a treatment for chronic constipation: A double-blind, placebo-controlled study. *American Journal of Gastroenterology, 85,* 261-265.

4. Ardron, M. E., & Main, A. N. (1990). Management of constipation [letter]. *British Medical Journal, 300,* 1400.

5. Battle, E. H., & Hanna, C.E. (1980). Evaluation of a dietary regimen for chronic constipation. *Journal of Gerontological Nursing, 6,* 527-532.

6. Bennett, R. G., & Greenough, W. B. (1990c). Difficile diarrhea: A common—and overlooked—nursing home infection. *Geriatrics, 45,* 77-87.

7. Benya, R., Layden, T. J., & Mobarhan, S. M. (1991). Diarrhea associated with tube feeding: The importance of using objective criteria. *Journal Clinical Gastroenterology, 13,* 167-172.

8. Berk, M. S. (1969). Comparative study of bowel control in nursing home patients. *Medical Times, 97,* 106-112.

9. Bloom, H. G., & Bottone, E. J. (1990). Aeromonas hydrophila diarrhea in a long-term care setting. *Journal of the American Geriatrics Society, 38,* 804-806.

10. Brinson, R. R., & Kolts, B. E. (1987). Hypoalbuminemia as an indicator of diarrheal incidence in critically ill patients. *Critical Care Medicine, 15,* 506-509.

11. Brinson, R. R., & Kolts, B. E. (1988). Diarrhea associated with severe hypoalbuminemia: A comparison of a peptide-based chemically defined diet and standard enteral alimentation. *Critical Care Medicine, 16,* 130-136.

12. Broatch, D. L., Wilson, A., & Thompson, J. (1968). The treatment of constipation in the elderly. *Nursing Times, 64,* 1631-1632.

13. Brocklehurst, J. C., Kirkland, J. L., Martin, J., et al. (1983). Constipation in long-stay elderly patients: Its treatment and prevention by lactulose, poloxalkol-dihydray-anthroquinolone and phosphate enemas. *Gerontology, 29,* 181-184.

14. Broholm, K. A. (1973). A controlled trial of a new combined preparation for the treatment of constipation in geriatric patients. *Geriatric Clinics, 15,* 25-31.

15. Burgio, L. D., Jones, L. T., & Engel, B. T. (1988). Studying incontinence in an urban nursing home. *Journal of Gerontology Nursing, 14,* 40-45.

16. Castle, S., Samuelson, M., Cantrell, M., et al. (1988). The efficacy of prophylactic docusate therapy in institutionalized geriatric patients [abstract]. *Journal of the American Geriatrics Society, 36,* 586.

17. Choi, M., Yoshikawa, T. T., Bridge, J., et al. (1990). Salmonella outbreak in a nursing home. *Journal of the American Geriatrics Society, 38,* 531-534.

18. Ciocon, J. O., Silverstone, F. A., Graver, L. M., et al. (1988). Tube feedings in elderly patients: Indications, benefits, and complications. *Archives of Internal Medicine, 148,* 429-433.

19. Clark, A. N. G., Scott, J. F. (1976). Wheat bran in dyschezia in the aged. *Age and Ageing, 5,* 149-154.

20. Clarke, M., & Wakefield, L. M. (1975). Food choices of institutionalized vs. independent living elderly. *Journal of American Dietetic Association, 66,* 600-604.

21. Coale, M. S., & Robson, J. R. (1980). Dietary management of intractable diarrhea in malnourished patients. *Journal of the American Dietetics Association, 76,* 444-450.

22. Connell, A. M., Hilton, C., Irving, G., et al. (1965). Variation of bowel habit in two population samples. *British Medical Journal* (Clinical Research) 2, 1095-1099.

23. Dodge, J., Bachman, C., & Silverman, H. (1988). Fecal incontinence in elderly patients. *Post Graduate Medical Journal, 83,* 258-270.

24. Donald, I. P., Smith, R. G., Cruikshank, J. G., et al. (1985). A study of constipation in the elderly living at home. *Gerontology, 31,* 112-118.

25. Edes, T. E., Walk, B. E., & Austin, J. L. (1990). Diarrhea in tube-fed patients: Feeding formula not necessarily the cause. *American Journal of Medicine, 88*, 91-93.
26. Eisenberg, P. (1989). Enteral nutrition: Indications, formulas, and delivery techniques. *Nursing Clinics of North America, 24*, 315-338.
27. Fagerman, K. E. (1992). Limiting bacterial contamination of enteral nutrition solutions: 6-year history with reduction of contamination at two institutions. *Nutritional Clinic Practice, 7*, 31-36.
28. Farber, B. F., Brennen, C., Puntereri, A. J., et al. (1984). A prospective study of nosocomial infections in a chronic care facility. *Journal of the American Geriatrics Society, 32*, 499-502.
29. Feller, A. G., Caindec, N., Fudman, I. W., et al. (1990). Effects of three liquid diets on nutrition-sensitive plasma proteins of tube-fed elderly men. *Journal of the American Geriatrics Society, 38*, 663-668.
30. Finlay, M. (1988). The use of dietary fibre in a long-stay geriatric ward. *Journal of Nutrition for the Elderly, 8*, 19-30.
31. Fischer, M., Adkins, W., Hall, L., et al. (1985). The effects of dietary fibre in a liquid diet on bowel function of mentally retarded individuals. *Journal of Mental Deficiency Research, 29*, 373-381.
32. Frank, H. A., & Green, L. C. (1979). Successful use of a bulk laxative to control the diarrhea of tube feeding. *Scandinavian Journal of Plastic Reconstructive Surgery, 13*, 193-194.
33. Frankenfield, D. C., & Beyer, P. L. (1989). Soy-polysaccharide fiber: Effect on diarrhea in tube-fed, head-injured patients. *American Journal of Clinical Nutrition, 50*, 533-538.
34. Frankenfield, D. C., & Beyer, P. L. (1991). Dietary fiber and bowel function in tube-fed patients. *Journal of the American Dietetics Association, 91*, 590-599.
35. Fredstrom, S. B., Baglien, K. S., Lampe, J. W., et al. (1991). Determination of the fiber content of enteral feedings. *Journal of Parenteral and Enteral Nutrition, 15*, 450-453.
36. Goldstein, M. K., Brown, E. M., Holt, P., et al. (1989). Fecal incontinence in an elderly man. *Journal of the American Geriatrics Society, 37*, 991-1002.
37. Guenter, P. A., Settle, R. G., Perlmutter, S., et al. (1991). Tube feeding-related diarrhea in acutely ill patients. *Journal of Parenteral and Enteral Nutrition, 15*, 277-280.
38. Guerrant, R. L., Hughes, J. M., Lima, N. L., et al. (1990). Diarrhea in developed and developing countries: Magnitude, special settings, and etiologies. *Reviews of Infectious Diseases, 12*, S41-S50.
39. Gurwitz, J. H., Noonan, J. P., & Sanchez, M. (1992). Barium enemas in the frail elderly. *American Journal of Medicine, 92*, 41-44.
40. Hamilton, J. W., Wagner, J., Burdick, B. B., et al. (1988). Clinical evaluation of methylcellulose as a bulk laxative. *Digestive Diseases and Sciences, 33*, 993-998.
41. Hart, G. K., & Dobb, G. J. (1988). Effect of a fecal bulking agent on diarrhea during enteral feeding in the critically ill. *Journal of Parenteral and Enteral Nutrition, 12*, 465-468.
42. Heather, D. J., Howell, L., Montana, M., et al. (1991). Effect of a bulk-forming cathartic on diarrhea in tube-fed patients. *Heart and Lung, 20*, 409-413.
43. Henderson, C. T. (1988). Nutrition and malnutrition in the elderly nursing home patient. *Clinics in Geriatric Medicine, 4*, 527-547.
44. Henderson, C. T. (1991). Safe and effective tube feeding of bedridden elderly. *Geriatrics, 46*, 56-66.

45. Henderson, C. T., Trumbore, L. S., Mobarhan, S., et al. (1992). Prolonged tube feeding in long-term care: Nutritional status and clinical outcomes. *Journal of the American College of Nutrition, 11,* 309-325.
46. Heymsfield, S. B., Roongspisuthipong, C., Evert, M., et al. (1988). Fiber supplementation of enteral formulas: Effects on the bioavailability of major nutrients and gastrointestinal tolerance. *Journal of Parenteral and Enteral Nutrition, 12,* 265-273.
47. Hoffmeister, J. A., & Dobbie, R. P. (1977, January). Continuous control pump-tube feeding of the malnourished patient with Isocal. *American Surgeon,* pp. 6-11.
48. Hope, A. K. (1983). The relief of constipation in the elderly. *Australian Nursing Journal, 12,* 45-48.
49. Hope, A. K., & Down, E. C. (1986). Dietary fibre and fluid in the control of constipation in a nursing home population. *Medical Journal of Australia, 144,* 306-307.
50. Hull, C., Greco, R. S., & Brooks, D. L. (1980). Alleviation of constipation in the elderly by dietary fiber supplementation. *Journal of the American Geriatrics Society, 28,* 410-414.
51. Jones, B. J. M., Lees, R., Andrews, J., et al. (1983). Comparison of an elemental and polymeric enteral diet in patients with normal gastrointestinal function. *Gut, 24,* 78-84.
52. Justice, C. L., Howe, J. M., & Clark, H. E. (1974). Dietary intakes and nutritional status of elderly patients. *Journal of American Dietetics Association, 65,* 639-646.
53. Kamm, M. A., Hawley, P. R., & Lennard-Jones, J. E. (1988). Outcome of colectomy for severe idiopathic constipation. *Gut, 29,* 969-973.
54. Kelly, T. W. J., Patrick, M. R., & Hillman, K. M. (1983). Study of diarrhea in critically ill patients. *Critical Care Medicine, 11,* 7-9.
55. Keohane, P. P., Attrill, H., Love, M., et al. (1984). Relation between osmolality of diet and gastrointestinal side effects in enteral nutrition. *British Medical Journal, 288,* 678-680.
56. Kinnunen, O., & Salokannel, J. (1987). Constipation in elderly long-stay patients: Its treatment by magnesium hydroxide and bulk-laxative. *Annals of Clinical Research, 19,* 321-323.
57. Kinnunen, O., & Salokannel, J. (1989). Comparison of the effects of magnesium hydroxide on a bulk laxative on lipids, carbohydrates, vitamins A and E, and minerals in geriatric hospital patients in the treatment of constipation. *Journal of Internal Medicine Research, 17,* 442-454.
58. Klos, S. E., Drinka, P., & Goodwin, J. S. (1991). The utilization of fecal occult blood testing in the institutionalized elderly. *Journal of the American Geriatrics Society, 39,* 1169-1173.
59. Kochen, M. M., Wegscheider, K., & Abholz, H. H. (1985). Prophylaxis of constipation by wheat bran: A randomized study in hospitalized patients. *Digestion, 31,* 220-224.
60. Kohn, C. L., & Keithley, J. K. (1989). Enteral nutrition: Potential complications and patient monitoring. *Nursing Clinics of North America, 24,* 339-353.
61. Krachenfels, M. M. (1987). Home tube feedings: Gastrointestinal complications. *Home Healthcare Nurse, 5,* 41-42.
62. Kreusky, B., Maurer, A. H., Malmud, L. S., et al. (1989). Cisapride accelerates colonic transit in constipated patients with colonic inertia. *American Journal of Gastroenterology, 84,* 882-887.
63. Lamy, P. P., & Krug, B. H. (1978). Review of laxative utilization in a skilled nursing facility. *Journal of the American Geriatrics Society, 226,* 544-549.

64. Lederle, F. A., Busch, D. L., Mattox, K. M., et al. (1990). Cost-effective treatment of constipation in the elderly: A randomized double-blind comparison of sorbitol and lactulose. *American Journal of Medicine, 89,* 597-601.

65. Lennard-Jones, J. E. (1985). Pathophysiology of constipation. *British Journal of Surgery, 72*(Suppl), 7-8.

66. MacLennan, W. J., Pooler, A.F.W.M.A (1975). Comparison of sodium picosulphate ("Laxoberal") with standardized senna ("Senekot") in geriatric patients. *Current Medical Research and Opinion, 2,* 641-647.

67. Madoff, R. D., Williams, J. G., & Caushaj, P. F. (1992). Fecal incontinence. *New England Journal of Medicine, 326,* 1002-1007.

68. Mamtani, R., Cimino, J. A., Kugel, R., et al. (1989). Brief communication: A calcium salt of an insoluble synthetic bulking laxative in elderly bedridden nursing home residents. *Journal of the American College of Nutrition, 8,* 554-556.

69. McBurney, M. I., & Thompson, L. U. (1991). Dietary fiber and total enteral nutrition: Fermentative assessment of five fiber supplements. *Journal of Parenteral and Enteral Nutrition, 15,* 267-270.

70. McCallum, G., Ballinger, B. R., & Presley, A. S. (1978). A trial of bran and bran biscuits for constipation in mentally handicapped and psychogeriatric patients. *Journal of Human Nutrition, 32,* 369-372.

71. McCamman, S., Beyer, P. L., & Rhodes, J. B. (1977). A comparison of three defined formula diets in normal volunteers. *American Journal of Clinical Nutrition, 30,* 1655-1660.

72. Miller-Kovach, K., & Farmer, N. (1989). The effect of a fiber containing isotonic formula (FCIF) on correcting diarrhea in patients with demonstrated intolerance to a low residue, isotonic formula (LRIF) [abstract]. *Journal of the American Dietetics Association, 89,* A-62.

73. Milne, J. S., & Williamson, J. (1972). Bowel habit in older people. *Gerontol Clinic, 14,* 56.

74. Morgentaler, A., & Koufman, C. N. (1990). Treatment of an impacted fecalith with electrohydraulic lithotripsy [letter]. *New England Journal of Medicine, 322,* 855-856.

75. Muller-Lissner, S. A. (1987). Bavarian Constipation Study Group: Treatment of constipation with cisapride and placebo. *Gut, 28,* 1033-1038.

76. National Cancer Institute. (1987). *Diet, nutrition and cancer prevention: A guide to food choices* (NIH Publ. No. 87-2878, National Institutes of Health, Public Health Service, U.S. Department of Health and Human Services). Washington, DC: U.S. Government Printing Office.

77. Nicolle, L. E., McIntyre, M., Zacharias, H., et al. (1984). Twelve-month surveillance of infections in institutionalized elderly men. *Journal of the American Geriatrics Society, 32,* 513-519.

78. Noelker, L. S. (1987). Incontinence in elderly cared for by family. *Gerontologist, 27,* 194-200.

79. Norman, D. C., Castle, S. C., & Cantrell, M. (1987). Infections in the nursing home. *Journal of the American Geriatrics Society, 35,* 796-805.

80. Odes, H. S., Madar, Z., Trop, M., et al. (1986). Pilot study of the efficacy of spent grain dietary fiber in the treatment of constipation. *Israel Journal of Medical Sciences, 22,* 12-15.

81. Ott, L., & Young, B. (1991). Nutrition in the neurologically injured patient. *Nutrition in Clinical Practice, 6,* 223-229.

82. Payne-James, J. J., Rana, S. K., Bray, M. J., et al. (1992). Retrograde (ascending) bacterial contamination of enteral diet administration systems. *Journal of Parenteral and Enteral Nutrition, 16,* 369-373.

83. Peck, A., Cohen, C. E., & Mulvihill, M. N. (1990). Long-term enteral feeding of aged demented nursing home patients. *Journal of the American Geriatrics Society, 38*, 1195-1198.

84. Pers, M., & Pers, B. (1983). A crossover comparative study with two bulk laxatives. *Journal of Internal Medicine Research, 11*, 51-53.

85. Pesola, G. R., Hogg, J. E., Eissa, N., et al. (1990). Hypertonic nasogastric tube feedings: Do they cause diarrhea? *Critical Care Medicine, 18*, 1378-1382.

86. Pesola, G. E., Hogg, J. E., Yonnios, T., et al. (1989). Isotonic nasogastric tube feedings: Do they cause diarrhea? *Critical Care Medicine, 17*, 1151-1155.

87. Pinho, M., Yoshioka, K., & Keighley, M. R. B. (1990). Long-term results of anorectal myectomy for chronic constipation. *Diseases of the Colon and Rectum, 33*, 795-797.

88. Podell, S. K. (1989). Intermittent tube feedings and gastroesophageal reflux control in head-injured patients. *Journal of the American Dietetics Association, 89*, 102-103.

89. Primrose, W. R., Capewell, A. E., Simpson, G. K., et al. (1987). Prescribing patterns observed in registered nursing homes and long-stay geriatric wards. *Age and Ageing, 16*, 25-30.

90. Pringle, R., Pennington, M. J., Pennington, C. R., et al. (1984). A study of the influence of a fiber biscuit on bowel function in the elderly. *Age and Ageing, 13*, 175-178.

91. Puxty, J. A. H., & Fox, R. A. (1986). Golytely: A new approach to fecal impaction in old age. *Age and Ageing, 15*, 182-184.

92. Qvitzau, S., Matzen, P., & Madsen, P. (1988). Treatment of chronic diarrhea: Loperamide versus ispaghula husk and calcium. *Scandinavian Journal of Gastroenterology, 23*, 1237-1240.

93. Read, N. W., Abouzekry, L., Read, M. G., et al. (1985). Anorectal function in elderly patients with fecal impaction. *Gastroenterology, 89*, 959-966.

94. Ryan, C. A., Tauxe, R. V., Hosek, G. W., et al. (1986). Escherichia coli 0157:H7 diarrhea in a nursing home: Clinical, epidemiological, and pathological findings. *Journal of Infectious Diseases, 154*, 631-638.

95. Sanders, J. (1978). Lactulose syrup assessed in a double-blind study of elderly constipated patients. *Journal of the American Geriatrics Society, 26*, 236-239.

96. Sandler, R. S., Jordan, M. C., & Sheeton, B. J. (1990). Demographic and dietary determinants of constipation in the U.S. population. *American Journal of Public Health, 80*, 185-189.

97. Sandman, P. O., Adolfsson, R., Hallmans, G., et al. (1983). Treatment of constipation with high-bran bread in long-term care of severely demented elderly patients. *Journal of the American Geriatrics Society, 31*, 289-293.

98. Sandstrom, B., Andersson, H., Bosaeus, I., et al. (1983). The effect of wheat bran on the intake of energy and nutrients and on serum mineral levels in constipated geriatric patients. *Human Nutrition Clinical Nutrition, 37*, 295-300.

99. Sempos, C. T., Johnson, N. E., Elmer, P. J., et al. (1982). A dietary survey of 14 Wisconsin nursing homes. *Journal of the American Dietetics Association, 81*, 35-40.

100. Slavin, J. L., Nelson, N. L., McNamara, E. A., et al. (1985). Bowel function of healthy men consuming liquid diets with and without dietary fiber. *Journal of Parenteral and Enteral Nutrition, 9*, 317-321.

101. Smallwood, R. (1984). Bran and bowel habit. *Medical Journal of Australia, 141*, 447-450.

102. Smith, R. G., Currie, J. E. J., & Walls, A. D. F. (1978). Whole gut irrigation: A new treatment for constipation. *British Medical Journal* (Clinical Research), 2, 396-397.

103. Snape, W. J. (1989). The effect of methylcellulose on symptoms of constipation. *Clinical Therapeutics, 11*, 572-579.
104. Snustad, D., Lee, V., Abraham, I., et al. (1991). Dietary fiber in hospitalized geriatric patients: Too soft a solution for too hard a problem. *Journal of Nutrition in the Elderly, 10*, 49-63.
105. Sonnenberg, A., & Koch, T. R. (1989). Epidemiology of constipation in the United States. *Diseases of the Colon and Rectum, 32*, 1-8.
106. Stone, J. M., Nino-Murcia, M., Wolf, V. A., et al. (1990). Chronic gastrointestinal problems in spinal cord injured patients: A prospective analysis. *American Journal of Gastroenterology, 85*, 1114-1119.
107. Surawicz, C. M., Elmer, G. W., Speelman, P., et al. (1989). Prevention of antibiotic-associated diarrhea by *Saccharomyces boulardii*: A prospective study. *Gastroenterology, 96*, 981-988.
108. Thomas, D. R., Benner, R. G., Laughon, B. E., et al. (1990). Postantibiotic colonization with Clostridium difficile in nursing home patients. *Journal of the American Geriatrics Society, 38*, 415-420.
109. Tinetti, M. E., Stone, L., Cooney, L., et al. (1989). Inadequate barium enemas in hospitalized elderly patients. *Archives of Internal Medicine, 149*, 2014-2016.
110. Valle-Jones, J. C. (1985). An open study of oat bran meal biscuits ("Lejfibre") in the treatment of constipation in the elderly. *Current Medical Research Opinion, 9*, 716-720.
111. Viall, C., Porcelli, K., Teran, J. C., et al. (1990). A double-blind clinical trial comparing the gastrointestinal side effects of two enteral feeding formulas. *Journal of Parenteral and Enteral Nutrition, 14*, 265-269.
112. Wigzell, F. W. (1969). The health of nonagenarians. *Gerontology, 11*, 1137.
113. Williamson, J., & Connolly, M. (1975). A comparative trial of a new laxative. *Nursing Times, 71*, 1705-1707.
114. Yoshika, K., & Keighley, M. R. (1989). Clinical results of colectomy for severe constipation. *British Journal of Surgery, 76*, 600-604.
115. Zimmaro, D. M., Rolandelli, R. H., Koruda, M. J., et al. (1989). Isotonic tube feeding formula induces liquid stool in normal subjects: Reversal by pectin. *Journal of Parenteral and Enteral Nutrition, 13*, 117-123.

Table 6.2 Intervention Studies of Fiber in the Treatment of Constipation

Reference Location	Type of Facility (and subjects)	Study Design (sample size)	Fiber/Agent Used	Subject Mean Age (range)	Duration of Study	Outcome
Clark & Scott, 1976 England	Geriatric long-stay ward	Pre- and posttreatment comparison (N=25)	Wheat bran (5-25 gm per day)	Women, 80 yrs Men, 83 yrs	9 wks	Bran decreased laxative use. In men there was increased frequency of BM and increased stool size. Less effect in women.
McCallum et al., 1978 Dundee	Psychiatric hospital and mental handicap ward (senile dementia or profound mental handicap)	Randomized trial of three treatment regimens with crossover (N=23)	Bran biscuits (30 gm bran per day) or unrefined bran (10 gm per day) or senekot syrup (10 cc)	50.3 yrs (19-96)	9 wks	No difference between the three treatment groups in frequency of BM, consistency of stools, or need for enemas.
Andersson et al., 1979 Sweden	Geriatric ward (wheelchair bound or partially ambulatory)	Comparison of two consecutive treatment regimens (N=10)	Bulk laxative (12 gm per day) or coarse wheat bran (10-20 gm per day)	75 yrs (66-87)	16 wks	Compared to bulk laxative, subjects on bran had decreased intestinal transit time and decreased need for additional laxative therapy.
Battle & Hanna, 1980 Tennessee	Psychiatric long-term care ward (ambulatory)	Controlled trial (N=12)	All-Bran cereal (26.7 gm dietary fiber per day) or usual diet	58.6 yrs (50-67)	6 wks	Bran decreased laxative use and cost. No change in blood chemistries.
Hull et al., 1980 New Jersey	Long-term care facility	Pre- and posttreatment comparison (N=entire 300-bed facility)	Bran ± prune juice supplemented diet (8-11 gm dietary fiber)	79.6 yrs	1 yr	Laxative use was virtually eliminated with decreased costs and increased bowel regularity.

184

Study	Setting	Design	Intervention	Age	Duration	Results
Hope, 1983 Australia	NH	Pre- and posttreatment comparison (N=14)	High-fiber biscuits and bran-apple-prune supplement (3-25 gm per day) +1,500 cc fluid	80.8 yrs	27 wks	Supplements decreased laxative use. There was no change in BM frequency.
Sandman et al., 1983 Sweden	Institutionalized patients at a psychogeriatric clinic (demented)	Pre- and posttreatment comparison (N=33)	WASA fiber high-bran bread (dietary fiber=22%, 6 pieces per day)	74.9 yrs	10 wks	Increased BM frequency, decreased laxative use, and decreased diarrhea.
Sandstrom et al., 1983 Sweden	Geriatric ward (wheelchair bound or partially ambulatory)	Randomized trial with two treatment groups (N=10)	Wheat bran (20 gm per day) or enzymatically treated wheat bran (15 gm per day)	81 yrs (70-89)	13 wks	No decreased intake of energy or nutrients or decrease in serum Ca, Mg, Zn, or Fe on either bran supplement.
Pringle et al., 1984 Dundee, Scotland	Long-stay geriatric ward	Placebo-controlled trial with crossover (N=53)	Course bran fiber biscuit (<5-10 mg per day)	80.8 yrs	4 mos	A daily consumption of 7.5 gm or more of bran resulted in increased stool weight, decreased stool-free days, and decreased laxative prescriptions.
Kochen et al., 1985 Germany	Two general medical wards in an acute hospital	Randomized trial (N=200 randomized; but 58 refusers and dropouts)	Wheat bran (40 gm per day)	Men, 60 yrs Women, 63.3 yrs		No difference in incidence of constipation or use of laxatives.
Hope & Down, 1986 Australia	NH	Pre- and posttreatment comparison (N=30)	Bran and other high-fiber foods (25 gm dietary fiber) and 1,500 cc fluid per day	83.5 yrs	1 yr	Supplements increased frequency of BM, eliminated need for laxatives, and decreased need for nursing intervention. No effects on minerals (possibly except vitamin D and Zn).

continued

Table 6.2 Continued

Reference Location	Type of Facility (and subjects)	Study Design (sample size)	Fiber/Agent Used	Subject Mean Age (range)	Duration of Study	Outcome
Kinnunen & Salokannel, 1987, 1989	Long-stay ward	Randomized trial of two treatments with crossover (N=64)	Magnesium hydroxide (average dose= 25 cc/day) or bulk laxative (Laxamucil, average dose 9 gm/day)	81 yrs (all ≥64)	16 wks	Magnesium hydroxide group had more frequent BM, less need for additional laxatives, and more normal stool consistency. No significant differences in plasma lipids, minerals, or vitamins A and E.
Finlay, 1988 England	Long-stay geriatric ward (all subjects on fiber-enriched diet through-out the study)	Randomized controlled trial (N=12 with constipation, 2 with diarrhea)	Bran added to breakfast porridge (1.5-4.5 gm per day) or fiber-enriched diet without bran supplement	80 yrs	12 wks	No overall increase in frequency of BM with bran. There was improved "regularization of bowel function" and improved quantity, consistency, and "effective clearing" of stool.
Mamtani et al., 1989 New York	NH (mentally alert, bedridden)	Randomized trial of two treatments with crossover (N=32)	Synthetic fiber laxative (calcium polycarbo-phil) or psyllium (Fibercon= Metamucil)	77 yrs	6 wks	Subjects preferred the synthetic fiber laxative. There was no difference between treatment groups in number, ease of passage, or consistency of stools.

| Ardron & Main, 1990 England (letter) | Geriatric unit in a hospital | Crossover trial (placebo-treatment-placebo) (N=20) | Wheat bran (10 gm per day) | 77 yrs | 9 wks | Bran increased stool weight and consistency and decreased number of days without stools. Frequent and distressing fecal incontinence in 10/20 subjects on bran. |
| Snustad et al., 1991 Virginia | 10-bed geriatric evaluation and rehabilitation unit in an acute care hospital | Randomized double-blind trial (N=46) | Fiber-enriched cookies (10 gm fiber per day) | Control group, 78.1 yrs Treatment group, 75.5 yrs | 1-3 wks | Treatment group had no decrease in laxative use and no increase in frequency of bowel movements. |

187

Table 6.4 Intervention Studies of Nonfiber Drug Treatment of Constipation

Reference Location	Type of Facility (and subjects)	Study Design (sample size)	Agent(s) Used	Subject Mean Age (range)	Duration of Study	Outcome
Broatch et al., 1968 Scotland	Geriatric unit	Stage 1= randomized double-blind, placebo controlled trial (N=21) Stage 2= randomized crossover trial (N=20)	Bisacodyl *or* bisacodyl plus dioctyl sodium sulphosuccinate (stool softener)	Elderly	Stage 1= 34 days Stage 2= 24 days	Bisacodyl plus stool softener increased frequency of BM and had greater patient preference.
Berk, 1969 Massachusetts	Nursing home (confined to bed or chair)	Consecutive treatment comparison trial (N=42)	Bisacodyl suppository (10 mg) *or* packaged phosphate enema *or* soapsuds enema	Elderly	3 doses of each agent	Bisacodyl suppository was associated with superior bowel evacuations, less discomfort, less nursing time, and greater patient satisfaction.
Broholm, 1973 Sweden	Geriatric unit	Consecutive treatment comparison trial (N=35)	Danthron and stool softener preparation (Dorbanex) *or* multiple therapy with casanthranol, dioctyl sodium sulphosuccinate, and bisacodyl	81 yrs (62-92)	8 wks	Similar results in the two treatment regimens.

Study	Setting	Design	Treatment	Age	Duration	Results
MacLennan et al., 1975 England	Long-stay hospital	Randomized trial of two treatments (N=50)	Sodium picosulfate (Laxoberol, 10 mg) or senna (Senekot, 15mg)	Treatment A, 77 yrs Treatment B, 78 yrs	2 wks	Both agents were equally effective as laxatives, with wide variation in individual patient response.
Williamson & Connolly, 1975 Scotland	Long-stay hospital	Randomized trial of two treatments (N=50)	Sodium picosulphate (Laxoberal 10 mg) or danthon and fecal softener (Dorbanex 10 mg)	75.6 yrs (55-91)	6 wks	Increased frequency of BM with either agent but more side effects in the Laxoberal group.
Sanders, 1978 Michigan	Nursing home	Randomized controlled trial of two treatments (N=37)	Lactulose syrup (50%, 15-30 ml at bedtime) or glucose syrup (control)	Treatment group, 84.7 yrs Control group, 86.8 yrs	8-12 wks	Lactulose group had increased frequency of BM, decreased abdominal symptoms, decreased fecal impactions, and decreased need for enemas.
Brocklehurst et al., 1983 England	Long-stay ward	Randomized controlled trial of two treatments (N=37)	Lactulose syrup (50%, up to 40 cc per day) or Porbanex (up to 10 cc per day) or control (regular toileting and enemas)	Group mean ages were 82, 80, and 83 yrs (range 67-98)	4 wks	Both treatment groups had decreased intestinal transit time compared to control but continued to require enemas for bowel evacuation.

continued

Table 6.4 Continued

Reference Location	Type of Facility (and subjects)	Study Design (sample size)	Agent(s) Used	Subject Mean Age (range)	Duration of Study	Outcome
M. Pers & B. Pers, 1983 Sweden	Hospital (7 subjects were bedridden, 9 could sit, 4 could walk)	Randomized comparison of two treatments with crossover (N=20)	2 stimulant laxative regimens: Agiolax (15 mg senna glucoside) or Lunelax comp (25 mg senna glucoside A&B)	Men, 81 yrs Women, 85 yrs (all ≥60)	5 wks	Bowel frequency was higher with Lunelax. No difference in enemas required or side effects.
Castle et al., 1988 California (abstract)	Nursing home	Randomized double-blind placebo-controlled trial with crossover (N=15)	Docusate calcium	Elderly	Not reported	No difference in number of BM, use of additional cathartics, or stool consistency between treatment and placebo.
Lederle et al, 1990 Minnesota	VA medical center outpatients and nursing home residents	Randomized double-blind trial of two treatments with crossover (N=30)	Lactulose syrup or 70% sorbitol (0-60 mg per day).	72 yrs (65-85)	14 wks	No difference between treatments in frequency of BM, severity of constipation, or other symptoms except more nausea with lactulose. Sorbitol was less expensive.

Table 6.5 Intervention Studies on Gastrointestinal Complications of Tube Feedings

Reference Location	Facility (or population)	Study Design	Formula	Age	Duration	Outcome
Fischer et al., 1985 Wisconsin	Long-term care facility (constipated, tube-fed, nonambulatory residents)	Randomized controlled trial with crossover (N=28)	Soy polysaccharide added to tube feedings (15.6-17.4 gm dietary fiber per day)	Three groups with mean ages: 15.5, 20.7, and 19.2 yrs	6-11 wks	Fiber-supplemented tube feedings did not significantly increase BM frequency or stool weight and did not decrease intestinal transit time.
Hart & Dobb, 1988 Australia	Hospitalized intensive care unit patients	Blinded, placebo-controlled, randomized trial of fiber added to enteral feedings (N=68)	Lactose-free formula (Osmolite) with either fiber (Ispaghula husk, Fybogel, 7 gm/day) or placebo	47.1±20.8 yrs (fiber) 48.5±18.6 yrs (placebo)	3-18 days	Fiber did not affect the occurrence of diarrhea. A weak correlation was found between diarrhea and the number of antibiotics and positive nonenteric bacterial cultures.
Heymsfield et al., 1988 New York	University hospital, stable medical inpatients	Randomized trial with crossover of four different enteral formulas administered by nasoenteral feeding (Phase A, N=6; Phase B, N=8)	Phase A: Fiber-free formula (Ensure) or fiber-supplemented formula (Susta II, 12.4 gm soy polysaccharide/ 200 Kcal) Phase B: Susta II or Enrich (38.5 gm soy polysaccharide/ 2,000 Kcal)	50.7 yrs (range 22-70)	2-4 wks	Fiber-supplemented formulas reduced absorption of organic compounds and minerals, but these changes were not clinically significant. Fiber increased stool weight. Subjects on fiber-free formula had loose or watery stools. Subjects on fiber-supplemented formula had firm or hard stools.

continued

Table 6.5 Continued

Reference Location	Facility (or population)	Study Design	Formula	Age	Duration	Outcome
Frankenfield & Beyer, 1989 Kansas	Hospitalized intensive care unit patients (well-nourished head injury patients)	Randomized double-blind trial with crossover (N=9)	Tube feeding with (Enrich) or without (Ensure) soy polysaccharide fiber (14 gm/liter, mean=33±2 gm per day)	31±14 yrs	10 days	Fiber-containing formula did not independently affect stool weight, stool consistency, or incidence of diarrhea. All these tended to improve over time regardless of feeding formula.
Guenter et al., 1991 Pennsylvania	Acutely ill hospitalized patients requiring tube feeding	Randomized trial of fiber-free or fiber-supplemented formula (N=100)	Fiber-free formula (Osmolite HN) or fiber-supplemented formula (soy polysaccharide 14.4 gm/L)	Fiber-free group: 66.2±2.7 Fiber group: 65.0±2.3	At least 5 days of formula	Diarrhea occurred more often in patients on antibiotics, and was associated with C. difficile toxin and low serum albumin. Fiber-supplemented subjects had less diarrhea, although this difference was not statistically significant.
Heather et al., 1991 Oregon	Hospitalized patients in an intensive care unit	Randomized trial of a bulk-forming cathartic in tube-fed patients (N=49)	Bulk-forming psyllium cathartic (Hydrocil, 3 teaspoons per day)	Not reported	6 days	Subjects on Hydrocil had firmer stool consistency. No difference in stool frequency.
Jones et al., 1983 England	Hospitalized patients	Randomized trial of two tube formula diets in patients requiring tube feeding (N=70)	Elemental diet (Vivonex HN) or isonitrogenous isocaloric polymeric diet (Clinifeed 400)	55.1±3.1 days (Vivonex) 15.2±3.1 (Clinifeed)	14.3±1.5 days (Vivonex) 15.2±2.0 days (Clinifeed)	The incidence of gastrointestinal side effects (i.e., diarrhea and vomiting) was not different between the two formulas. Diarrhea was often due to antibiotic.

192

Study	Population	Design	Formula	Age	Duration	Results
Keohane et al, 1984 England	Hospitalized patients	Double-blind randomized trial of three tube feeding regimens (N=118)	Group 1: Hypertonic diet (Clinifeed 400) Group 2: Hypertonic diet diluted initially, then full strength Group 3: Isotonic diet (Clinifeed Iso)	Not reported	Mean 8.7 days (range 3-35 days)	All groups had similar incidence of nausea, bloating, and cramps. Diarrhea was significantly associated with concurrent treatment with antibiotics.
Brinson & Kolts, 1988 Florida	Hospitalized intensive care unit patients with hypoalbuminemia	Blinded, randomized controlled trial of two tube-fed formulas (N=12)	A standard isotonic enteral formula (Osmolite HN) or peptide-based feeding formula (Vital HN)	Mean 49.1 yrs Range 22-73 yrs	2-3 wks	No difference in stool frequency or fecal weight. On Osmolite HN, stools were significantly more watery, which resolved when formula was changed to vital HN.
Miller-Kovach & Farmer, 1989 Ohio (abstract)	Acute hospital	Pre- and post comparison in small sample of tube-fed patients with diarrhea (N=6)	Fiber-containing isotonic formula (Profiber)	Not reported	4 days	Five of six patients with diarrhea or tube feedings had resolution of diarrhea when switched to fiber-containing formula.

continued

Table 6.5 Continued

Reference Location	Facility (or population)	Study Design	Formula	Age	Duration	Outcome
Feller et al., 1990 Wisconsin	Nursing home (demented, bedridden, male residents with gastrostomy tubes)	Baseline observation on Isocal, then randomized trial of two alternate formulas, with crossover (N=10)	Isocal followed by a peptide-based mixture (Peptamen *or* an amino acid based preparation, Vivonex TEN)	Median: 69 yrs (range 61-80)	12 wks	No gastrointestinal side effects observed with any of the formulas (i.e., no vomiting, diarrhea, or abdominal distress). A shift to Vivonex caused a significant decline in serum plasma proteins.
Viall et al., 1990 Ohio	Nonsurgical hospitalized patients requiring enteral nutrition	Controlled randomized double-blind trial of two enteral feeding formulas (N=23)	Soy hydrolysate (study formula) *or* casin formula (control formula)	73.2 yrs (54-92)	6 days	No difference in incidence of diarrhea between groups. The soy formula group had somewhat fewer bowel movements and less vomiting.

7

Nutritional Problems in the Nursing Home Population: Opportunities for Clinical Interventions

ADIL A. ABBASI, M.D.
SAILENDRA N. BASU, M.D.
ABBAS PARSA, M.D.
LUCA ALVERNO, M.D.
DANIEL RUDMAN, M.D.

In this chapter, we present material leading to three conclusions. First, nutritional deficiencies are common underlying causes for adverse clinical outcomes within the nursing home (NH) population. Second, these nutritional deficiencies are frequently not recognized. Third and most important, opportunities exist to improve clinical outcomes within NHs by preventing or correcting these nutritional deficiencies; but this is possible only if the significance and reversible nature of the deficiencies are recognized.

PRINCIPLES OF CLINICAL NUTRITION

A review of certain basic principles of clinical nutrition serves as a useful starting point (56). Our food, composed of recently living plant and animal tissue, has all the chemical complexity of living organisms. Many food components are physiologically indispensable,

Supported by PHS grant ID 31 PE 95008-03, NIH grant RR-03326, and by grants from the Department of Veterans Affairs, the Alzheimer's Disease Foundation, and the Retirement Research Foundation. The authors also wish to acknowledge the valuable help of Karen Isaacson, R.D., Dr. Ken Shay, and Dr. Ruth Hartmann in preparing this chapter.

but only a few are nutritionally indispensable (i.e., must be supplied by the diet). The identification of the second group has been the goal of several generations of nutrition scientists. The problem is not only theoretical but practical as well; it sometimes becomes necessary to nourish patients by a simplified, even synthetic diet, either enterally or parenterally. The correct formulation of such "elemental" diets is dependent on our understanding of essential nutrients.

Identification of the essential nutrients became feasible when nutrition investigators developed purified diets. An animal or person under study was fed a mixture consisting only of known, purified nutrients. If the transition from mixed foods to the restricted diet caused a failure of growth or other indication of illness, one or more essential nutrients must have been withdrawn. Useful indicators sensitive to the withdrawal of an essential nutrient in healthy growing subjects (animal or human) have been body weight gain and nitrogen retention, and in healthy adult subjects, maintenance of zero nitrogen balance and constant body weight. The purified restricted diet, furthermore, often caused lesions specific for the withdrawal of a particular essential nutrient, for example, rachitic bone (vitamin D), scorbutic skin (vitamin C), beriberi opisthotonos (vitamin B_1), and canine blacktongue (niacin). In this way, it was recognized in the early 20th century that crude lipid and water-soluble extracts of liver were required for the growth and integrity of rats fed highly purified diets. Two or more essential factors (fat-soluble and water-soluble vitamins, among others) were subsequently demonstrated in each of these extracts. Each factor corrected a different component of the disorder induced by the purified diet. For most (but not all) nutrients, signs of nutritional deficiency are more likely caused by protracted rather than short-term consumption of the restricted diet. For example, only by prolonged feeding of purified diets was the essentiality of polyunsaturated fatty acids and the trace elements revealed.

The essential nutrients that have been identified in this fashion can be divided into macronutrients (more than 100 mg/day required in humans) and micronutrients (less than 100 mg/day required in humans). They can also be divided into organic factors (protein, essential fatty acids, vitamins) and inorganic factors (water, minerals, trace elements). The catalog of the 40 essential nutrients includes 23 organic compounds (9 essential amino acids, 13 vitamins, 1 fatty acid), 15 elements, water, and an energy source (56) (see Table 7.1).

For each essential nutrient, there are three dosage thresholds: minimum daily requirement (MDR), recommended daily allowance

Table 7.1 Catalogue of the 40 Known Essential Nutrients

Essential Amino and Fatty Acids	*Vitamins*	*Elements*	*Other*
Amino acids	Thiamine	Sodium	Water
L-threonine	Niacin	Potassium	Energy sources
L-valine	Riboflavin	Calcium	
L-isoleucine	Pyridoxine	Magnesium	
L-leucine	Folic acid	Chloride	
L-lysine	B$_{12}$	Phosphorus	
L-tryptophan	Ascorbic acid	Iron	
L-methionine-cyst(e)ine	Biotin	Copper	
L-phenylalanine-tyrosine	Pantothenic acid	Zinc	
L-histidine	Vitamin A	Chromium	
	Vitamin D	Manganese	
Fatty acids	Vitamin E	Selenium	
Linoleic acid	Vitamin K	Molybdenum	
		Iodine	
		Fluoride	

SOURCE: Rudman and Williams (1985).

(RDA), and maximal daily tolerance. The MDR is determined in a group of healthy subjects of specified age, sex, and physiologic status (e.g., level of physical activity, whether pregnant or lactating) and represents the mean value, in the subjects tested, of the lowest amount of the nutrient that will prevent clinical or chemical manifestations of a deficiency illness. The RDA, the amount estimated to prevent deficiency in at least 97% of the population, takes into account the interindividual variation in MDR and is usually 30% to 100% higher than the MDR. The maximal daily tolerance reflects the fact that every dietary component, essential or nonessential, will cause illness if sufficient excess is taken for a sufficient time period.

NUTRITIONAL DEFICIENCIES IN THE NURSING HOME POPULATION: PREVALENCE AND CONSEQUENCES

In the two decades after World War II, comments appeared frequently in the literature concerning nutritional problems of the elderly population. The resulting concern led to a series of systematic surveys of the nutritional status of older Americans. Two strategies were used. Some investigators focused on the nutritional intakes

Table 7.2 Nutritional Status of Community-Living Healthy and Institutionalized Elderly

| | Community Living (Healthy)[1] | | Institutionalized[2] | |
	Low Intakes	Subnormal Nutritional Indicators	Low Intakes	Subnormal Nutritional Indicators
Calories	29-33%	3%	5-18%	30-66%
Protein	2-15%	3%	0-33%	15-60%
Calcium	37%	0-54%	2%	
Iron	—	4%	5-35%	10-31%
Magnesium				
Vitamin A	11%	—	5-13%	0-18%
Vitamin D	72%	15%	63-77%	48%
Ascorbic acid	5%	4-24%	0-40%	0-83%
Thiamin	8%	2-5%	7-30%	4-23%
Riboflavin	4%	2-3%	0-34%	2%
Pyridoxine	85%	18%	57-100%	28-49%
Folate	77%	8-9%	37%	7-57%
Niacin	0%	13%	0%	33%
Vitamin B12	31%	3-31%	—	0-20%
Zinc	76%	—	21%	
Phosphorus	3%			
Vitamin E	44%	4%	—	3-40%
Biotin	—	1%	—	0%
Pantothenic acid	—	4%	—	3%

NOTES: 1. See References 4-10,21-24,40,42,47. 2. See References 2,3,12,30,33,40,41,51,58,62,65,66,70,71.

of the study groups as measured by diet recall or diet diary. Other observers measured the anthropometric and biochemical indicators of nutritional status. (See also Rudman & Feller, 1989.)

When the study group was a random sample of the entire elderly population, with its wide range of clinical conditions, the resulting data understandably portrayed great variability in nutritional status. A more coherent picture, however, was provided by surveys on more sharply defined elderly subgroups.

In Table 7.2, Columns 1 and 2 summarize surveys of independent community-living elderly (4-10,21-24,40,42,47). In about one third of the subjects, energy intake was below the RDA. Consumption of minerals and vitamins was below the RDA in up to 50% of subjects, and the blood levels were subnormal in 10% to 30%. Yet body weight, adipose mass, and muscle mass were rarely depleted, and protein intake was generally adequate. The interpretation of these findings is that the diminishing energy expenditure of the elderly leads to a lower energy requirement and therefore to a reduced food intake. But unless the nutrient density of the diet is simultaneously increased, subclinical mineral and vitamin deficiencies will tend to occur. Because the U.S. diet tends to be high in protein, however, the intake of protein usually remains adequate even at the lower level of calorie consumption.

The nutritional picture in the NH subgroup of U.S. elderly was less favorable (Table 7.2, Columns 3 and 4)(41,40,12,70,58,66,30,2,65,62, 3,33,71,51). Intakes were frequently low for both calories and protein. From 30% to 50% of the residents were substandard in body weight, midarm muscle circumference, and serum albumin level, indicating widespread protein-calorie undernutrition (PCU). Blood levels were frequently low for both water-soluble and fat-soluble vitamins.

The adverse effect of PCU on clinical outcome in the acutely ill general hospital population of all ages has been recognized since the 1970s. Only recently, however, has the linkage between PCU and death rate in the NH been documented. In 1986, Phillips reported a reciprocal correlation of midarm muscle circumference and albumin level to the mortality rate in the NH. Dwyer et al. (1987) reported that the recent loss of weight was a sensitive predictor of death in residents.

The present authors conducted an epidemiologic survey in 1985 in the 200-bed NH of the North Chicago Veterans Affairs (VA) Medical Center (55). At the beginning of the surveillance year, a 67-item clinical data base was compiled, including diagnoses; drugs; and measures of nutritional, metabolic, hematologic, hepatic, and renal function. Deaths were recorded during the year of observation. Correlations were then sought between the items of the annual data base and mortality.

Fifty-five deaths occurred during the year, for which infection was usually the immediate cause (50 cases) and chronic organic brain disorder was most commonly an underlying cause (42 cases). Of the 67 attributes in the data base, only 7 were significant predictors of death in the univariate analysis: age, functional level, and five nutrition-related variables (triceps skinfold, midarm muscle circumference, albumin, cholesterol, and hematocrit). The decedents were older, more dependent, depleted in adipose and muscle, hypoalbuminemic, and hypocholesterolemic.

For each mortality-related nutritional indicator, there was a threshold at which the risk of death increased (Table 7.3). For albumin, cholesterol, or hematocrit, the threshold occurred within the conventional

Table 7.3   Relation of Death Rates to Mortality-Related Patient
Attributes in North Chicago VA Nursing Home, 1985

Attribute	Annual Death Rate
Body weight as % of ideal	
>100	9.8%
90-100	11.3%
80-89	14.3%
<80	26.3%
Hematocrit (%)	
<37	37%
37-39	14%
39-41	27%
>41	4%
Cholesterol (mg/dl)	
<156	67%
157-180	0%
181-202	10%
>203	11%
Albumin (g/dl)	
>4.0	11.1%
3.5-3.99	43.4%
<3.5	50%

SOURCE: Adapted from Rudman et al. (1987).

"normal range." Thus, death rate rose significantly when the albumin
concentration declined below 4.0 g/dl, when the cholesterol level declined below 160 mg/dl, or when the hematocrit declined below 41%.
Evidently, the "desirable ranges" for nutritional indicators (and perhaps for other clinical tests) in the nursing home elderly are not the
same as the normal ranges, which are usually defined as the 95%
confidence limits in the general population of overtly healthy adults.

When multivariate analysis was applied to the seven mortality-
related variables, the statistical model selected cholesterol first and
hematocrit second. These analyses demonstrated the dire prognostic
significance of a serum cholesterol level below 160 mg/dl in the NH
patient.

CAUSES OF UNDERNUTRITION IN NURSING HOMES

In general, the causes of PCU can be arranged in two categories:
those causing inadequate intake and those causing increased nutritional requirements (e.g., recurrent infections). Analysis of data on

PCU from Third World countries suggests both types of mechanisms are usually involved (53,46). In contrast to the population of the Third World where poverty is the main cause of inadequate food intake, inadequate food intake of U.S. NH patients occurs despite the adequate food supply, which is mandated by law (31). These rules call for the provision to residents of meals providing at least one RDA of each essential nutrient in an attractive environment under sanitary conditions and under the supervision of qualified dieticians.

Normal eating, however, requires more than the serving of complete nutrition. The psychosocial setting must be suitable for the feeding process. Taste, smell, cognition, attention, manual dexterity, and the ability to chew and swallow are all required. Normal swallowing follows efficient mastication; proceeds through the oral, pharyngeal, and esophageal stages; and totally excludes food and secretions from the larynx (72,35). Moreover, mood affects appetite and eating habits (19).

Many of these eating functions are altered in NH patients. The changes in taste buds and olfactory nerve with advancing age influence the thresholds for recognition and discrimination, altering established food preferences (60). Chewing is slower and less effective, a regression that is aggravated by loss of teeth (18). From 30% to 80% of residents are edentulous (25), and about a third have depressed mood (11,52). Loss of manual dexterity is a common prelude to chronic institutionalization (74). In the study by Siebens et al. (1986) paralysis or contracture caused impaired arm function in about 30% of the NH cases, and oral and pharyngeal types of neurogenic dysphagia affected 20% and 40%. The dementing illnesses eventually lead to neurogenic dysphagia in most of the advanced cases (69,49,15,64). Other common causes of low food intake in long-term care institutions are anorexigenic drugs and chronic medical disorders. Finally, the environment in the NH may not be conducive to eating (39,48,14).

For the various reasons cited above, many NH residents are unable or unwilling to eat and are labeled "eating dependent." In the 1986 study by Siebens et al., 40% required assistance in eating. Until dysphagia or anorexia becomes advanced, eating dependency can be compensated in many individuals by assisted feeding, provided there is adequate staff. Indeed, a number of studies have shown that individuals receiving feeding assistance had better nutritional status judged by body weight and serum albumin level than those individuals apparently capable of independent eating (63,43,45).

An additional risk factor for diminished food intake by some NH residents arises from a lowered energy requirement caused by the gradual decline in the basal metabolic rate (44) and a low level of physical activity. Because energy balance is the main determinant of hunger, the hypometabolic NH patient desires and eats less food. Although caloric needs are met, the consumption of other essential nutrients may be suboptimal unless the nutrient density of the food is increased (61,28).

In the same population of NH patients whose ability or desire to eat is limited, there are factors operating that tend to increase the nutritional requirements. Some chronically institutionalized patients with brain disease are hyperactive (agitated, wandering, pacing) or affected by involuntary movements (17). A more pervasive mechanism, however, is the high rate of infection. "Point-in-time" surveys show 15%-20% of NH residents have active infection in the urinary tract, respiratory tract, skin, or eye (20). Infectious processes cause confusion, anorexia, and hypophagia in the elderly (76), as well as the catabolic response of negative nitrogen balance (8). Hospitalization of a NH patient is frequently associated with weight loss (57). The capacity for post-illnesses repletion is often inadequate because of the various limitations on food intake discussed above. Infectious illnesses, even without fever, cause a negative nitrogen balance that may last for a month afterward (8). The nutritional requirements to repair these catabolic periods are about 50% above maintenance (59). When wasted children (as evident from studies on children with PCU in the Third World countries) are provided adequate nutrition (for example, when convalescing from infection, after a period of famine, or both), they respond with hyperphagia and "catch-up" growth (1,73). Anorexic, dysphagic, confused, apraxic NH patients may lack this capacity to mount a hyperphagic response. Moreover, the NH dietary staff may not provide the extra food above the RDA that is needed during a period of restorative hyperphagia. Each recurrent infection, which may occur as often as every 3 months, therefore tends to lower the patient to the next degree of PCU.

EVIDENCE FOR MODIFIABLE CAUSES OF NH UNDERNUTRITION

The consensus concerning the high prevalence of PCU in the NH and its adverse consequences is clear and concerning. To what extent are the causes of NH PCU intrinsic (endogenous, the unmodifiable consequences of diseases and old age) and to what extent are they extrinsic (environmental)? The answers could have significant im-

Table 7.4   Demographic Statistics of Three Nursing Homes

Location	Nursing Home A Urban	Nursing Home B Urban	Nursing Home C Urban
Size	400	200	190
Male/female	95/5	93/7	94/6
Length of stay			
<6 months	24%	38%	20%
>6 months	76%	62%	80%
Medical/neurologic	64%	82%	60%
Psychiatric	36%	18%	40%
Schizophrenia	29%	11%	30%
Affective	6%	5%	8%
Other	1%	2%	2%
Functional level			
1	0%	0%	0%
2	44%	39%	46%
3	43%	45%	40%
4	13%	16%	14%
Age			
<50	4%	6%	3%
50-60	13%	14%	12%
60-70	41%	38%	41%
70-80	28%	25%	29%
80-90	8%	9%	9%
>90	6%	8%	6%

NOTE: Functional level 1=independent, resides in community; 2=nursing home, requires no assistance in ADL; 3=nursing home, requires partial assistance in ADL; 4=nursing home, requires total care.

pact on the choice of intervention strategies and the allocation of clinical resources.

The authors have conducted a pilot study, the findings of which indicate a substantial contribution of extrinsic causes. From 1987 to 1989, a comparison was made of the following indicators of adverse outcomes in three VA NHs (labeled A, B, and C): the point-in-time prevalences of underweight and hypoalbuminemia, the point-in-time prevalence of bedsores, and the frequency of deterioration in ADLs over a 6-month period. These indicators are all sensitive to both case mix and to quality of care. The three institutions had similar proportions of independent, partially dependent, and totally dependent patients (see Table 7.4). Chronic psychiatric patients constituted 18% to 40% of the patients in the three NHs.

Frequencies of undernutrition, bedsores, and deteriorating ADLs differed greatly between the three facilities, despite the similarity in proportions of dependent and independent patients (Table 7.5). NH A had the highest initial frequency of undernutrition and bedsores, and the highest rate of deterioration in ADLs over a 6-month period. The prevalences of body weight less than 90% and serum albumin below 3.5 g/dl were about 40% and 15% respectively; 10% of the patients had bedsores; 30% of the independent or partially dependent patients deteriorated substantially in ADLs during a 6-month period of observation. Moreover, in NH A these figures were similar for the psychiatric and for the medical/neurologic patients. The corresponding figures were lowest in NH C. In this facility, the adverse outcomes occurred in less than 8% of the psychiatric and medical/neurologic patients. In NH B, the figures were generally intermediate between facilities A and C, but the outcome profile was more favorable for the psychiatric than for the medical/neurologic patients.

The high frequencies of adverse outcomes in NH A, and the similarly poor outcome profile for psychiatric and nonpsychiatric patients there, might suggest that the quality of care in this facility was inferior to that in NH C, where all the adverse outcomes under study were uncommon. Nevertheless, it will be desirable to adjust the crude frequencies for severity of illness before these indicators could be used definitively to evaluate quality of care. The wide differences between the psychiatric populations of the three NHs regarding the occurrences of underweight, bedsores, and the decline of ADLs suggest that a monitoring of these unfavorable somatic outcomes may be a useful addition to quality assurance programs in long-term psychiatric facilities, where quality surveillance currently focuses mainly on behavioral elements.

The "focused review" is another way to investigate the question of what proportion of NH PCU is due to modifiable, extrinsic causes rather than to unmodifiable, intrinsic causes. In a nursing home where PCU is prevalent, individual cases can be reviewed with an appropriate instrument to ascertain whether the undernutrition was modifiable or unmodifiable. The authors have carried out such a study in a 200-bed VA NH in which the prevalences of underweight (body weight less than 80% of ideal) and of hypoalbuminemia (less than 3.5 g/dl) were 32% and 21% respectively. As a first step, the writers prepared from a review of the pertinent literature (36,48,49, 61-67) a classification of unavoidable and avoidable causes of protein-calorie undernutrition (Table 7.6) and a specific list of 15 avoidable causes (Table 7.7). Table 7.7 also describes how each modifiable cause can be detected and corrected. Noteworthy are the following

Table 7.5 Proportions of Patients With Adverse Outcome Indicators in Three Nursing Homes

Indicator	Nursing Home A						Nursing Home B				Nursing Home C	
	10/87 to 4/88		4/88 to 10/88		10/88 to 4/89		10/88 to 4/89		4/89 to 10/89		10/88 to 4/89	
	P	MN	P	MN	P	MN	P	MN	P	MN	P	MN
1. Body weight <90% of ideal	.39 (55/140)	.39 (99/253)	.40 (55/138)	.40 (102/255)	.35 (50/144)	.40 (100/250)	.27 (10/36)	28% (50/164)	.24 (8/33)	.28 (45/162)	.03 (2/76)	.08 (9/114)
2. Body weight <80% of ideal	.15 (21/140)	.11 (28/253)	.14 (19/138)	.13 (33/255)	.12 (17/144)	.14 (35/250)	.07 (3/36)	12% (20/164)	.09 (3/33)	.11 (18/162)	0 (0/76)	.02 (2/114)
3. Serum albumin <3.5 g/dl	.11 (14/131)	.16 (38/236)	.11 (14/123)	.15 (35/235)	.13 (17/130)	.16 (37/230)	.07 (2/31)	.26 (37/230)	.06 (2/28)	.24 (38/158)	.02 (1/69)	.05 (5/92)
4. Bedsores+	.10 (14/140)	.12 (30/253)	.11 (15/138)	.11 (28/255)	.09 (13/144)	.10 (25/250)	0 (0/36)	.03 (5/164)	0 (0/33)	.04 (6/162)	.02 (1/76)	.04 (5/114)
5. Major loss of ADLs	.30 (38/125)	.32 (65/204)	.27 (31/116)	.33 (70/211)	.28 (36/130)	.30 (62/208)	0 (0/28)	.03 (4/143)	0 (0/24)	.04 (6/142)	0 (0/59)	.06 (6/96)

NOTE: P=Chronic nonorganic psychiatric patients; MN= Medical/neurologic patients; +=Bedsore Score 2 or greater; Major loss of ADLs=Proportion of patients for whom the sum of the four ADL scores deteriorated (i.e., increased) by four points or more during the 6-month period of observation; total care patients are excluded because their ADLs are already maximally impaired.

Table 7.6 Categories of Underweight or Weight Loss

Desirable weight loss
  Obesity, edema states

Undesirable underweight or weight loss
                    Undesirable but unmodifiable
  Incurable malignancy
  Inability to eat and refusal of tube feeding
  End stage pulmonary, cardiac, hepatic, or renal disease
  Advanced disease of the small intestine
                    Undesirable and modifiable

Inadequate feeding assistance	Suboptimal dining environment
Prescription of maintenance instead of repletion dietary intakes	Inadequate nutritional support during intercurrent illness
Limited menu choices	Depression
Inappropriate use of restricted diets	Medications causing hypophagia
Poor dental status	Swallowing disorders
Staff unawareness	Occult infection

points: multiple clinical services are involved; administrative-fiscal factors are influential; hypophagia is the major pathophysiologic mechanism; the avoidable causes can be detected by simple observation and in most cases can be corrected by educational intervention. With this classification and instrument, the authors now reviewed 30 charts of patients with body weight less than 80% of ideal. The focused review classified 10 out of the 30 cases as unmodifiable PCU (metastatic cancer, 7; advanced emphysema, 3). But in 20 of the cases, an unmodifiable cause could not be found, and instead, a variety of modifiable causes were identified: inadequate feeding assistance, inappropriate use of restricted or modified diets, suboptimal dining environment, limited menu choices, prescription of maintenance instead of repletion dietary intake, and staff unawareness of the presence of PCU.

After the focused review, an intervention was introduced. A nutrition support team (NST) comprising a physician, a dietician, and a nurse was established and consulted on patients with body weight less than 80% of ideal or serum albumin level below 3.5 g/dl who had been unresponsive to conventional management by the ward team to improve nutritional status. The "instrument" shown in Table 7.7 was used to search for modifiable cause(s) on each patient consulted and to guide the recommendations by the NST to the ward dietician and

Table 7.7 Fifteen Modifiable Causes of PCU in the Nursing Home

Cause	*Method of Identification*	*Corrective Action*
1. Staff unawareness	Lack of documentation of PCU in the chart by MD, RN or RD	Staff education
2. Inappropriate use of restricted diets	Patient receiving a restricted diet no longer indicated	Replace by ad lib diet
3. Use of drug(s) impairing ability or desire to eat	Review of medications	Discontinue or replace offending drug
4. Unmet need for eating assistance or eating self-help devices	Observation and calorie count	Provide the assistance or devices
5. Suboptimal technique of eating assistance	Observation	Retrain the nursing aide
6. Suboptimal dining environment	Observation	Improve the environment
7. Prescription of maintenance instead of repletion dietary intakes (either oral or enteral)	<1.5 RDA of calories and protein prescribed	Increase prescription to 1.5 RDA calories and protein
8. Inadequate nutritional support during intercurrent illnesses	Weight and/or albumin decline during intercurrent illness: inadequate nutritional support	Project MD will consult on each NHCU patient during intercurrent illness
9. Unrecognized febrile illness	Daily temperature reveals elevations	Identify and treat infection
10. Unrecognized or untreated depression	Geriatric depression score >15	Evaluate and treat
11. Unmet need for a modified diet	Clinical review	Prescribe indicated modified diet
12. Inadequate management of tube-feeding complications	Prescribed level of tube-feeding not being administered or absorbed due to diarrhea, aspiration, or mechanical complication	Correct management of the complication
13. Poor dental status	Oral examination	Prompt dental care
14. Unmet need for dysphagia workup	Clinical signs suggest dysphagia but workup not requested	Consult speech pathology for evaluation of swallowing
15. Suboptimal treatment of dysphagia	Recommendations of speech pathology not being followed	Speech pathologist retrains ward staff

nursing staff. Body weight and serum albumin concentration were recorded at the beginning and at the end of an 8-week intervention period. Patients were followed on a weekly basis by the NST and recommendations were modified as deemed necessary.

Eighteen patients were seen in consultation and ten (55%) were found to have one or more modifiable cause(s) of PCU. During the 8-week intervention, attempts were made to correct the identified modifiable causes. Five (50%) patients showed an average weight gain of 4.5 kg at the end of the intervention period, but no improvement in serum albumin was observed.

Results from the focused review and the intervention study led the authors to conclude that the prevalence of PCU in NHs can indeed be reduced by identifying and correcting modifiable causes of PCU. However, the underweight status is more readily improved than is the hypoalbuminemia.

NUTRITIONAL INTERVENTIONS IN NURSING HOMES

It is clear from the above discussion that PCU is a common problem in the institutionalized elderly, and that it is often preventable as well as potentially treatable. Nevertheless, the authors could find only five published interventional studies concerning NH malnutrition (13,36,37,5,38). Table 7.8 summarizes these reports. Because of the scarcity of publications in this area, several intervention studies done to improve the nutrition of geriatric patients in the hospital have also been included (75,10,6,34,68). In the publications summarized, the following points were notable: (a) nearly all led to favorable clinical results; (b) tube feeding was the most common intervention; (c) in other studies, a variety of simple oral dietary modifications were effective; (d) all of the interventions were aimed to improve low caloric intake.

Winograd and Brown (1990) suggested that aggressive oral refeeding with high-caloric foods (e.g., candy, chocolate bars) is an underutilized therapy for malnourished patients. They observed a gradual return of appetite, inclusion of other foods in the diet, improvement in ADLs, weight gain, and increases in serum albumin and total lymphocyte count. This approach is particularly useful for patients with poor oral intake who are not candidates for enteral nutritional support. Tomaiolo et al. (1981) used a different approach to improve the nutritional status of malnourished elderly hospitalized patients. Relatively tasteless supplements, namely polycose (Ross laboratories), Promix (Nubro), and Loralac (Mead Johnson), were used to improve the nutritional value and caloric density of foods selected by patients. This method markedly improved the daily caloric intake in most patients; foods and beverages prepared with tasteless supplements provided an additional average of 1200 cal/day. In addition, the serum levels of albumin and transferrin rose. Nitrogen balance studies confirmed that most patients were in positive nitrogen balance. Commercially available canned nutritional supplements are frequently prescribed to improve caloric intake. However, like Tomaiolo and associates, we have had only limited success in terms of increasing caloric intake using these supplements. On the other hand, adding tasteless supplements to the food chosen by the patients seems to be an effective method of achieving desired caloric intake in orally fed patients. Manning and Means (1975) outlined a self-feeding program for NH patients who require feeding assistance. This is a simple stepwise, nursing-oriented approach that not only improved food intake but also enhanced motivation and self-esteem. Coulston et al. (1990) addressed the inappropriate use of restricted diets in NHs. They showed that the custom of routinely prescribing diabetic diets for patients with noninsulin-dependent diabetes mellitus confined to chronic care facilities was often not necessary. The effectiveness of enteral nutritional support as a temporary means of replenishing nutritional deficits has been documented by a number of studies (36,37,6,34). Thus the literature review of intervention studies in Table 7.8 is consistent with the classification of avoidable causes in Tables 7.6 and 7.7, and with the findings of the authors' focused review, in leading to the conclusion that much of the occurrence of NH undernutrition is preventable.

CONCLUSIONS

PCU is not uncommon in NHs and in a substantial proportion of patients may be modifiable. PCU is associated with increased mortality, morbidity, and medical care expenditures. Future research should focus not only on the causes and consequences of PCU, but also on programs for prevention, early recognition, and more effective treatment.

Table 7.8 Summary of Publications for the Treatment of Protein Calorie Undernutrition

Reference	Study Group	Intervention	Duration (days)	Complication	Outcome
1. Winograd & Brown, 1990	Three hospitalized patients	Oral refeeding using sweets (candy bars, ice cream . . .)	14-21	None	Weight gain, improvement in serum albumin, and functional status were noted in all 3 patients. Oral intake also improved after 2-3 weeks of initial intervention.
2. Coulston et al., 1990	18 residents with noninsulin-dependent diabetes mellitus from two skilled nursing facilities	Diet was changed from diabetic diet to regular diet for 8 weeks and glycemic control and caloric intake monitored.	112	None	No significant change in blood glucose was noted during 8-week period when residents were on a regular diet as compared to when they were on a diabetic diet. Caloric intake increased when these residents were on a regular diet.
3. Brown et al., 1987	102 hospitalized patients on enteral nutritional support	Subjects divided into two groups. One managed by enteral nutrition support team, the other by the primary physician.	105	None	Team-managed patients received more calories, were supported for longer period of time, and had fewer tube feeding related complications.
4. Bastow et al., 1983	Randomized controlled study on patients (who underwent surgery for hip fracture) in an acute hospital and a rehabilitation hospital	Patients divided into 3 groups: normally nourished, mildly to moderately malnourished, and severely malnourished. Last 2 groups were given supplemental tube feeding at night.	Not known	None	Improvements in anthropometric and plasma protein measurements as well as clinical outcomes like rehabilitation time and hospital stay.

Study	Patients	Intervention	Duration	Complications	Results
5. Kaminski et al., 1982	102 hospitalized patients prospectively studied Mean age Grp I= 52 yrs (young), Grp II=76 yrs (old)	Enteral or parenteral nutritional support in two groups of hospitalized patients Measured somatic and visceral parameters	Grp I=38 (mean) Grp II=45 (mean)	None	No difference in the degree of improvement or maintenance of somatic or visceral parameters in the two groups
6. Lipschitz, 1982	35 elderly NH patients	Caloric intake increased by enteral nutritional support and/or oral supplements	21	None	Marked decrease in confusion. Improvement in functional status. Increase in serum albumin, TIBC, body weight, hemoglobin total lymphocyte count, and colony-forming unit-C.
7. Lipschitz et al., 1982	9 elderly malnourished NH patients ranging from 73-95 years	Increasing caloric intake by enteral hyperalimentation (7 subjects) and oral nutritional supplements (2 subjects)	21	None	Decreased confusion; weight gain; improved appetite and morbidity; increase in colony-forming unit-C.
8. Tomaiolo et al., 1981.	117 elderly hospitalized patients (mean age=73 years)	Increasing caloric intake using relatively tasteless supplements with regularly served meals	Not known	None	Improvement in serum albumin and transferrin. Improvement in nitrogen balance. No change in weight was noted.

REFERENCES

1. Ashworth, A., & Millward, D. J. (1987). Catch-up growth in children. *Nutrition Reviews, 44*, 157-163.
2. Asplund, K., Normark, M., & Pettersson, V. (1981). Nutritional assessment of psychogeriatric patients. *Age and Ageing, 10*, 87-94.
3. Baker, H., Frank, O., Thind, I. S., et al. (1979). Vitamin profiles in elderly persons living at home or in nursing homes, versus profile in healthy young subject. *Journal of the American Geriatrics Society, 27*, 444-450.
4. Baltes, M. M., & Zerbe, M. B. (1976). Re-establishing self feeding in a nursing home resident. *Nursing Research, 25*, 24-26.
5. Banerjee, A. K., Brocklehurst, J. C., Wainwright, H., et al. (1978). Nutritional status of long stay geriatric inpatients: Effects of a good supplement (Complan). *Age and Ageing, 7*, 237-243.
6. Bastow, M. D., Rawlings, J., & Allison, S. P. (1983). Benefits of supplementary tube feeding after fractured neck of femur: A randomized controlled trial. *British Medical Journal, 287*, 1589-1592.
7. Beaumont, D. M., & James, O.F.W. (1985). *Clinical Gastroenterology, 14*, 811-827.
8. Beisel, W. R. (1977). Magnitude of the host nutritional responses to infection. *American Journal of Clinical Nutrition, 30*, 1236-1247.
9. Bienia, R., Ratcliff, S., Barbour, G., et al. (1982). Malnutrition in the hospitalized geriatric patient. *Journal of the American Geriatrics Society, 30*, 433-436.
10. Brown, R. O., Carlson, S. D., Cowan, G.S.M., Jr., et al. (1987). Enteral nutritional support management in a university teaching hospital: Teams vs non-team. *Journal of Parenteral and Enteral Nutrition, 11*, 52-56.
11. Cheah, K. C., & Beard, O. W. (1980). Psychiatric findings in the population of a geriatric evaluation unit: Implications. *Journal of the American Geriatrics Society, 28*, 153-156.
12. Chen, L. H., & Fan-Chiang, W. L. (1981). Biochemical evaluation of riboflavin and vitamin B_6 status of institutionalized and non-institutionalized elderly in central Kentucky. *International Journal for Vitamin and Nutritional Research, 51*, 232-238.
13. Coulston, A. M., Mandelbaum, D., & Reaven, G. M. (1990). Dietary management of nursing home residents with non-insulin dependent diabetes mellitus. *American Journal of Clinical Nutrition, 51*, 67-71.
14. Davies, A. D., & Snaith, P. A. (1980). Mealtime problems in a continuing care hospital for the elderly. *Age and Ageing, 9*, 100-105.
15. Donner, M., & Silbiger, M. (1966). Cinefluorographic analysis of pharyngeal swallowing in neuromuscular disorders. *American Journal of the Medical Sciences, 251*, 600-616.
16. Dwyer, J. T., Coleman, K. A., Krall, E., et al. (1987). Changes in relative weight among institutionalized elderly adults. *Journal of Gerontology, 42*, 246-251.
17. Fauman, M. A. (1978). Treatment of the agitated patient with an organic brain disorder. *Journal of the American Medical Association, 240*, 380-382.
18. Feldman, R. S., Kapur, K. K., Alman, J. E., et al. (1980). Aging and mastication: Changes in performance and the swallowing threshold with natural dentition. *Journal of the American Geriatrics Society, 28*, 97-103.
19. Garfinkel, P. E., Garner, D. M., Kaplan, A. S., et al. (1983). Differential diagnosis of emotional disorders that cause weight loss. *Canadian Medical Association Journal, 129*, 939-945.

20. Garibaldi, R. A., Brodine, S., & Matsumiya, S. (1981). Infections among patients in nursing homes. *New England Journal of Medicine, 305,* 731-735.
21. Garry, P. J., Goodwin, J. S., & Hunt, W. C. (1982a). Nutritional status in a healthy elderly population: Riboflavin. *American Journal of Clinical Nutrition, 36,* 902-909.
22. Garry, P. J., Goodwin, J. S., & Hunt, W. C. (1984). Folate and vitamin B_{12} status in a healthy elderly population. *Journal of the American Geriatrics Society, 32,* 719-726.
23. Garry, P. J., Goodwin, J. S., Hunt, W. C., et al. (1982b). Nutritional status in a healthy elderly population: Vitamin C. *American Journal of Clinical Nutrition, 36,* 332-339.
24. Garry, P. J., Goodwin, J. S., Hunt, W. C., et al. (1982c). Nutritional status in a healthy elderly population: Dietary and supplemental intakes. *American Journal of Clinical Nutrition, 36,* 319-331.
25. Goldberg, A. F., Mattson, D. E., & Rudman, D. (1988). The relationship of growth to alveolar ridge atrophy in an older male nursing home population. *Special Care in Dentistry, 8,* 184-186.
26. Goodwin, J. S. (1989). Social, psychological and physical factors affecting the nutritional status of elderly subjects: Separating cause and effect. *American Journal of Clinical Nutrition, 50,* 1201-1209.
27. Henderson, C. T. (1988). Nutrition and malnutrition in the elderly nursing home patient. *Clinics in Geriatrics Medicine, 4,* 527-547.
28. Henriksen, B., & Cate, H. D. (1971). Nutrient content of food served versus food eaten in nursing homes. *Journal of the American Dietetics Association, 59,* 126-129.
29. Hogstel, M. O., & Robinson, N. B. (1989). Feeding the frail elderly. *Journal of Gerontological Nursing, 15*(3), 16-20.
30. Hontela, S., Vobecky, J., Shapcott, D., et al. (1983). Serum level of vitamins A, C, E, folate and iron in female psychogeriatric patients in comparison with their controls. *Nutrition Reports International, 27,* 1101-1111.
31. Joint Commission on Accreditation of Hospitals. (1986). *Long term care standards manual.* Chicago: Author. pp 9-14.
32. Jones, A. M. (1978). Overcoming the feeding problem of the mentally and physically handicapped. *Journal of Human Nutrition, 32,* 359-367.
33. Justice, C. L., Howe, J. M., & Clark, H. E. (1974). Dietary intakes and nutritional status of elderly patients: Study in a private nursing home. *Journal of the American Dietetics Association, 65,* 639-646.
34. Kaminski, M. V., Nasr, J. N., Freed, B. A., et al. (1982). The efficacy of nutritional support in the elderly. *Journal of the American College of Nutrition, 1,* 35-40.
35. Linden, P., & Siebens, A. A. (1983). Dysphagia: Predicting laryngeal penetration. *Archives of Physical Medicine and Rehabilitation, 64,* 281-284.
36. Lipschitz, D. A. (1982). Protein calorie malnutrition in the hospitalized elderly. *Primary Care, 9,* 531-543.
37. Lipschitz, D. A., & Mitchell, C. O. (1982). The correctability of the nutritional immune and hematopoietic manifestations of protein calorie malnutrition in the elderly. *Journal of the American College of Nutrition, 1,* 17-25.
38. Manning, A. M., & Means, J. G. (1975). A self feeding program for geriatric patients in a skilled nursing facility. *Journal of the American Dietetics Association, 66,* 275-276.
39. Miller, M. B. (1971). Unresolved feeding and nutrition problems of the chronically ill aged. *Gerontologist, 11,* 329-336.
40. Morgan, D. B., Newton, H. M., Schorah, C. J., et al. (1986). Abnormal indices of nutrition in the elderly: A study of different clinical groups. *Age and Ageing, 15,* 65-76.

41. Munice, H. L., Jr., & Carbonetto, C. (1982). Prevalence of protein-caloric malnutrition in an extended care facility. *Journal of Family Practice, 14,* 1061-1064.
42. Munro, H. N., McGandy, R. B., Hartz, S. C., et al. (1987). Protein nutriture of a group of free-living elderly. *American Journal of Clinical Nutrition, 46,* 586-592.
43. MacLennan, W. J., Martin, P., & Mason, B. J. (1975). Causes for reduced dietary intake in a long-stay hospital. *Age and Ageing, 4,* 175-180.
44. McGandy, R. B., Barrows, C. H., Spanias, A., et al. (1966). Nutrient intakes and energy expenditures in men of different ages. *Journal of Gerontology, 21,* 581-587.
45. Nguyen, N. H., Flint, D. M., Prinsley, D. M., et al. (1985). Nutrient intakes of dependent and apparently independent nursing home patients. *Human Nutrition and Applied Nutrition, 39,* 333-338.
46. Olson, R. E. (1975). In R. E. Olson (Ed.), *Protein-calorie malnutrition* (pp. 275-297). New York: Academic Press.
47. Omdahl, J. L., Garry, P. J., Hunsaker, L. A., et al. (1982). Nutritional status in a healthy elderly population: Vitamin D. *American Journal of Clinical Nutrition, 36,* 1225-1233.
48. Ostasz, J. (1986). Successful techniques for hand-feeding the elderly. *Geriatric Care, 18*(11), 11-12.
49. Palmer, E. D. (1974). Dysphagia in parkinsonism. *Journal of the American Medical Association, 229,* 1349.
50. Phillips, P. (1986). Grip strength, mental performance and nutritional status as indicators of mortality risk among female geriatric patients. *Age and Ageing, 15,* 53-56.
51. Pinchcofsky-Devin, G. D., & Kaminski, M. V., Jr. (1986). Correlation of pressure sores and nutritional status. *Journal of the American Geriatrics Society, 34,* 435-440.
52. Rovner, B. W., Kafonek, S., Filipp, L., et al. (1986). Prevalence of mental illness in a community nursing home. *American Journal of Psychiatry, 143,* 1446-1449.
53. Rudman, D. (1987). Protein and energy undernutrition. In Braunwald, E., Isselbacker, K. J., Petersdorf, R. G., et al. (Eds.), *Harrison's principles of internal medicine* (11th ed., pp. 393-397). New York: McGraw-Hill.
54. Rudman, D., & Feller, A. G. (1989). Protein-calorie undernutrition in the nursing home. *Journal of the American Geriatrics Society, 37,* 173-183.
55. Rudman, D., Mattson, D. E., Nagraj, H. S., et al. (1987). Antecedents of death in the men of a Veterans Administration nursing home. *Journal of the American Geriatrics Society, 35,* 496-502.
56. Rudman, D., & Williams, P. J. (1985). Pathophysiologic principles of nutrition. In L. H. Smith & S. O. Their (Eds.), *Pathophysiology: The biological principles of disease* (pp. 440-486) (2nd ed.). Philadelphia: Saunders.
57. Sahyoun, N. R., Otradovec, C. L., Hartz, S. C., et al. (1988). Dietary intakes and biochemical indicators of nutritional status in an elderly institutionalized population. *American Journal of Clinical Nutrition, 47,* 524-533.
58. Sandman, P. O., Adolfsson, R., Nygren, C., et al. (1987). Nutritional status and dietary intake in institutionalized patients with Alzheimer's disease and multi-infarct dementia. *Journal of the American Geriatrics Society, 35,* 31-38.
59. Scrimshaw, N. S. (1977). Effect of infection on nutrient requirements. *American Journal of Nutrition, 30,* 1536-1544.
60. Schiffman, S. S., & Covey, E. (1984). Changes in taste and smell with age: Nutritional aspects. In J. M. Ordy (Ed.), *Nutrition in gerontology* (pp. 43-64). New York: Raven.
61. Sempos, C. T., Johnson, N. E., Elmer, P. J., et al. (1982). A dietary survey of 14 Wisconsin nursing homes. *Journal of the American Dietetics Association, 81,* 35-40.

62. Shaver, H. J., Loper, J. A., & Lutes, R. A. (1980). Nutritional status of nursing home patients. *Journal of Parenteral and Enteral Nutrition, 4,* 367-370.
63. Siebens, H., Trupe, E., Siebens, A., et al. (1986). Correlates and consequences of eating dependency in institutionalized elderly. *Journal of the American Geriatrics Society, 34,* (192-198.
64. Silbiger, M., Pikielny, R., & Donner, M. (1966). Neuromuscular disorders affecting the pharynx. *Transactions of the American Neurological Association, 91,* 157-161.
65. Smith, J. L., Wickiser, A. A., Korth, L. L., et al. (1984). Nutritional status of an institutionalized aged population. *Journal of the American College of Nutrition, 3,* 13-15.
66. Stiedemann, M., Jansen, C., & Harrill, I. (1978). Nutritional status of elderly men and women. *Journal of the American Dietetics Association, 73,* 132-139.
67. Sullivan, D. H., Patch, G. A., Walls, R. C., et al. (1990). Impact of nutrition status on morbidity and mortality in a select population of geriatric rehabilitation patients. *American Journal of Clinical Nutrition, 51,* 749-58.
68. Tomaiolo, P. P., Enman, S., & Kraus, V. (1981). Preventing and treating malnutrition in the elderly. *Journal of Parenteral and Enteral Nutrition, 5,* 46-48.
69. Veis, S. L., & Logemann, J. A. (1985). Swallowing disorders in persons with cerebrovascular accident. *Archives of Physical Medicine and Rehabilitation, 66,* 372-375.
70. Vincent, M., & Gibson, R. S. (1982). Dietary intake of a group of chronic geriatric psychiatric patients. *Gerontology, 28,* 245-251.
71. Vir, S. C., & Love, A. H. (1979). Nutritional status of institutionalized and noninstitutionalized aged in Belfast, Northern Ireland. *American Journal of Clinical Nutrition, 32,* 1934-1947.
72. Wayler, A. H., Kapur, K. K., Feldman, R. S., et al. (1982). Effect of age and dentition status on measures of food acceptability. *Journal of Gerontology, 37,* 294-299.
73. Whitehead, R. G. (1977). Protein and energy requirements of young children living in the developing countries to allow for catch-up growth after infections. *American Journal of Clinical Nutrition, 30,* 1545-1547.
74. Williams, M. E., Hadler, N. M., & Earp, J. A. (1982). Manual ability as a marker of dependency in geriatric women. *Journal of Chronic Diseases, 35,* 115-122.
75. Winograd, C. H., & Brown, M. E. (1990). Aggressive oral refeeding in hospitalized patients. *American Journal of Clinical Nutrition, 52,* 967-968.
76. Yoshikawa, T. T. (1983). Geriatric infectious diseases: An emerging problem. *Journal of the American Geriatrics Society, 31,* 34-39.
77. Young, E. A. (1983). Nutrition, aging and the aged. *Medical Clinics of North America, 67,* 295-313.

8

Clinical Research on Falls in the Nursing Home

LAURENCE Z. RUBENSTEIN, M.D., M.P.H.
KAREN R. JOSEPHSON, M.P.H.

INTRODUCTION

Falls are a common and serious problem in the nursing home, causing considerable morbidity, mobility disturbance, and mortality. Interest in the problem of falling and the sophistication of fall-related research have greatly increased over the past 20 years. Research objectives have progressed from simply establishing the epidemiology and causes of falls, to identifying risk factors that predict which patients are most likely to fall, to designing and testing interventions to prevent falls. This chapter presents a systematic review of the literature on falls in the NH setting, synthesizes the available research data, and outlines research questions that remain to be answered.

EPIDEMIOLOGY

Incidence of Falls

Both the incidence of falls in older adults and the severity of complications rise steadily with age and with increased physical disability. Accidents are the fifth leading cause of death in older adults, and falls constitute two thirds of these accidental deaths. About three fourths of deaths due to falls in the United States occur in the 13% of the population aged 65 and older (24). Approximately

Table 8.1 Incidence of Falls and Fall-Related Injuries in Long-Term Care Facilities

Reference	Site[a]	Mean Age of Population	Annual Incidence per 1,000 Beds	Percent of Falls With Serious Injury	Percent of Falls With Fracture
Gryfe et al., 1977	BC	81%≥75	650	17%	6%
Pablo, 1977	CC	72	730	17%	0
Feist, 1978	NH	83	3,300	4%	3%
Cacha, 1979	NH	82	2,400	1%	NA[b]
Miller & Elliott, 1979	NH	82	1,400	NA	1%
Louis, 1983	NH	83	760	12%	NA
	NH	79	1,100	14%	NA
Colling & Park, 1983	NH	NA	2,600	5%	2%
Blake & Morfitt, 1986	BC	≥60	3,600	3%	NA
Berry et al., 1981	CC	68%≥70	1,500	5%	3%
Berryman et al., 1989	NH	≥65	2,000	NA	NA
Gross et al., 1990	NH/BC	82	220	15%	10%
Rubenstein et al., 1990	NH/BC	≥65	1,200	NA	2%
Gostynski, 1991	NH/BC	86	1,300	6%	2%
Neufeld et al., 1991	NH/BC	84	630	NA	5%
Svensson et al., 1991	NH	95%≥65	350	36%[c]	NA
Simple mean of all surveys			1,480		

NOTES: a. BC=Board and care facility; CC=Chronic care facility; NH=Nursing home.
b. NA=Data not available.
c. Percent of injurious falls in this study considered to be serious.

one third of older adults living at home will fall each year, and about 5% will sustain a fracture or require hospitalization. Among institutionalized populations the risk and consequences of falling are even greater. Each year about 1800 fatal falls occur in NHs. Among persons 85 years and older, one out of five fatal falls occurs in a NH (2). Incidence rates reported for institutionalized elderly persons are about three times the rate for community-living elderly persons, due both to the more frail nature of institutionalized populations and to the more accurate reporting of falls in institutional settings. Studies performed in institutional settings have reported annual fall incidence at 0.4 to 3.6 (mean = 1.4) falls per bed. These data are listed in Table 8.1. Variation between reported studies seem to reflect differences in case mix and ambulation levels, as well as a number of institutional differences, such as staffing levels and environmental factors.

Incidence of Fall-Related Morbidity

Despite the high fall rates among institutionalized populations, most falls fortunately do not cause serious injury. As shown in Table 8.1, only 1%-10% of falls result in fractures. Other serious injuries, such as head trauma, soft tissue injuries, and severe lacerations occur in 1%-17% of falls. However, once injured, the case fatality rate is much higher for elderly people than for younger people (24). NH patients have a disproportionately high incidence of hip fracture and have also been shown to have higher mortality rates following hip fracture than community-living elderly persons (45). Further, due to the high number of falls, residents of a given institution can experience a substantial number of injurious falls per year.

In addition to physical injuries, falls can have other serious consequences for NH residents. "Fear of falling" and the "postfall anxiety syndrome" have been reported to result in self-imposed functional limitations (43). Loss of confidence in the ability to ambulate safely can lead to further functional decline, depression, feelings of helplessness, and social isolation. The use of physical or chemical restraints by institutional staff to prevent high-risk persons from falling also clearly has negative impacts on functioning.

Situational Factors Associated With Falls

Numerous descriptive studies have attempted to characterize some of the situational factors (e.g., location, time of day, activity) associated with falls in long-term care facilities. The major findings from these studies are presented in Table 8.2. Fifteen of the 17 studies reviewed used nursing incident reports as their primary data source and two (36,23) relied on patient recall of the fall. Given the diversity of the patient populations surveyed and differences in how the data were reported, only general trends can be gleaned from the compilation of these findings.

The majority of studies reported the location of falls. The single most common site of falls was generally the bedroom, at the bedside. This finding is probably due to the fact that patients usually spend a great deal of unsupervised time in their bedroom. Falls in toilet or shower areas were less frequent, which may be related to the staff assistance that many patients receive during toileting and bathing or the relatively less time spent in those areas. There may be an increased risk of injury in the bathroom, however, given slippery tile floors, the possibility of water or urine on the floor, and multiple transferring activities. In one study, 50% of the *injurious* falls occurred in the bathroom (17). Few falls occurred outdoors, as would be expected from the limited unsupervised extrainstitutional activity among most NH residents.

Perhaps more informative than location are the activities most commonly associated with falls. Among those surveys that reported these data, the majority of falls occurred from a chair or wheelchair, or from the bed. It is unclear what percentage of falls were the result of normal transferring and what percentage were due to patients trying to escape from soft restraints or bed rails. Relatively few falls were associated with falling from the toilet. However, attempting to ambulate to or from the bathroom was reported to be associated with 44% of falls in one study (1) and 80% of fall-related fractures in another (10).

The data do not reveal any consistent association between time of day and increased fall rates. Most authors reported that peak fall times corresponded with peak activity times, often around mealtime, rising, and going to bed. Only three studies found higher rates of falls at night (5,17,36); two of these studies were conducted in residential homes for the aging, both of which had a more functional patient population than would be expected in a NH. Nighttime falls, however, have been reported to more often result in serious injury (10,17). Changing light levels at sunrise and dusk have also been hypothesized as contributing to falls (31).

Some studies have also reported that falls increase when nurse staffing is low, such as during breaks and at shift change (10,11,20, 34,42) and on the weekends (31), presumably due to lack of staff supervision. Only one study, however, actually showed a significant inverse correlation between number of falls and number of staff (5).

The frequency of falls occurring while patients were restrained ranged from 6% to 47% in the five surveys that reported these data. Falls occurred as a result of patients untying soft restraints and attempting to ambulate, or trying to climb over bed rails. Several studies reported impressions that falls by persons under restraint tended to be more serious.

CAUSES OF FALLS

Determination of the major causes of falls has been attempted in numerous studies. However, comparability of these data has been limited by several factors, including differences in diagnostic approaches used between studies, differences in study populations,

Table 8.2 Factors Related to Falls in the Institutional Setting

Reference	Site[a] # Beds	Survey Period	Number Falls	Location of Falls				Associated Activity				Miscellaneous Factors		
				Bed-room	Bath-room	Outside	Other/ Unspeci-fied	Walking	From Chair	From Bed	From Toilet	Peak Time of Day	Low Staffing	Re-straints Used[c]
Ashley et al., 1977 Canada	BC 200	5 yrs	651	59%	12%	5%	24%	44%	18%	19%	—	No specific times	—	—
Pablo, 1977 Canada	CC 186	3 yrs	544[b]	58%	23%	1%	18%	17%	30%	15%	15%	7a-7p	Yes	—
Feist, 1978 USA	NH 42	42 mo	490	—	—	—	—	—	—	—	—	6-9p	—	6%
Cacha, 1979 USA	NH 135	1 yr	319	—	—	—	—	17%	41%	8%	9%	11a-12p 8-9p	No	21%
Miller & Elliott, 1979 USA	NH 88	1 yr	203[b]	55%	8%	5%	32%	—	—	—	—	11a-12p 3-4p	Yes	15%
Morfitt, 1980 Great Britain	BC —	1 yr	96	32%	5%	8%	55%	—	—	—	—	11p-8a (25%)	—	—
Berry et al., 1981 Canada	CC 400	2 yrs	1803	42%	30%	—	28%	—	40%	—	—	Daytime	—	—
Foerster, 1981 USA	NH 242	10 wk	105	—	43%	—	57%	—	—	—	—	8a-4p 12-4a	No	—
Colling & Park, 1983 USA	NH 129	8 mo	214	78%	14%	3%	5%	—	—	—	—	9-11a 6-8p	Yes	—
Louis, 1983 USA	NH 115	2 yrs	253	70%	—	—	30%	—	—	—	—	6-7a 6-7p	No	—

220

Study, Country	Facility	N	Duration	Incidents									Time	Assoc.
Louis, 1983 USA	NH	190	3 mo	36	47%	—	—	53%	—	—	—	—	6-7a 5-6p	Yes
Dimant, 1985 USA	NH	—	29 mo	310[b]	64%	8%	2%	26%	46%	31%	17%	7%	3-4p	Yes
Blake & Morfitt, 1986 Great Britain	BC	60	16 mo	296[b]	62%	4%	—	34%	—	—	—	—	10p-6a	Yes
Haga et al., 1986 Japan	BC	—	1 yr	204	11%	8%	40%	41%	—	—	—	—	Daytime	—
Gross et al., 1990 USA	NH	178	1 yr	40	73%	—	—	27%	28%	40%	30%	3%	10a-12p	Yes
Gostynski, 1991 Switzerland	BC	79	1 yr	102	61%	14%	8%	17%	—	—	—	—	8-10a 10-12p	—
Neufeld et al., 1991 USA	NH	514	1 yr	323	54%	19%	—	27%	39%	33%	—	23%	Daytime Evening	—

NOTES: a. BC=Board and care facility; CC=Chronic care facility; NH=Nursing home.
b. Study included incidents/accidents besides falls (i.e., burns, cuts, scraps), although falls accounted for the majority of incidents.
c. Yes=Significant association between staffing levels and fall rates; No=No association found.

Table 8.3 Comparison of Causes of Falls in Nursing Home and Community-Living Populations: Summary of Studies That Carefully Evaluated Elderly Persons After a Fall and Specified a "Most Likely Cause"

| | Nursing Home | | | | | Community-Living (N=7 studies,[a] 2,312 falls) |
Cause of Falls	Rubenstein (N=77)	Lipsitz (N=70)	Svensson (N=827)	Gostynski (N=102)	Total (N=1,076)	
"Accident"/environment-related	27%	6%	16%	17%	16%	41% (23-53%)[b]
Gait/balance disorder, weakness	39%	34%	25%	20%	26%	13% (2-29%)
Dizziness/vertigo	—	6%	30%	15%	25%	8% (0-19%)
Drop attack	—	—	—	3%	0.3%	13% (0-25%)
Confusion	—	—	14%	—	10%	2% (0-7%)
Postural hypotension	16%	11%	—	—	2%	1% (0-6%)
Visual disorder	3%	4%	5%	—	4.5%	0.8% (0-4%)
Syncope	—	3%	—	—	0.2%	0.4% (0-3%)
Other specified causes[c]	10%	34%	10%	12%	12%	17% (2-39%)
Unknown	5%	1%	—	34%	4%	6% (0-16%)

NOTES: a. Brocklehurst et al. (1978); Clark (1968); Exton-Smith (1977); Lucht (1971); Morfitt (1983); Robbins et al. (1989); Sheldon (1960).
b. Mean percent,calculated from the total number of falls in the studies reviewed. Ranges indicate the percentage reported in each of the studies. Percentages do not total 100% because some studies reported more than one cause per fall.
c. This category includes arthritis, acute illness, drugs, alcohol, pain, epilepsy, and falling from bed.

different classification methods (e.g., single best diagnosis versus multiple diagnoses used for classifying each fall, varying importance placed on coexisting environmental hazards), variable patient recall, and the characteristic multifactorial causes for falls (e.g., tripping due to both gait disorder and poor vision). Nonetheless, these studies provide some useful general information about the nature of falling in the elderly population.

Table 8.3 lists the major causes of falls and their relative frequencies as described in four studies of NH patients and compares these to summary data from seven studies of community-living populations. As can be seen in the table, the distribution of causes clearly differs between populations studied. Frail, high-risk, institutionalized populations tend to have higher incidence of falls due to gait disorders, weakness, dizziness, and confusion, whereas community-living populations tend to have more environment-related falls.

In the NH the broad category of weakness and gait problems was the most common cause for falls, accounting for about a quarter of reported falls. Muscle weakness is an extremely common finding among the aged population. Studies have reported the prevalence of grossly detectable lower extremity weakness to range from 48% among community-living older persons (7), to 57% among residents of an intermediate care facility (57), to over 80% among NH residents (47). Muscle weakness, especially plantarflexor and dorsiflexor weakness, is also a common cause of gait deviations. Gait disorders affect 20%-50% of the elderly population (51), and nearly three quarters of NH patients require assistance with ambulation or are unable to ambulate (39). Case-control studies performed in NHs reported that over two thirds of fallers have substantial gait disorders, a prevalence 2.4 to 4.8 times higher than among nonfallers (47,57).

The sensation of dizziness is an extremely common complaint among elderly fallers and was the attributed cause in 25% of reported NH falls. This symptom is often difficult to evaluate, since the description of dizziness means different things to different people and can arise from very diverse etiologies, including vestibular dysfunction, postural hypotension, and medication effects.

So-called accidents, or falls stemming from environmental hazards, constitute a major categorical cause of reported falls—16% of NH falls and 41% of community falls. However, true accidents are difficult to verify, and many falls in this category may actually stem from interactions between environmental hazards or hazardous activities and increased individual susceptibility to hazards from accumulated effects of age and disease. Among impaired patients, even normal activities of daily living might be considered hazardous if they are performed without assistance or modification. Most normal older people have stiffer, less coordinated, and more dangerous gaits than do younger people. Posture control, speed of body-orienting reflexes, muscle strength and tone, and height of stepping all decrease with aging and impair ability to avoid a fall after an unexpected trip or while reaching or bending. Age-associated impairments of vision, hearing, and memory also tend to increase the number of trips and stumbles.

Confusion and cognitive impairment is a frequently cited cause of falls and may reflect an underlying systemic or metabolic process causing both the confusion and the fall (e.g., electrolyte imbalance, fever). Dementia can increase falls by impairing judgment, visuospatial perception, and ability to orient oneself geographically. Wandering activities of demented patients are often associated with falls. Falls also occur when demented patients attempt to get out of wheelchairs or climb over bed rails.

Orthostatic (postural) hypotension, usually defined as a drop of 20 mm or more of systolic blood pressure after standing, has a 5% to 25% prevalence among "normal" elderly people living at home (46). It is even more common among persons with certain predisposing risk factors, including autonomic dysfunction, hypovolemia, low cardiac output, parkinsonism, metabolic and endocrine disorders, and medications (particularly sedatives, antihypertensives, vasodilators, and antidepressants) (33). The orthostatic drop may be more pronounced on arising in the morning, since the baroceptor response is diminished after prolonged recumbency, after meals, and after ingestion of nitroglycerin (28,26). Yet despite its high prevalence, orthostatic hypotension is only a relatively infrequently identified cause of falls, particularly outside institutions. This is perhaps because of its transient nature, making it harder to detect after the fall, or because most persons with orthostatic hypotension feel lightheaded and deliberately find a seat to avoid falling.

Drop attacks are defined as falls associated with sudden leg weakness but without loss of consciousness or dizziness. Sudden change in head position is often a precipitating event. This syndrome has been attributed to transient vertebrobasilar artery insufficiency, although it is probably due to more diverse pathophysiologic mechanisms.

Syncope, defined as a sudden loss of consciousness with spontaneous recovery, is a serious but less common cause of falls. However, it is probably more common than the mean figure listed in Table 8.3, because several of the studies specifically excluded patients with syncope. Syncope results from decreased cerebral blood flow or occasionally from metabolic causes such as hypoglycemia or hypoxia. The most frequent etiologies in elderly persons are cardiac arrhythmias, orthostatic hypotension, vasovagal reactions, and—a large category—"syncope of unknown cause."

Other specified causes of falls include visual problems, arthritis, acute illnesses, disorders of the central nervous system, drug side effects, and alcohol intake. Drugs frequently have side effects that result in impaired mentation, stability, and gait. Especially important are agents with sedative, antidepressant, and antihypertensive effects, particularly diuretics, vasodilators, and beta blockers (19,38). Overuse of alcohol is an underreported but common problem in the elderly. Although less likely to be a problem within the NH than in the community, alcohol is an occult cause of instability, falls, and serious injury. Other less common causes of falls include seizures, anemia, hypothyroidism, unstable joints, foot problems, and severe osteoporosis with spontaneous fracture.

RISK FACTORS FOR FALLS

Because a single specific cause for falling often cannot be identified and because falls are usually multifactorial in origin, many investigators have performed epidemiologic case-control studies to identify specific risk factors that place individuals at increased likelihood of falling. The idea underlying these studies is that by identifying risk factors early, preventive strategies can be devised and instituted. Table 8.4 lists the major fall risk factors identified from several institutional studies that compared fallers and nonfallers. Once again, these data are difficult to synthesize due to differences in study design, study populations, and data collection methods.

Of the 10 studies reviewed, 4 performed physical examinations on both fallers and nonfallers (57,55,47,29); the remaining studies relied on data abstracted from medical chart reviews. Comparison of fallers with nonfallers revealed that lower extremity weakness was a significant risk factor in four of these studies, increasing the odds of falling an average of fivefold (range 3.5 to 8.4). Gait and balance impairments were found to be a significant risk factor in three studies, associated with about a threefold increased risk of falling (range 2.4 to 5.4), as was visual impairment (range 3.3 to 4.5). Postural hypotension was found to be a significant risk factor in one study (57), but only had borderline significance in another (47). Similar findings were reported for the relationship between cognitive impairment and falls, but this risk factor also had an association with injurious falls (range 5.2 to 7.4) (56).

Functional impairment has also been shown to be a significant risk factor for falls. Using an assistive device increased the risk of falling about threefold (range 2.0 to 4.6). Inability to perform basic activities of daily living (ADL), and self-reported limitations in mobility were associated with a three- and fivefold increased risk of falling, respectively.

Several other case-control studies have looked at the association between falls and medication use. In one study, patients taking four or more prescription medications had a significantly greater risk of falling (47). Specific classes of medications found to increase the risk of falling in NH patients include: psychotropic drugs (19,38), sedatives (19,27,52), cardiac drugs (19,38,27,58), and nonsteroidal antiinflammatory drugs (38).

The relationship between medical diagnoses and falls has been repeatedly studied, but this association is fairly weak. In two studies, fallers had a significantly greater number of established medical

Table 8.4 Risk Factors for Falls or Fall-Related Injuries Identified in Case-Control Studies

Reference Year Published Number of Subjects Study Design[a] Endpoint (Fall vs. Injury)	Wells et al. 1985 N=77 Retro Fall	Tinetti et al. 1986 N=79 Prosp Fall	Granek et al. 1987 N=368 Retro Fall	Tinetti 1987 N=79 Prosp Injury	Robbins et al. 1989 N=149 Retro Fall	Kerman & Mulvihill 1990 N=147 Retro Fall	Lipsitz et al. 1991 N=126 Retro Fall	Myers et al. 1991 N=178 Retro Fall/Injury	Svensson et al. 1991 N=588 Retro Injury	Tinetti et al. 1992 N=397 Prosp Injury
Physical Examination										
Muscle weakness	—	5.4	—	3.5	8.4*	—	4.9	—	—	—
Gait impairment	—	2.4	—	NS	+	—	4.8	—	—	—
Balance impairment	—	5.4	—	NS	+*	—	3.9	+	+*	—
Postural hypotension	—	3.4	—	NS	‡	—	NS	—	NS	—
Cognitive impairment	—	2.0†	—	NS	‡	—	—	—	—	5.2-7.4
Visual impairment	—	3.5	—	NS	NS	—	NS	4.5*	NS	3.3
Functional Level										
Impaired ADL	—	3.1	—	§	+	—	—	—	+	NS
Use assistive device	—	4.6	—	NS	2.0	—	—	NS	+	NS
Mobility limitation	—	5.3	—	NS	NS	—	—	—	+	NS
Drugs										
Number of drugs	+	—	+	—	+*	+	—	—	+*	—
Sedative/Hypnotic	NS	3.2	2.6	NS	NS	1.5	NS	36.6*	+	NS
NSAID	NS	—	2.4	—	NS	NS	NS	15.8*	NS	—
Vasodilators	NS	—	2.1	—	NS	NS	NS	5.0*	NS	—
Major tranquilizers	NS	—	1.8‡	—	NS	NS	NS	NS	+	—

Diagnosis								
Antidepressants	NS	†	NS	5.7*	NS	2.6	—	NS
Analgesic	NS	NS	NS	2.7	NS	—	—	—
Antihypertensives	†	NS	NS	NS	NS	NS	—	—
Cardiac	NS	NS	NS	NS	2.5	NS	—	—
Arthritis	NS	NS	NS	—	NS	2.3	NS	—
Incontinence	NS	NS	—	12.4*	—	—	NS	—
Depression	NS	NS	NS	—	NS	2.3	§	NS
Parkinson's	NS	†	NS	—	NS	NS	NS	†*
Dizziness	NS	†*	—	—	NS	—	NS	—

NOTES: a. Numbers indicate relative risks for prospective studies (Prosp) and odds ratios for retrospective studies (Retro).
†=Significant risk factor (p<.05), odds ratio not reported.
*=Risk factor confirmed in multivariate analysis.
‡=Risk factor of borderline significance (.1>p>.05).
§=Risk factor is negatively correlated with falls.
NS=Risk factor is not significant (p>.1).

diagnoses than the nonfaller comparison patients (47,58). Certain medical diagnoses that have been identified as a significant risk factor for falls in NHs include arthritis (19,38), incontinence (47), and depression (19). Interestingly, depression was negatively correlated with injurious falls in one study (56).

Other case-control studies have examined the relationship between single risk factors and falls. For example, Whipple et al. (1987) examined knee and ankle strength, and reported that weakness at both joints was found to be significantly more common among institutionalized fallers than nonfallers. They also performed gait analysis of 49 NH patients and found that fallers had significantly slower gait speed and shorter stride length than nonfallers (61).

Perhaps as important as identifying individual risk factors is appreciating the interaction and probable synergism between multiple risk factors. Several studies have shown that the risk of falling increases dramatically as the number of risk factors increases (57,47,38). In their survey of patients residing in three intermediate care facilities, Tinetti et al. (1986) reported that the percentage of patients who fell rose from 0% for patients with less than four risk factors, to 31% for those with four to six risk factors, and to 100% for patients with more than six risk factors. (Risk factors included mobility score, vision, hearing, mental status, morale, orthostatic blood pressure, medications, functional status.) Myers et al. (1991) estimated the relative odds of falling for NH patients with various combinations of risk factors identified from logistic regression. In this study, the relative odds of falling were 15 times greater for patients who were ambulatory and were taking sedative or hypnotic medications, and 18 times greater for patients with a history of falls and visual impairment.

In a study by Robbins et al. (1989) involving both an institutionalized and outpatient population, many individual risk factors were significantly correlated with falls. Multivariate analysis enabled simplification of the model to the point that maximum predictive accuracy for falls could be obtained by use of only three risk factors in a branching logic, algorithmic fashion. Using this model (Figure 8.1), the predicted 1-year risk of falling ranged from 12% for persons with none of the three risk factors to 100% for persons with all three risk factors (i.e., hip weakness assessed manually, unstable balance, and taking four or more prescribed medications).

As even among frail elderly patients the majority of falls do not result in serious injury, several research groups have attempted to identify those risk factors specifically associated with injurious falls, rather than falls per se. Among ambulatory intermediate care resi-

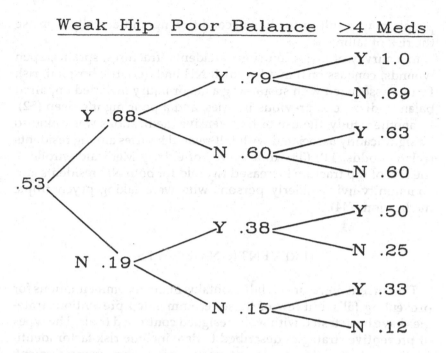

Figure 8.1. Algorithm Predicting the Likelihood of Falling in a 1-Year Period Based on Presence or Absence of Three Major Risk Factors Derived From Multivariate Analysis

SOURCE: Robbins et al. (1989).
NOTE: Risk factors include: hip weakness (weak hip), low balance score (poor balance), taking more than four medications (>4 medications). Y indicates yes; N, no. Numbers at right indicate proportion of patients who fell.

dents who fell, Tinetti (1987) found that the risk of sustaining an injury was greatest for functionally independent, nondepressed patients with lower extremity weakness. In another study conducted in 12 NHs, Tinetti et al. (1992) found that female gender, poor vision and hearing, disorientation, number of falls, and use of mechanical restraints were independently associated with both falls and fall-related injuries. A particularly noteworthy finding was that the risk of a fall-related injury was 10 times greater for patients who had been restrained at some time during the 1-year study period than for those who had not been restrained. Both falls and serious injuries significantly increased as restraint use increased. This observation challenges the assumption that restraints provide protection from falls. The authors suggest that intermittent use of restraints in frail older people may result in further deconditioning and actually increase the risk of falling.

In a survey of major injurious accidents (fractures, sprains, open wounds, concussions) in a Swedish NH and geriatric hospital, risk factors associated with sustaining a major injury included impaired balance, dizziness, previous injuries, and a poor night's sleep (52). In another study, the use of hypotensive medications was found to be significantly associated with fall-related injuries among residents (relative odds, 4.0) (38). In a survey of elderly Medicaid enrollees, the risk of hip fracture increased twofold for both NH residents and community-living elderly persons who were taking psychotropic medications (44).

PREVENTION OF FALLS

The current literature on falls contains many recommendations for preventing falls, but few of these recommended prevention strategies have been tested with well-designed controlled trials. The types of preventive strategies described to date include risk factor identification and referral for treatment, postfall comprehensive assessment, exercise programs for high-risk persons, environmental assessment, nursing interventions, alarm systems, and protective devices.

Based upon the evidence summarized in the previous section that patients at high risk of falling can be easily identified, the inclusion of a fall risk assessment into the periodic physical examination has been frequently recommended for geriatric patients, especially for frail subpopulations (57,47). To identify the most important risk factors, it has been suggested that this screening assessment include at least several specific items: postural blood pressure measurement, visual acuity testing, manual muscle testing of the lower extremities, balance and gait evaluation, functional and mental status evaluations, and a review of medications and dosing. Despite its logic and appeal, the efficacy of screening NH patients for fall risk factors on admission or periodically as a fall prevention strategy remains to be tested.

Evaluation of patients after a fall by a special fall consultation team is another prevention strategy being developed in institutional and outpatient settings, but again, few evaluative data are available. The purpose of the postfall assessment is to prevent recurrent falls by identifying the direct or contributing causes of a patient's recent fall that may be amenable to medical therapy or other corrective inter-

Table 8.5   Primary and Secondary Causes for Falls in a Long-Term Care
Institution (N=77)

Cause	Primary	Secondary	Total
Weakness	35%	31%	66%
Environmental hazard	27%	5%	32%
Orthostatic hypotension	16%	26%	42%
Drug effect	5%	17%	22%
Acute illness	5%	10%	15%
Gait/balance disorder	4%	49%	53%
Poor vision	3%	33%	36%
Neuropathy	—	21%	21%
Cognitive impairment	—	8%	8%
Arrhythmia	—	7%	7%
Urinary tract infection	—	7%	7%
Other*	—	20%	20%
Unknown	5%	—	—
	100%		

SOURCE: Adapted from Rubenstein et al. (1990).
* NOTE: "Other" included weight loss, positive stool guaiac test for occult blood, impaired vision
and hearing, incontinence, and vertigo. There was a mean of 3.3 contributory causes per fall.

vention. A descriptive study published by a multidisciplinary falls
consultation team in a NH provides preliminary evidence that a
postfall assessment uncovers new diagnoses and leads to a reduction
in future falls (40).

Recently, a randomized trial of a postfall assessment intervention
was published (48). In this study, 160 NH patients who had fallen
were randomly assigned within 7 days of a fall to receive either a
comprehensive postfall assessment (N = 79) or usual care (N = 81).
The postfall assessment performed by a nurse practitioner included
a detailed physical examination, environmental assessment, and
referrals for specific treatment and preventive interventions. The
probable primary causes of the fall as well as multiple secondary risk
factors were identified for each intervention subject (Table 8.5). Many
remediable problems (e.g., weakness, environmental hazards, orthostatic hypotension, drug side effects, gait dysfunction) were detected. At the end of a 2-year follow-up period, there were trends for
intervention subjects to have lower fall and mortality rates (9% fewer
falls and 17% fewer deaths), but these did not reach statistical significance. Strikingly, the intervention group did experience significant reductions in hospitalizations (26%) and hospital days (52%)
compared to controls (Figure 8.2). This study strongly suggests that

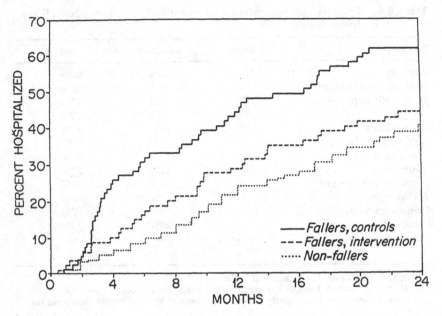

Figure 8.2. Proportion of Nursing Home Patients Hospitalized During the 2 Years After Randomization: Comparison of Fallers Receiving the Intervention (*N*=79), Fallers in the Control Group (*N*=81), and Ambulatory Nursing Home Residents Who Did Not Fall During the Entire Study Period (*N*=309)
SOURCE: Adapted from Rubenstein et al. (1990).

falls are markers of underlying disorders easily identifiable by a careful postfall assessment, which in turn can be treated with reduction in disability.

Intervention programs to ameliorate single specific fall risk factors (e.g., weakness, gait and balance impairments) as a means of preventing falls have been increasingly established and described. These interventions are quite varied in content and include exercise programs, educational programs to improve medication prescribing, and environmental assessment programs. Although some of these interventions are currently being studied for their effectiveness in reducing falls, no results specific to falls have been published as yet. The expectation that these types of intervention programs will be successful in preventing falls is based upon data from published studies with similar designs that have shown that the specific risk factors can be reversed or improved (e.g., muscle weakness, instability, polypharmacy).

Results of exercise interventions to improve muscle strength, gait, and balance have only recently been attempted in chronically ill or institutionalized populations. Although the results from these studies have been encouraging, the effect on fall rates has not been documented. In a descriptive study of community-living veterans with chronic illness (35), subjects who attended a 16-week exercise program showed significant improvement in cardiovascular fitness, hip flexibility, and abdominal strength. A randomized trial of an exercise program for community-living older adults with chronic illness and functional limitations showed greater improvement in treadmill performance, balance, and strength among the exercise group, although these differences did not reach statistical significance (54). A recent study of frail NH residents with a mean age of 90 years also reported remarkable increases in muscle strength following an 8-week high-intensity weight-training program (16). The 10 subjects averaged a 174% increase in knee extensor strength, a 9% increase in midthigh muscle area, and a 48% increase in mean tandem gait speed. In addition, two subjects stopped using a cane during ambulation. Currently, several exercise interventions supported by the National Institutes of Health (NIH) are in progress in NH settings and will provide data on the effect of exercise on fall rates and functional status.

Numerous interventions to improve prescribing practices and reduce the incidence of polypharmacy in NHs have been conducted (22) (see also Chapter 2). In the majority of these studies, the intervention has consisted of a consultant pharmacist reviewing medication orders and providing recommendations to physicians and nurses. Positive outcomes demonstrated by these interventions include reductions in number of drugs prescribed per patient (25,53) and the number of doses taken per patient (62).

Environmental assessment has been another promising fall prevention strategy, both as a means of identifying and removing potential hazards (e.g., clutter, poor lighting, throw rugs) and for modifying the environment to improve mobility and safety (e.g., installation of grab bars, raised toilet seats, lowered bed height). Although there are no published studies that prove the value of environmental assessment and modification, several are under way and should produce data soon.

Nursing interventions are probably the most widely used fall prevention strategy in institutional settings. Fortunately, there has been a move away from the "traditional" nursing intervention of physical restraints, as recent research has shown that the adverse affects of physical restraints on functional status and quality of life are in many cases worse than the potential risk of falls (11,13,30,34), and restraints may even be a risk factor for falling (56). The primary intent of most current nursing interventions is to identify patients at admission who are at high risk for falling and to institute appropriate precautions. To assist in the identification of such high-risk patients, fall assessment tools have been developed and described in the literature (4,49,63). Using these tools, the nursing staff assesses such patient factors as mental status, history of falls, ambulation status, medications, physical status, continence, and sensory deficits. A patient's fall risk status is determined by either the number of risk factors present or by a summary score (4,49). Once a patient has been identified as being at high risk for falling, a nursing care plan is usually developed that includes interventions aimed at injury prevention. Such interventions include indicating on the medical chart and the patient's door that the patient is at high risk for falls; moving high-risk patients to rooms that are close to the nursing station to increase observation; periodic reassessment of patients following new episodes of illness or change in medication; lowering bed rails and bed height for patients who climb out of bed; increasing nurse-to-patient ratio; and fall prevention education for patients and staff.

Few data have been published to support the validity of assessment tools or the effectiveness of these types of prevention programs. However, one recent study (49) reported high reliability and validity of a scored fall assessment tool developed to identify hospitalized patients at high risk of falling. Implementation of this tool, along with standardized nursing care plans for high-risk patients and installation of new safety equipment (safety vests, bed alarm system), resulted in an average 20% decrease in falls over the first year of the program.

Technologic devices that alert caregivers to patient movement or protect patients from fall injuries are also currently being developed and marketed. The most widely available devices are various alarm systems that are activated when patients try to get out of bed or ambulate unassisted. These devices are a possible alternative to restraints for many high-risk patients. One such alarm system (Ambularm®) was pilot-tested on an orthopedic and a general medicine hospital ward. Preliminary 5-month data indicated that patient falls were reduced 33% and 45%, respectively (60). An infrared scanning system that activates an alarm in the nursing station when a patient sits up or gets out of bed was found to reduce the incidence of nighttime falls from 2.8 to 1.0 falls per month when installed on a psychogeriatric unit (12). Video recording systems are also being used as a means of providing closer monitoring of patient activities. Injury-prevention alternatives, such as ceiling-mounted inertia-reel safety harnesses and hip protective pads (64), are also currently being tested but are not generally available.

One consideration complicating formulation of fall prevention strategies is the two-edged effect of physical activity on falls. Activity is, and should be, encouraged as a positive goal leading to higher function and quality of life, but activity also facilitates the opportunity for falling. Although not well studied, active individuals may have more falls overall but may also have fewer falls per unit of activity. Moreover, active individuals tend to have less serious fall complications. This interaction between falls, activity levels, frailty, and injury needs to be studied much more carefully.

FUTURE RESEARCH

The current research on falls in the NH strongly supports the complex multifactorial etiology of falls and the notion that the presence of certain risk factors substantially increases the risk of falls and fall-related injuries. However, few if any data exist to demonstrate whether risk factors so identified can be effectively reversed in such a way as to reduce subsequent risk of falling without jeopardizing independence and quality of life. It is toward this goal that future research should be directed. Currently, the National Institutes of Health are sponsoring eight intervention studies designed to reduce the loss of functional capacities and to prevent fall-related injuries (FICSIT). Three of these studies are being conducted in NH settings. These FICSIT studies are collecting common data on falls and injuries, demographics, cognition, quality of life, and physical functioning. Although no results are currently available from these trials, the accumulation of these data will undoubtedly advance our understanding of falls.

Priorities for future research on falls have been outlined in a report to the Institute of Medicine (41). Specific research strategies relevant to institutionalized populations that have been given high priority include randomized fall prevention trials, prospective studies focusing on the interrelationship between falls and risk factors, and studies that address specific methodological issues. Suggested research studies within each category are outlined in Table 8.6.

In conclusion, our understanding of the mechanisms and impacts of falls among elderly people living in NHs continues to improve. It

Table 8.6   Priorities for Future Research on Falls

Randomized Intervention Trials
  Multiple risk factor reduction programs
  Exercise and rehabilitation programs for improving strength, balance, and gait
  Diagnosis/treatment strategies for neurologic, musculoskeletal, and sensory
    disorders
  Strategies to improve use of hypnotic-anxiolytic drugs
  Alternatives to restraints
  Educational programs for staff

Prospective Natural History Studies
  Determining the interrelationship between falls, physical and environmental risk
    factors, and situational factors
  Reassessing risk factors at regular intervals
  Identifying risk factors for the subgroup of falls causing injury
  Identifying contributing risk factors in high-risk subgroups (i.e., patients with
    dementia or neurologic disorders)
  Determining the psychological and functional effects of falls
  Determining the effects of falls on staff attitudes and patient care practices

Studies of Methodological Issues
  Assessing reliability of fall surveillance methods (e.g., incident reporting,
    accelerometers, video systems)
  Developing accurate quantification of physical activity to account for the
    interaction between fall risk and activity
  Developing standard classification methods for describing causes and
    consequences of falls
  Developing methods to quantify the economic costs of falls in nursing homes

---

SOURCE: Adapted from Nevitt (1990).

is apparent that a large proportion of falls are probably preventable with careful medical and environmental evaluation and intervention. Although further research is still warranted, there is substantial evidence to indicate that a vigorous diagnostic, therapeutic, and preventive approach is appropriate in all older patients who fall, as well as in those simply at high risk of falling. Many promising interventions are currently being tested, and results are eagerly awaited.

REFERENCES

1. Ashley, M. J., Gryfe, C. I., & Amies, A. (1977). A longitudinal study of falls in an elderly population: 2. Some circumstances of falling. *Age and Ageing, 6,* 211-220.
2. Baker, S. P., & Harvey, A. H. (1985). Falls injuries in the elderly. *Clinics in Geriatric Medicine, 1,* 501-507.

3. Berry, G., Fisher, R. H., & Lang, S. (1981). Detrimental incidents, including falls, in an elderly institutional population. *Journal of the American Geriatrics Society, 29,* 322-324.
4. Berryman, E., Gaskin, D., Jones, A., et al. (1989, July/August). Point by point: Predicting elders' falls. *Geriatric Nursing,* pp. 199-201.
5. Blake, C., & Morfitt, J. M. (1986). Falls and staffing in a residential home for elderly people. *Public Health, 100,* 385-391.
6. Brocklehurst, J. C., Exton-Smith, A. N., Lempert-Barber, S. M., et al. (1978). Fractures of the femur in old age: A two-center study of associated clinical factors and the cause of the fall. *Age and Ageing, 7,* 2-15.
7. Cacha, C. A. (1979). An analysis of the 1976 incident reports of the Carillon nursing home. *American Health Care Association Journal, 5,* 29-33.
8. Campbell, A. J., Borrie, M. J., & Spears, G. F. (1989). Risk factors for falls in a community-based prospective study of people 70 years and older. *Journal of Gerontology, 44,* M112-117.
9. Clark, A.N.G. (1968). Factors in fracture of the female femur: A clinical study of the environmental, physical, medical and preventive aspects of this injury. *Gerontologia Clinica, 10,* 257-270.
10. Colling, J., & Park, D. (1983). Home, safe home. *Journal of Gerontological Nursing, 9,* 175-192.
11. Dimant, J. (1985). Accidents in the skilled nursing facility. *New York State Journal of Medicine, 85,* 202-205.
12. Dubner, N. P., & Creech, R. (1988). Using infrared scanning to decrease nighttime falls on a psychogeriatric unit. *Hospital and Community Psychiatry, 39,* 79-81.
13. Evans, L. K., Strumpf, N. E., & Williams, C. (1991). Redefining a standard of care for frail older people: Alternatives to routine physical restraint. In P. R. Katz, R. L. Kane, & M. D. Mezey (Eds.), *Advances in long-term care* (Vol. 1, pp. 81-101). New York: Springer.
14. Exton-Smith, A. N. (1977). Functional consequences of aging: Clinical manifestations. In A. N. Exton-Smith & J. Grimley Evans (Eds.), *Meeting the challenge of dependency* (pp.41-57). London: Academic Press.
15. Feist, R. R. (1978). A survey of accidental falls in a small home for the aged. *Journal of Gerontological Nursing, 4,* 15-17.
16. Fiatarone, M. A., Marks, E. C., Ryan, N. D., et al. (1990). High-intensity strength training in nonagenarians. *Journal of the American Medical Association, 263,* 3029-3034.
17. Foerster, J. (1981). A study of falls: The elderly nursing home resident. *Journal of the New York State Nursing Association, 12,* 9-17.
18. Gostynski, M. (1991). Häufigkeit, Umstände und Konsequenzen von Sturzen institutionalisierter Betagter: Eine Pilotstudie. *Soz Praventivmed, 36,* 341-345.
19. Granek, E., Baker, S. P., Abbey, H., et al. (1987). Medications and diagnoses in relation to falls in a long-term care facility. *Journal of the American Geriatrics Society, 35,* 503-511.
20. Gross, Y. T., Shimamoto, Y., Rose, C. L., et al. (1990). Monitoring risk factors in nursing homes. *Journal of Gerontological Nursing, 16,* 20-25.
21. Gryfe, C. I., Amies, A., & Ashley, M. J. (1977). A longitudinal study of falls in an elderly population: 1. Incidence and morbidity. *Age and Ageing, 6,* 201-210.
22. Gurwitz, J. H., Soumerai, S. B., & Avorn, J. (1990). Improving medication prescribing and utilization in the nursing home. *Journal of the American Geriatrics Society, 38,* 542-552.

23. Haga, H. Shibata, H., Shichita, K., et al. (1986). Falls in the institutionalized elderly in Japan. *Archives of Gerontology and Geriatrics, 5*, 1-9.
24. Hogue, C. C. (1982). Injury in late life: 1. Epidemiology; 2. Prevention. *Journal of the American Geriatrics Society, 30*, 183-190.
25. Hood, J. C., Lemberger, M., & Stewart, R. B. (1975). Promoting appropriate therapy in a long-term care facility. *Journal of the American Pharmacy Association, 15*, 32.
26. Jónsson, P. V., Lipsitz, L. A., Kelley, M., et al. (1990). Hypotensive responses to common daily activities in institutionalized elderly: A potential risk for recurrent falls. *Archives of Internal Medicine, 150*, 1518-1524.
27. Kerman, M., & Mulvihill, M. (1990). The role of medication in falls among the elderly in a long-term care facility. *Mount Sinai Journal of Medicine, 57*, 343-347.
28. Lipsitz, L. A., & Fullerton, K. J. (1986). Postprandial blood pressure reduction in healthy elderly. *Journal of the American Geriatrics Society, 34*, 267-270.
29. Lipsitz, L. A., Jónsson, P. V., Kelley, M. M., et al. (1991). Causes and correlates of recurrent falls in ambulatory frail elderly. *Journal of Gerontology, 46*, M114-122.
30. Lofgren, R. P., MacPherson, D. S., Granieri, R., et al. (1989). Mechanical restraints on the medical wards: Are protective devices safe? *American Journal of Public Health, 79*, 735-738.
31. Louis, M. (1983). Falls and their causes. *Journal of Gerontological Nursing, 9*, 142-156.
32. Lucht, U. (1971). A prospective study of accidental falls and injuries at home among elderly people. *Acta Socio-Medica Scandinavica, 2*, 105-120.
33. Mader, S. L., Josephson, K. R., & Rubenstein, L. Z. (1987). Low prevalence of postural hypotension among community-dwelling elderly. *Journal of the American Medical Association, 258*, 1511-1514.
34. Miller, M. B., & Elliott, D. F. (1979). Accidents in nursing homes: Implications for patients and administrators. *In M. B. Miller (Ed.), Current issues in clinical geriatrics* (pp. 97-137). New York: Tiresias.
35. Morey, M. C., Cowper, P. A., Feussner, J. R., et al. (1989). Evaluation of a supervised exercise program in a geriatric population. *Journal of the American Geriatrics Society, 37*, 348-354.
36. Morfitt, J. M. (1980). Residential homes for the elderly—which are the safest? *Public Health, London, 94*, 223-228.
37. Morfitt, J. M. (1983). Falls in old people at home: Intrinsic versus environmental factors in causation. *Public Health, 97*, 115-120.
38. Myers, A. H., Baker, S. P., Van Natt, M. L., et al. (1991). Risk factors associated with falls and injuries among elderly institutionalized persons. *American Journal of Epidemiology, 133*, 1179-1190.
39. National Center for Health Statistics, Hing, E., Sekscenski, E., & Strahan, G. (1989). *The National Nursing Home Survey: 1985 summary for the United States. Vital and health statistics* (Series 13, No. 97. DHHS Pub. No. [PHS] 89-1758. Public Health Service). Washington, DC: U.S. Government Printing Office.
40. Neufeld, R. R., Tideiksaar, R., Yew, E., et al. (1991). A multidisciplinary falls consultation service in a nursing home. *Gerontologist, 31*, 120-123.
41. Nevitt, M. C. (1990). Falls in older persons: Risk factors and prevention. In R. L. Berg & J. F. Cassells (Eds.), *The second fifty years: The promotion and prevention of disease* (pp. 263-290). Institute of Medicine Division of Health Promotion and Disease Prevention. Washington, DC: National Academy Press.
42. Pablo, R. Y. (1977). Patient accidents in a long-term-care facility. *Canadian Journal of Public Health, 68*, 237-246.

43. Pawlson, L. G., Goodwin, M., & Keith, K. (1986). Wheelchair use by ambulatory nursing home residents. *Journal of the American Geriatrics Society, 34,* 860-864.

44. Ray, W. A., Griffin, M. R., & Schaffner, W. (1987). Psychotropic drug use and the risk of hip fracture. *New England Journal of Medicine, 316,* 363-369.

45. Rhymes, J., & Jaeger, R. (1988). Falls: Prevention and management in the institutional setting. *Clinics in Geriatric Medicine, 4,* 613-622.

46. Robbins, A. S., & Rubenstein, L. Z. (1984). Postural hypotension in the elderly. *Journal of the American Geriatrics Society, 32,* 769-774.

47. Robbins, A. S., Rubenstein, L. Z., Josephson, K. R., et al. (1989). Predictors of falls among elderly people: Results of two population-based studies. *Archives of Internal Medicine, 149,* 1628-1633.

48. Rubenstein, L. Z., Robbins, A. S., Josephson, K. R., et al. (1990). The value of assessing falls in an elderly population: A randomized clinical trial. *Annals of Internal Medicine, 113,* 308-316.

49. Schmid, N. A. (1990). Reducing patient falls: A research-based comprehensive fall prevention program. *Military Medicine, 155,* 202-207.

50. Sheldon, J. H. (1960). On the natural history of falls in old age. *British Medical Journal, 2,* 1685-1690.

51. Sudarsky, L. (1990). Geriatrics: Gait disorders in the elderly. *Current Concepts in Geriatrics, 322,* 1441-1446.

52. Svensson, M. L., Rundgren, A., Larsson, M., et al. (1991). Accidents in the institutionalized elderly: A risk analysis. *Aging, 3,* 181-192.

53. Thompson, J. F., McGhan, W. F., Ruffalo, R. L., et al. (1984). Clinical pharmacists prescribing drug therapy in a geriatric setting: Outcome of a trial. *Journal of the American Geriatrics Society, 32,* 154-159.

54. Thompson, R. F., Crist, D. M., Marsh, M., et al. (1988). Effects of physical exercise for elderly patients with physical impairments. *Journal of the American Geriatrics Society, 36,* 130-135.

55. Tinetti, M. E. (1987). Factors associated with serious injury during falls by ambulatory nursing home residents. *Journal of the American Geriatrics Society, 35,* 644-648.

56. Tinetti, M. E., Liu, W. L., & Ginter, S. F. (1992). Mechanical restraint use and fall-related injuries among residents of skilled nursing facilities. *Annals of Internal Medicine, 116,* 369-374.

57. Tinetti, M. E., Williams, T. F., & Mayewski, R. (1986). Fall risk index for elderly patients based on number of chronic disabilities. *American Journal of Medicine, 80,* 429-434.

58. Wells, B. G., Middleton, B., Lawrence, G., et al. (1985). Factors associated with the elderly falling in intermediate care facilities. *Drug Intelligence and Clinical Pharmacy, 19,* 142-145.

59. Whipple, R. H., Wolfson, L. I., & Amerman, P. M. (1987). The relationship of knee and ankle weakness to falls in nursing home residents: An isokinetic study. *Journal of the American Geriatrics Society, 35,* 13-20.

60. Widder, B. (1985, September/October). A new device to decrease falls. *Geriatric Nursing,* p. 287.

61. Wolfson, L., Whipple, R., Amerman, P., et al. (1990). Gait assessment in the elderly: A gait abnormality rating scale and its relation to falls. *Journal of Gerontology, 45,* M12-19.

62. Young, L. Y., Leach, D. B., Anderson, D. A., et al. (1981). Decreased medication costs in a skilled nursing facility by clinical pharmacy services. *Contemporary Pharmacy Practice, 4,* 233-237.

63. Young, S. W., Abedzadeh, C. B., & White, M. W. (1989, November). A fall-prevention program for nursing homes. *Nursing Management*, pp. 80Y-80FF.

64. Zylke, J. W. (1990). Research focuses not only on where, why, how of falls, but also on preventing them. *Journal of the American Medical Association, 263*, 2022-2023.

9

The Assessment and Control of Pain in the Nursing Home

BRUCE A. FERRELL, M.D.

INTRODUCTION

That the proper assessment and management of pain is an important problem among elderly people is only recently acknowledged in the medical literature (1,8,12,20). In the past, pain research has been essentially limited to younger patients, patients in acute care settings, and patients with cancer. Pain assessment and management remain understudied in the nursing home (NH) population. Thus, strategies for pain control among elderly NH residents remain based largely on anecdotal experiences rather than on empirically derived data (1,8). Because elderly people are at such great risk for chronic and often painful illnesses, it is unfortunate and ironic that pain is so often underrecognized and undetected in the geriatric population.

Pain should be an important concern in NH care. It is the most common symptom of disease and the symptom most likely to lead to accurate diagnosis and effective treatment of the underlying processes (18). Pain is also associated with increased dependency, health care utilization, and cost (16). Most important, pain and its management have major implications for quality of care and quality of life among NH residents (10).

Effective pain management may present unique problems in the NH setting. Multiple sources for pain and the high prevalence of cognitive impairment make pain assessment problematic in this population (9). Elderly patients are more sensitive to side effects of analgesic drugs, and polypharmacy can be a substantial problem. Control policies, such as triplicate prescription requirements and

access to effective nonpharmacologic techniques, may represent significant barriers to pain management (32). Solutions to these problems are
not obvious from the present medical literature and pose substantial
challenges to clinicians and researchers in the NH setting.

EPIDEMIOLOGIC DATA

Pain is a common complaint among elderly people, especially
those in long-term care facilities. The overall prevalence of chronic
pain complaints has been difficult to describe, even among the
general population. The Nuprin® Pain Report was a nationwide
cross-sectional survey of the adult U.S. population, conducted by the
Harris organization in the early 1980s. This telephone survey que-
ried subjects about pain during the previous year. Findings suggested that prevalence rates for pain lasting more than 3 months
were 5% for headache, 9% for backache, 5% for muscle pain and 10%
for joint pain. Although no total prevalence rate was reported, the
morbidity decreased with age in each of these categories except joint
pain (30). In a postal survey, Von Korff et al. (1988) studied a random
sample of 1,500 enrollees of a group health cooperative aged 15-75.
Subjects were asked to report pain problems that had lasted more
that 1 day or had occurred several times in a year. The prevalence
rates for pain condition in the previous 6 months were: headache
26%, backache 41%, abdominal pain 17%, facial pain 12%, and chest
pain 12%. No age-associated analysis was reported (31). A county
postal survey in Sweden surveyed a random sample of 1,009 subjects
aged 18-84. Although the authors admitted the 80-84 age group was
less likely to respond to the postal survey, with telephone follow-up
they achieved an 82% response rate. This study measured pain
intensity and pain distress by querying patients about pain that
might occur in 10 common locations. "Obvious pain" complaints
were defined by both pain intensity and distress reports greater than
3 on 6-point ordinal scales. Results suggested that 43.9% of subjects
had "obvious pain" for 1-6 months duration and 39.9% for over 6
months' duration. Ten to twenty percent reported pain of musculoskeletal origin; 8%, facial; and 4%, chest or abdominal. Pain was
more common in the middle age group (45-64 years; $p < 60.001$) and
not apparently related to sex, marital status, living arrangements, or
employment. This study also described several ADL limitations reported by respondents. Difficulty in dressing was reported by 6.4%;
walking up and down stairs, 12%; dancing or running, 25%. The

prevalence of ADL impairment was no higher among the elderly group than younger groups (4). Finally, a community-based survey in Burlington, Ontario, of 500 randomly selected households, conducted interviews with over 800 subjects. In this study the age-associated morbidity for pain was doubled (250 per thousand vs. 125 per thousand) among those over age 60, compared to those less than 60. Subjects were asked to focus on pain that had occurred in the last 2 weeks and required either taking medications or contacting a health care provider (6).

In long-term care facilities, the prevalence of pain is even higher and may approach 70%-80% of institutionalized elderly (10,15,27). Previous national NH surveys in the United States have not addressed pain as a problem, and our understanding of pain in NHs remains based on only three small epidemiologic studies in the British literature. Table 9.1 presents these studies and illustrates some of the difficulties facing future epidemiologic research in the NH.

First, the definition of pain remains poorly standardized. The language of questionnaires can have a dramatic effect on identifying which patients have significant pain (sensitivity of the instrument). The high prevalence of visual, hearing, and motor impairments may impede use of instruments established in younger populations. Cognitive impairment, delirium (common among acutely ill elderly), and dementia (occurring in as many as 50% of institutionalized elderly) represent serious barriers to pain assessment for which no solution exists in the literature. In contrast, a variety of techniques have been published for the assessment of pain among cognitively undeveloped children (1). Extrapolation from pediatric scales as well as traditional approaches to pain assessment, including the use of visual analog scales, verbal descriptor scales, and numerical scales, have not been psychometrically tested in the elderly population.

Sampling remains a serious problem. Given the heterogeneity of NHs and residents, subjects from a single NH probably do not represent the entire NH population. Because of the problems mentioned above with assessment, subjects with significant cognitive impairment have usually been systematically excluded from studies. Finally, sample sizes need to be large enough to detect the true heterogeneity of sources and description in this population.

Previous studies have relied strongly on medical records and patient recall for information about etiology of pain, functional correlates, and current treatments. This has continued despite the notorious inaccuracy of NH medical records and the tendency to attribute pain to previously existing conditions. An example of the

Table 9.1 Epidemiologic Studies of Pain Among Nursing Home Residents

	Ferrell et al., 1990	Lau-Ting & Phoon, 1988	Roy & Thomas, 1986
Sample and Selection	N=103, all residents of 3 selected wards from a single 311-bed facility	N=630, all residents from 5 nongovernment NHs	N=100, selected from a single 400-bed facility; criteria included: age≥65, ambulatory, oriented to time and place, no cancer, not receiving psychiatric therapy, not suffering debilitating diseases
Exclusions	4% refused 2% unavailable 5% severe dementia	14% extreme ill health, hospitalization, or communication barriers; 24% incomplete data	3% refused
Age	Mean=88.4 years	28% ≥80 years	34%≥80 years
Sex	83% females	52.3% females	62% females
Definition of Pain	Pain of any cause, at least "some of the time"	"Do you have arthritic aches and pains often?"	"Current pain-related problem"
Prevalence of Pain	71%	49%	83%
Functional Correlates	77% reported pain interference in daily activities; weak correlation between pain and Katz ADL score (r<.10)	Not reported	74% reported pain interference with daily living; function not quantitated

244

Psychologic Correlates	Weak correlation between pain and GDS score (r<.20)	Not reported	Not reported
Cognitive Correlates	Weak correlation between pain and FMMSE score (r<.10)	Not reported	Not reported
Causes of Pain	Low back 40% Peripheral arthritis 31% Previous fractures 14% Neuropathies 11% Leg cramps 9% Claudication 8% Headache 6% Neoplasm 3%	Arthritis 100%	Back, joint, muscle 88% Headache 12%
Current Treatments	Drug therapy 84% Physical therapy 42% Heating pad 15%	Not reported	Drug therapy 84%

limited use of NH medical record review is the observation that physicians often routinely prescribe aspirin or acetaminophen and bowel preparations, regardless of a documented indication for their use.

Finally, previous studies have been cross-sectional, providing little insight into the overall outcomes of chronic pain or its natural history in this population. Future studies will have to attend to these important issues.

PSYCHOLOGY OF PAIN IN ELDERLY PEOPLE

Pain is a universal sensation, yet an individual experience (9). Moreover, pain is distressing at any age. The interaction between pain and emotion has been an important area of research for many years. The emotional component of pain perception has important implications for pain assessment as well as treatment outcomes. The multidisciplinary model of pain management, which remains the most effective strategy for chronic pain control, regards psychologic (affective) components of pain sensation as important as nociceptive components (22,29). Thus, attention to the emotional issues usually associated with chronic pain experiences should be underscored.

Psychologic issues in pain management are probably similar between younger and older patients (29). Barsky et al. (1991) have shown hypochondriasis to be no more common among elderly than younger individuals. Indeed, several authors have suggested that elderly people are often stoic about pain and its functional correlates (10,11). Middaugh et al. (1988) reported psychological profiles, dropouts, and treatment outcomes to be similar among selected older and younger patients from a multidisciplinary pain clinic. Sorkin et al. (1990) corroborated these findings, maintaining that for treatment purposes, similarities between younger and older chronic pain patients are more important than differences.

The association between chronic pain and depression has been well established empirically (13,23,26). Investigators have shown that chronic pain patients report more depression than do other individuals. This holds true whether or not patients are elderly and despite the presence or absence of a definable medical cause for the pain (23,19). Conversely, depressed persons of all ages have been shown to exhibit more pain complaints than nondepressed persons (7). The majority of these investigations examined patients with specific pain complaints such as low back pain or headaches as well as generalized pain complaints. However, few have explored other functional variables such as overall health, functional, and medical characteristics that may moderate the pain-depression relationship.

In an attempt to define these complex interactions, Parmelee et al. (1991) found a significant correlation between pain and depression among a general NH population, which remained robust when controlled for overall health and functional status. This study found these relationships strongest among subjects with localized pain complaints where a specific physiologic pain disorder might be attributable. No age- or sex-associated differences were noted in these relationships. The authors point out that these observations are similar to findings of depression among younger populations with chronic pain (23).

PAIN MANAGEMENT IN THE NURSING HOME

Analgesic drugs remain the most common strategy for pain management in NH settings (10). Despite the fact that pharmacologic pain management may entail special problems among elderly patients, few studies have been conducted to describe drug effects among elderly subjects in the NH. For the most part, information has been derived from younger populations and from those with cancer pain. Analgesic medications are considered in two broad categories: nonopiate and opiate drugs. Adjuvant analgesic drugs (medications without inherent analgesic properties, such as antidepressants, anticonvulsants, and tranquilizers) may also enhance overall pain management under certain circumstances. Although a review of individual drugs is beyond the scope of this chapter, several important generalizations should be considered.

Analgesic drugs vary widely with respect to analgesic activity and side effect profiles among elderly people. Analgesic drugs are safe and effective among elderly people when used appropriately (8). Elderly persons appear to be as sensitive (or more sensitive) to the analgesic properties of many drugs than younger patients. For example, short-term studies have shown elderly subjects to be particularly sensitive to the analgesic properties of opiate drugs (3,14). Elderly patients often experience increased peak pain relief and longer duration of action from many opiate drugs (3). This has been shown for postoperative pain as well as chronic cancer pain (14). At least one study has shown enhanced analgesia for elderly women even when morphine is given epidurally (25). These studies have documented altered pharmacokinetics of morphine in elderly people, which may account for these observations. Thus elderly patients may achieve pain relief from smaller doses of opiate drugs than required by younger patients.

Elderly people are also more likely to experience side effects from most pain medications. Although consultant pharmacists have been utilized to assure more appropriate analgesic prescribing in the NH, it remains to be shown whether this practice will have an effect in reducing adverse drug effects (17). Nonsteroidal antiinflammatory drugs (NSAIDs) can result in gastric side effects, renal impairment, and bleeding more often in elderly than younger subjects. Other NSAID side effects are also more common in elderly people, including headaches, confusion, and constipation. Although possibly related to pharmacokinetic and pharmacodynamic changes associated with aging, the reason for NSAID sensitivity among elderly patients remains to be fully explained (5).

For opiate analgesics, the risk for drowsiness, delirium, and respiratory depression remains a serious threat, especially among opiate-naive patients (persons not previously exposed to opiate drugs) (21). Tolerance does occur among elderly patients, with the side benefit of reducing drowsiness and respiratory depression with prolonged use. To what extent tolerance contributes to increased drug requirement remains debatable. It has been observed that tolerance to analgesics develops much more slowly than tolerance to other side effects; thus effective doses have been observed for many months. Previous studies reporting serious problems with analgesic tolerance among cancer patients have often been confounded by rapidly advancing disease associated with increased analgesic requirements (21).

Adjuvant analgesic drugs are medications without analgesic properties themselves, although they exhibit some efficacy for treating certain pain syndromes. For example, antidepressants are helpful in the management of underlying depression that may complicate pain management. Tricyclic antidepressants and anticonvulsants have been shown efficacious for some neuropathic pains such as chronic herpes zoster or diabetic neuropathy (24). Minor tranquilizers may be helpful in controlling anxiety and helping patients get a good night's sleep. Unfortunately, side effect profiles for these drugs are also greater among elderly patients (28). Additional research is needed to define the risks and benefits for many of these strategies in the NH setting.

CONCLUSION

Recently, attention has been shifting toward populations who are at particular risk of undermanagement of pain. The Agency for Health Care Policy and Research (1) acknowledged that elderly people have been systematically excluded from most previous pain research. As geriatric and gerontologic research becomes more focused on functional and quality of life outcomes, pain management will become a logical target for future intervention trials. Although the identification of a quantifiable biological marker for pain will remain the "Holy Grail" in pain research, valid and reliable proxy measures such as functional status, pain questionnaires, coping, and behavioral observations need to be investigated in this setting. Increased attention should be paid toward pain management strategies for arthritis and nonmalignant and nonterminal pain syndromes. New drugs with milder side effect profiles are urgently needed. Nonpharmacologic pain management strategies should certainly be explored. And finally, long-term outcomes of various pain management strategies need to be evaluated and compared in the NH population.

REFERENCES

1. Acute Pain Management Guideline Panel. (1992, February). *Acute pain management: Operative or medical procedures and trauma. Clinical guideline* (AHCPR Pub. No. 92-0032). Rockville, MD: Agency for Health Care policy and Research, Public Health Service, U.S. Department of Health and Human Services.
2. Barsky, A. J., Frank, C. B., & Cleary P. D. (1991). The relation between hypochondriasis and age. *American Journal of Psychiatry, 148*(7), 923-928.
3. Bellville, J. W., Forrest, W. H., Miller, E., et al. (1971). Influence of age on pain relief from analgesics: A study of postoperative pain. *Journal of the American Medical Association, 217*(13), 1835-1841.
4. Brattberg, G., Thorslund, M., & Wilkman, A. (1989). Prevalence of pain complaints in a general Population: The results of a postal survey in a county of Sweden. *Pain, 37,* 215-222.
5. Butt, J. H., Barthel, J. S., & Moore, R. A. (1988). Clinical spectrum of upper gastrointestinal effects of nonsteroidal anti-inflammatory drugs: Natural history, symptomatology and significance. *American Journal of Medicine, 84*(2A), 4-14.
6. Cook, J., Rideout, E., & Browne, G. (1989). The prevalence of pain complaints in a general population. *Pain, 18,* 299-314.
7. Dwarkin, S. R., Von Korff, M., & Le Resche, L. (1990). Multiple pain and psychiatric disturbance: An epidemiologic investigation. *Archives of General Psychiatry, 47,* 239-244.
8. Ferrell, B. A. (1991). Pain management in elderly people. *Journal of the American Geriatrics Society, 39,* 64-73.

9. Ferrell, B. A., & Ferrell, B. R. (1989). Assessment of chronic pain in the elderly. *Geriatric Medicine Today, 8*(5), 123-134.
10. Ferrell, B. A., Ferrell, B. R., & Osterweil, D. (1990). Pain in the nursing home. *Journal of the American Geriatrics Society, 38*(4), 409-414.
11. Foley, K. (1985). Treatment of cancer pain. *New England Journal of Medicine, 113,* 84-95.
12. From the NIH: Pain in the elderly: Patterns change with age. (1979). *Journal of the American Medical Association, 241,* 2191-2192.
13. Haley, W. E., Turner, J. A., & Romano, J. M. (1985). Depression in chronic pain patients: Relation to pain, activity and sex differences. *Pain, 23,* 337-343.
14. Kaiko, R. F., Wallenstein, S., Roger, A. G., et al. (1982). Narcotics in the elderly. *Medical Clinics of North America, 66*(5), 1079-1089.
15. Lau-Ting, C., & Phoon, W. O. (1988). Ache and pains among Singapore elderly. *Singapore Medical Journal, 29,* 164-167.
16. Lavanski-Shulan, M., Wallace, R. B., Khout, F. J., et al. (1985). Prevalence and functional correlates of low back pain in the elderly: The Iowa +65 rural health survey. *Journal of the American Geriatrics Society, 33*(1), 23-28.
17. Lischer, D. E., & Cooper, J. W. (1981). The consultant pharmacist and analgesic/anti-inflammatory drug usage in a geriatric long-term facility. *Journal of the American Geriatrics Society, 29*(9), 429-432.
18. Maciewicz, R., Martin, J. B. (1987). Pain: Pathophysiology and management. In E. Braunwald, K. J. Isselbacher, R. G. Petersdorf, et al. (Eds.), *Harrison's principles of internal medicine.* New York: McGraw-Hill.
19. Magni, G., Fabrizio, S., & De Leo, D. (1985). Pain as a symptom in elderly depressed patients. *European Archives of Psychiatry and Neurological Science, 235,* 143-145.
20. Melding, P. S. ((1991). Is there such a thing as geriatric pain? *Pain, 46,* 119-121.
21. Melzack, R. (1990). The tragedy of needless pain. *Scientific American, 262*(2), 27-33.
22. Middaugh, S. J., Levin, R. B., Kee, W. G., et al. (1988). Chronic pain: Its treatment and geriatric and younger patients. *Archives of Physical Medicine and Rehabilitation, 69,* 1021-1026.
23. Parmelee, P. A., Katz, I. R., & Lawton, M. P. (1991). The relation of pain to depression among institutionalized aged. *Journal of Gerontology, 46*(1), P15-P21.
24. Portenoy, R. K. (1988). Drug treatment of pain syndromes. *Seminars of Neurology, 7*(2), 139-149.
25. Ready, B. L., Chadwick, H. S., & Ross, B. (1987). Age predicts effective epidural morphine dose after abdominal hysterectomy. *Anesthesiology and Analgesia, 66,* 1215-1218.
26. Roy, R. (1987). A psychosocial perspective on chronic pain and depression in the elderly. *Social Work in Health Care, 12*(2), 27-36.
27. Roy, R., & Thomas, M. (1986). A survey of chronic pain in an elderly population. *Canadian Family Physician, 32,* 513-516.
28. Salzman, C. (1984). *Clinical geriatric psycho-pharmacology.* New York: McGraw-Hill.
29. Sorkin, B. A., Rudy, T. E., Hanlon, R. B., et al. (1990). Chronic pain in old and young patients: Differences appear less important than similarities. *Journal of Gerontology, 45*(2), P64-P68.
30. Sternbach, R. A. (1986). Survey of pain in the United States: The Nuprin pain report. *Journal of Clinical Pain, 2,* 49-54.
31. Von Korff, M., Dwarkin, S. F., Le Resche, L., et al. (1988). An epidemiologic comparison of pain complaints. *Pain, 32*(2), 173-183.
32. Zullich, S. G., Grasela, T. H., Jr., Fredler-Kelly, J. B., et al. (1992). Impact of triplicate prescription program on psychotropic prescribing patterns in long term care facilities. *Annals of Pharmacotherapy, 26,* 539-546.

10

The Management of Depression
in the Nursing Home

JAMES RANDY MERVIS, M.D.
KENNETH D. COLE, PH.D.
STEVEN LLOYD GANZELL, PH.D.

Depression experienced by patients in nursing homes (NHs) can range from mild, transient dysphoric feelings lasting for a day to profound withdrawal and despondency that can persist for months or even years. In an effort to estimate the extent of more serious problems with depression in these settings, we will review a number of studies documenting the epidemiology of depression in the NHs. Then we will turn our attention to studies on various treatment approaches to depression in both a psychiatric and a psychological manner as well as more novel approaches.

EPIDEMIOLOGY OF DEPRESSION IN NURSING HOMES

Early studies investigating the prevalence of depression typically used a psychiatric interview, perhaps bolstered by a chart review and consultations with staff. For example, in the earliest study listed in Table 10.1, Kay et al. (1964), working in residential homes of different levels of care in Great Britain, found that the diagnosis of neurotic depression was the most common (17%) of the psychiatric diagnosis in these settings using criteria from the first Diagnostic Statistical Manual (DSM-I). Concomitantly, they found a rate of "neurosis and

The authors are grateful for the assistance and collaboration of Richard Paradise and Nancy Pachana, Ph.D.

Table 10.1 Nursing Home Prevalence Studies

Study	N	Instrument	Criteria	Findings	Comment
1. Kay et al., 1964	78	Psychiatrist interview	Psychiatric diagnosis (DSM-I)	17% depressive neurosis	Found prevalence of "neurosis" 26% in community
2. Lowther & McLeod, 1974	200	Psychiatrist interview	Psychiatric diagnosis (DSM-II)	9% depression	40.5% dementia 7% misc. psych. disorder
3. Teeter et al., 1976	74	Psychiatrist interview Chart review Interview with relatives and staff	Psychiatric diagnosis by SW (DSM-II)	25.7% primary depression	Almost 2/3 of psychiatric disorders not diagnosed 24.3% secondary depression
4. Hyer & Blazer, 1982	156	Psychiatric interview	DSM-III	15-25% "suggestive of major depression"	50% depressive symptoms of lesser severity
5. Snowdon & Donnelly, 1986	206	Modified GDS	DSM-III	26% depression	Depression correlated with shorter length of stay
6. Spagnoli et al., 1986	368	Psychiatric interview CARE	Feighner criteria (28)	30% depression	Dementia 36% (50% for either or both) Depression correlated with disability, loss, marital status
7. Rovner et al., 1986	50	Semistructured interview and chart review	DSM-III	6% depression	10% total primary psychotic
8. Lesher, 1986	51	GDS and structured psychiatric interview	Research, diagnostic criteria (88)	14% (definite)	Validated GDS for long-term care settings
9. Chandler & Chandler, 1988	65	Geropsychiatric interview	DSM-III-R	1.5% major depressive disorder (1 out of 65)	72% dementia syndromes 12% with "behavioral problems" of anxiety/depression
10. Burns et al., 1988	526	Questionnaire Staff nurse interview Chart review	Organic disorders vs. others	5% severe depression	24% "other mental disorders," of these, 23.7% were depressed

allied disorders" that was 26% in the community. In an Edinburgh residential home 10 years later, Lowther and McLeod (1974) diagnosed 9% of the inhabitants with depression and over 40% with dementia. Depressed males outnumbered females by a 2:1 ratio, but Ames (1991) observed that this may partly be due to the fact that more than twice as many women were diagnosed with dementia.

Working in a similar fashion in Minneapolis, Teeter et al. (1976) determined that 85% of a random sample of patients in two proprietary NHs had a primary psychiatric diagnosis. Forty-six percent had "chronic brain syndrome"; 22% were given a primary diagnosis of depressive neurosis; and 4% were diagnosed with psychotic depression, yielding a total of 25.7% primary depressives. An additional 24.3% were assigned a secondary diagnosis of depression. It is notable that almost two thirds of the psychiatric disorders had not been previously diagnosed.

Using DSM-III criteria, Hyer and Blazer (1982) evaluated higher functioning intermediate care patients in five NHs and determined that 15%-25% had symptoms suggestive of major depression and 50% had depressive symptoms of lesser severity. Lesher (1986), in a validation study of the Geriatric Depression Scale (GDS), a 30-item, self-response questionnaire with higher scores indicating severity of depression, found that 14% of a sample of 51 met the diagnostic criteria for major depression by Research Diagnostic Criteria (RDC) (88) and an additional 35% had "depressive features" (mean GDS scores were 21.1 and 12.6, respectively).

Studying three private and three publicly funded NHs in Sydney, Australia, Snowdon and Donnelly (1986) took the GDS, modified 4 questions to better relate to NH life, and reported that a cutoff score of 14 yielded 86% sensitivity and 87% specificity in classifying those patients who had fulfilled the DSM-III criteria for major depression in earlier work. Of the 339 patients studied, 61% completed the GDS. Over one quarter (26.2%) scored equal or greater than 14 on their hybrid GDS, with almost 40% scoring 11 or more. For those who had been in the NH less than 3 months, the mean GDS was 13.9; it lowered to 9.9 for those from 3 months to 2 years, and to 9.2 for those over 2 years.

As the authors themselves recognize, the GDS is a screening instrument and not a diagnostic tool. This can be misunderstood by epidemiologists and clinicians alike. Some researchers may mistake a cutoff score on the depression scale as sole evidence for a major depressive episode, whereas clinicians may spend too much time documenting fluctuations in dysphoric affect rather than systematically investigating it.

In Milan, Italy, Spagnoli et al. (1986) evaluated 368 patients in 9 geriatric institutions, including skilled NHs, old people's homes, and residential homes. They used the Intervista Psicogeriatrica, which included an organic brain syndrome scale and the depression scales from the Comprehensive Assessment and Referral Evaluation (CARE) (40), including 19 items scored from 0 to 29, corresponding to "not depressed" to "severely depressed." Using a cutoff score of 11 with 278 respondents, the authors determined an estimated prevalence of 30%. Positive correlates of depression were disability and marital status; negative correlates included length of stay for men (higher depression associated with shorter time at the NH). A response of "once married" was robustly and independently correlated with high depression scores. The authors note that admission to a NH is preceded by many losses.

In another investigation published the same year, Rovner et al. (1986) explored a random sample of 50 patients of a proprietary intermediate nursing facility. Although they found a very high prevalence of dementia (78%), only 6% were assessed to have major depression. Over one third (36%) of the patients were found to have depression related to primary degenerative or vascular dementia. "Behavioral problems" were categorized separately, independent of diagnosis; a mild depression identified by a screening device in one study may be loosely equivalent to coded maladaptive behaviors, such as "self-destructive," in this work.

In Iowa City, Chandler and Chandler (1988) similarly presented "behavioral problems" of 65 NH patients in a table, confining their DSM-III-R classifications to more severe diagnoses reached by use of a semistructured interview administered by the first author, a geropsychiatrist. Although they uncovered a 37% occurrence of dementia of probable Alzheimer type and a total of 72% with dementia syndromes, only one in the sample was deemed to have major depression. Organic personality syndrome covered 14% of the sample; organic psychotic disorders included another 12%. A total of 8 patients (12%) were coded as having behavioral problems of "anxiety or depression." The authors found fewer primary psychotic disorders (3%) than did Rovner et al. (10%), perhaps because of the addition of the diagnosis of organic affective disorder to the types of presentations that Rovner and colleagues would have called major depressions or perhaps due to greater diagnostic accuracy.

In their preliminary findings from the 1984 National Nursing Home Survey Pretest, Burns et al. (1988) present findings on a sample of 526 patients in 112 NHs in Atlanta, Boston, Denver, and

Toledo. Utilizing a chart review together with nurse interviews and the Current Resident Questionnaire, they divided the sample into three categories: OMD (other mental disorder), OBS (organic brain syndrome, which superseded OMD diagnoses), and no mental disorder. Although 39% were assessed to have OBS, an additional 29% were in the OMD category, which was largely comprised of mental retardation (25.4%), depression (23.7%), schizophrenia (21.9%), anxiety (16.7%), and other psychosis (12.3%). Diagnoses were duplicated across patients, lengthening the list. Still, 23.7% of the OMD patients had depression as at least one of their diagnoses, which translates to about 27, or 5% of the original sample of 526. Burns and colleagues noted that the OBS and "no diagnosis" groups tended to be in their 80s, whereas the OMD group was 10 years younger on average. The researchers agreed that the NHs are not staffed to provide coordinated mental health treatment and that there is little financial incentive for them to do so, leading the researchers to call for more innovative approaches to providing mental health services in NHs to replace the typical overreliance on neuroleptics and other psychotropic medications.

At the Philadelphia Geriatric Center, Katz et al. (1989) screened patients from two long-term care facilities with a mental status questionnaire, the Geriatric Depression Scale, and an instrument tailored from the Schedule of Affective Disorders and Schizophrenia (88). Patients who exhibited symptoms consistent with major depression were evaluated by a psychiatrist 2-3 weeks later to confirm the diagnosis. Forty-three percent of the 51 patients scored 11 or more on the GDS. Of these, 31% were deemed as having "significant dysphoria," and 20% were diagnosed with major depression. Besides dysphoria, the most prominent symptoms of major depression were apathy, withdrawal, and disengagement. At a 6-month followup of 45 patients, 27% were dysphoric and 18% had a major depression, with a consistent percentage scoring 11 or more on the GDS. At a cutoff of 11, the GDS had an 84% sensitivity and 95% specificity; with a cutoff of 14, it yielded a 80% sensitivity and a 100% specificity. Although the above percentages do not represent the same people across the 6 months, individual trackings of GDS scores show that only six of the high scorers at Time 1 improved, revealing how persistent depressive mood can be in chronic care settings.

Using the Zung Self-Rating Depression Scale to screen 920 patients of 32 Japanese "nursing homes" (which included residential facilities), Horiguchi and Inami (1991) found a prevalence of 61% for all levels of depression compared with the 36% in the community. Using cutoff scores of 70, 60, and 50, respectively, in medical NHs they found rates of 11% severe, 24% moderate, and 37% mild depression. Problems with the Zung scale include the heavy loading of this scale for somatic complaints and dysfunction, prevalent in both the elderly and infirm.

A recently published Australian study surveyed the patients of 24 NHs using the Canberra Interview for the Elderly (CIE) and draft ICD-10 with standard DSM-III-R criteria (67). Those scoring 18 or above on the Mini-Mental State Examination were interviewed with the CIE (165 of 323 patients). Utilizing the CIE with the DSM-III-R criteria, these authors found the prevalence of major depression to be 9.7%. Using the ICD-10 criteria, 6.7% of the sample suffered from a mild, 6.7 % a moderate, and 6.1% from a severe depressive episode.

Some of the same group at the Philadelphia Geriatric Center screened patients of a large NH and congregate apartment complex with a checklist tailored from the Schedule for Affective Disorders and Schizophrenia (SADS) as well as the GDS (65). Observer ratings of depression were completed by interviewers and staff. Those deemed to be suffering from symptoms of a possible major depression were referred for clinical evaluations in psychology and psychiatry. The data for the NH patients were divided into "new admissions" and "veterans." Among the cognitively intact patients, the prevalence of possible major depression was 9.5% for the new admissions and 9.3% for the veterans. Less depressed patients were assessed to be suffering from dysthymia, adjustment disorder with depressed mood, and "other dysphoric states." The prevalence of possible major depression coinciding with cognitive impairment for new admissions was quite high (20.7%); for veterans it was 7.5%. Prevalences of lower level depression among the cognitively impaired were 11.2% for new admissions and 23.6% for veterans. The high-rise apartment dwellers were more likely to display symptoms of a low level depression than the NH patients.

Rovner and colleagues (1990, 1991) evaluated 454 consecutive new admissions to eight proprietary NHs. This group used the Modified Present State Exam (75), which is a semistructured interview for rating the intensity and duration of abnormalities in mood, neurovegetative functioning, perception, and thinking. Family and nursing staff interviews, as well as chart reviews, were also utilized. Fifty-seven (12.6%) of the patients were classified with major depression by DSM-III-R criteria; 82 (18.1%) had "depressive symptoms," levels of depression not meeting DSM-III-R criteria for major depression. Participants with depressive disorder and depressive symptoms were less often demented, had higher levels of cognitive function, and tended to be less disabled in activities of daily living than their nondepressed counterparts. Major depression, rather than depressive symptoms, was a potent risk factor for mortality, increasing the probability of death after 1 year by 59%. At 1-year follow-up, 141 of the original 454 patients (31%) had died. Over 47% with depressive disorders had died, compared with 30% of the nondepressed and 24% with only depressive symptoms. No differences were found between depressives who were treated with medication and those who were not.

Causes of death associated with depression included poor nutrition from anorexia, inadequate rest from insomnia, immobility, and perhaps immune system dysfunction. Causes of depressive disorder included loss of health, decreased mobility and independence, separation from home and family, premorbid vulnerability to illness, and associated medications. Patients were especially at risk with the following diseases: left frontal stroke, Alzheimer's disease, and cancer. The authors estimate that there are almost half a million persons in U.S. NHs with depressive disorders and depressive symptoms that are potentially treatable (79). They recommend appropriate treatment including adoption of acceptable standards of psychiatric care that can be provided in an effective and affordable manner.

In summary, across the studies using more replicable strategies, the prevalence of major depression in many different types of NH settings is about 10%. For more minor depressive symptoms suggesting a diagnosis of dysthymia, adjustment disorder, or bereavement processes, the prevalence seems to average around 18%-20%, placing the total prevalence of depressive states at close to one third. One is struck by the wide range of prevalences depicted in Table 10.1, which undoubtedly is a function of the mix of patients the NH attracts and the wide variance in quality of environment. Moreover, the screening instruments and criteria utilized for diagnoses of depressive disorders vary from study to study.

As described in the articles reviewed, the GDS is commonly used to screen for depression in long-term care settings. Together with the Beck Depression Inventory (BDI), the GDS was found to be a valid screening instrument for geriatric outpatients with good sensitivity (.86) and specificity (.83) with the typical cutoff score of 14 (64). Use of the GDS in NH populations was supported by Lesher (58), who found that a cutoff score of 14 yielded sensitivity rates of 100% for major depression and 55% for "depressive features" with specificity rates of 81%. Cognitively impaired subjects were screened out of the study with a mental status questionnaire. However, Lesher felt that the GDS may be overly sensitive to day-to-day affect and subjective well-being, which are also influenced by low levels of life satisfaction, demoralization, and mourning as well as depressive conditions. Also, the elderly can report several depressive characteristics but then not reach diagnostic criteria for depressive disorders on a clinical interview (39).

More recent work questions the GDS as a screening instrument in NHs. In a sample of 70, Kafonek et al. (1989) found 15 (21.4%) depressed on psychiatric examination. The GDS cutoff scores of 14 on the 66 who could complete the instrument correctly identified 7 (sensitivity = 47%) of these depressives; 13 higher scorers were not depressed on examination (specificity = 75%). Sensitivities of family recollections and nursing observations were stronger than the GDS in this sample. However, removing cognitively impaired patients from the sample improved the sensitivity to 75%, which underscores the importance of using this screening instrument only with organically intact patients.

The diagnosis of depression in patients in long-term care facilities is often difficult. A review of the literature reveals inadequacies in available screening instruments. Future research needs to be directed toward improving the reliability and sensitivity of diagnostic instruments, with the goal of improving the recognition of patients suffering from a treatable depression. The next section will deal specifically with somatic treatments for depression.

SOMATIC TREATMENTS

Although treatment issues of depression have been extensively studied in the general population, there are few studies that deal specifically with the treatment of depressed patients who reside in long-term treatment facilities. In this section, we review studies concerned with somatic treatment modalities of depression, including pharmacologic agents and electroconvulsive therapy.

The elderly are much more inclined to receive a greater amount and variety of medications than a younger population for a variety of reasons. A recent study reviewing the medical records of 91 patients in a teaching NH showed that 24% of these patients received psychoactive medication continuously over a 5-year period, often in combination with other psychoactive drugs (57). During this period, 70% of the patients were exposed to a psychotropic medication.

Twenty-nine percent of the patients were diagnosed as suffering with major affective disorder. Despite an estimated 1.5 million patients in NHs who are exposed to these medications, very few studies specifically investigate the efficacy and adverse effects on this patient population. We will review this literature as well as other pertinent research that uses elderly depressed patients as the primary subjects.

Cyclic antidepressants have been the first line of pharmacologic treatment for major depressive disorder for almost 40 years. The efficacy of the tricyclic antidepressants in the treatment of major depression in elderly individuals is quite favorable. Sorenson et al. (1978) found a response rate of 90% in a group of patients over age 65 treated with nortriptyline. Rockwell et al. (1988) reviewed recent controlled studies comparing various antidepressant responses in population groups of patients older than 60 years. Most of the studies compared the tertiary amine compounds to the newer generation antidepressants. Both groups of medication were found to be effective in treating depression in the elderly. The reader can also refer to Plotkin et al. (1987) and Alexopoulos (3) for reviews of recent antidepressant drug studies in the elderly. The majority of these studies were done with geriatric outpatients.

There are few studies that specifically identify NH patients as the source for research subjects. Katz et al. (1990) recently treated a group of 35 patients living in a residential care setting with nortriptyline in a well-designed double-blind study. Seven had to discontinue the study because of adverse effects, either secondary to medication side effects or concurrent medical problems. Seven of the 12 taking the medication exhibited marked improvement. Only 1 of the 11 taking placebo was rated as experiencing marked improvement. Other significant findings were that patients with low serum albumin and those patients with a high level of disability had a lower rate of response.

Though depression often can be successfully treated, the adverse effects of antidepressants can be detrimental to the treatment of the medically compromised NH patient (see Chapter 2). Four major side effects that must be considered are anticholinergic side effects, hypotension, sedation, and cardiac rate and rhythm changes (83). Research specifically investigating these side effects in the depressed NH patient has been neglected. Certainly more studies of this population are warranted.

One of the most severe adverse effects of tricyclic antidepressants is a central anticholinergic syndrome characterized by confusion, agitation, and even delirium (94). This side effect, somewhat unusual in younger populations, is common in older individuals and is thought to be due to a generalized cholinergic depletion associated with aging. Not only do heterocyclic antidepressants have anticholinergic properties, but antipsychotic, antihistaminic, and antiparkinsonism medications, as well as many nonprescription hypnotics, have these properties as well. The presence of delirium following the initiation of pharmacotherapy strongly indicates the presence of an anticholinergic syndrome. Although often encountered clinically, there are no studies looking at the frequency of a delirium resulting from the use of antidepressants.

Sedation is also a common side effect of antidepressant pharmacotherapy. Although sedation can sometimes be a beneficial side effect, it can have deleterious or even disastrous consequences in NH patients. Overly sedated patients often become amotivational, bed bound, and severely withdrawn. These patients are at high risk for skin breakdown and resulting decubiti, a serious management problem in most NHs. Additionally, these patients are at increased risk for physiological deconditioning because of difficulties in feeding and maintaining activities of daily living. One of the most serious side effects in the elderly taking antidepressants is orthostatic hypotension (35). Elderly patients are at great risk for orthopedic injury as a result of falls. Falls are a serious contributor to morbidity and mortality in the elderly population (see Chapter 8).

The elderly are often at risk to develop cardiac side effects from most antidepressants that are given in the NH (73). There are no studies looking at the incidence of these side effects, which if unmonitored can cause measurable mortality and morbidity.

Aside from the troublesome side effects of some of the tricyclic antidepressants, there are patients who will not respond to the drugs' antidepressant properties (36). Often a patient becomes a nonresponder when not given an adequate trial, either due to too small a dose of medication or too short a time period of taking the medication. According to Quitkin et al. (1984), a therapeutic trial should last at least 6 weeks. Quitkin and colleagues found that a significant number (40%) of patients who had not responded at 4 weeks of treatment eventually exhibited signs of improvement at 6 weeks.

New antidepressants with less harmful side effects and more efficacious therapeutic properties than tricyclics are being developed. Feighner and Cohen (1985) and Feighner et al. (1988) found fluoxetine (Prozac) to be effective in a geriatric population. Fluoxetine has few anticholinergic side effects or adverse cardiac side effects, which may make this a valuable drug in the NH. The main problems encountered in treatment of the elderly are the drug's weight-reducing and activating properties. There are several other serotinergic uptake inhibitors that also may be useful in the elderly; these include Fluvoxamine, which is currently available in Europe but not in the United States. Future research will help further delineate the specific serotinin reuptake inhibitors' promising role in the treatment of psychiatric disorders in the elderly.

A variety of agents including lithium, thyroid supplement, monoamine oxidase inhibitors, and psychostimulants have been reported to be effective adjuvants of tricyclic antidepressants (24). Lithium is very effective for the treatment and prophylaxis of the manic phase, and the prophylaxis for the depressive phase of bipolar affective disorder. Yet it is not very effective in the treatment of unipolar depression. Several studies not dealing specifically with the elderly have shown lithium to be an effective adjuvant in unipolar patients who were unresponsive to tricyclic antidepressants alone (59,43). Triiodothyronine (T3) has been reported to successfully potentiate tricyclic antidepressants in 9 of 12 patients by Goodwin et al. (1982). Gitlin et al. (1987) found T3 to be of no benefit in a well-designed study of 16 tricyclic nonresponders. Of the psychostimulants, methylphenidate can increase tricyclic serum levels, yet must be used carefully to avoid the possible induction of insomnia and agitation. Buspirone, an azaspirodecanedione marketed as an anxiolytic, has recently been shown to improve antidepressant response in seven of eight subjects taking fluoxetine (47). The moderate doses of buspirone used (10 mg t.i.d.) caused minimal adverse affects. The effectiveness of buspirone as an adjuvant and as an antidepressant itself needs further study, as this agent appears to have a very low side effect profile.

Treatment with bright light has been found to be effective in the treatment of seasonal affective disorders (78). Exposure to sunlight and other environmental interventions may have significant effects on the outcome of the treatment of depression in the NH, yet these interventions would be difficult to measure.

The monoamine oxidase inhibitors (MAOIs) are effective for tricyclic antidepressant treatment resistant and atypical depressions as well as for many patients with unipolar and bipolar depressions (49). Still, they are infrequently prescribed by clinicians because of fears of potential side effects, associated drug interactions, and the specific dietary precautions that need to be followed. A recent review of seven studies examining MAOIs in the elderly by Rockwell et al. (1988) showed the MAOIs to be effective and safe for treatment of depression in tricyclic resistant cases as well as in demented patients. Georgotas et al. (1986) found phenelzine to be effective in 65% of a group of elderly patients with a treatment-resistant depression, again with few adverse effects.

Combinations of a tricyclic and an MAOI have been used successfully (12). The combination of these two drugs is less dangerous than initially thought, yet serious side effects have been reported. The most dangerous side effect of the MAOIs in the elderly patient is orthostatic hypotension. Other adverse effects are insomnia or sedation, depending on the MAOI prescribed (71). MAOIs are known to increase appetite (72). This side effect can be used to benefit the often malnourished depressed NH patient. MAOIs have much weaker anticholinergic side effects than the tricyclic antidepressants. As with the tricyclic antidepressants, few studies evaluate either the efficacy or the side effects of the monoamine oxidase inhibitors in the NH.

There is a specific role for psychostimulants in the treatment of depressed NH patients. One of the most common problems encountered in the NH is determining whether a patient's medical illness or a possible coexisting endogenous depression is causing a patient to become more apathetic and withdrawn and to have a decreased desire to eat and drink. Several studies have shown that the psychostimulants methylphenidate and dextroamphetamine can be useful in the psychomotorically retarded, apathetic, medically ill patient as well as the depressed patient (see Table 10.2). These are patients who often cannot tolerate the anticholinergic, cardiac, and sedative side effects of the tricyclic antidepressants.

Stimulants have also been found to be helpful in treating demented patients with a concurrent depressive episode (13). Patients who have just initiated traditional antidepressant treatment also may benefit from a brief trial of stimulants during the usual 2- to 3-week lag time it usually takes for the antidepressant to become effective. This is due to the rapid onset of action of the stimulants, usually within 24 to 48 hours. Nonresponders to tricyclic antidepressants are often denied a trial of psychostimulants, yet could also benefit from their effects (21).

Few studies have dealt specifically with using psychostimulants with elderly persons. Table 10.2 contains studies published since 1975 using psychostimulants for the treatment of depression in elderly subjects. Most show the efficacy of the drugs to be more favorable than had been previously thought. These studies all report a low incidence of side effects. None of the studies or case reports describes any decrease in the patient's appetite, which is generally of great concern. More controlled clinical studies are certainly warranted to help delineate the usefulness and efficacy of these drugs, especially when used to augment antidepressant therapy in elderly populations.

Electroconvulsive therapy (ECT) has been used as an effective treatment for depression for over 50 years. The use of ECT has been limited due to various reasons, including a general misunderstanding of the technique of the procedure. The technique has changed dramatically since the early 1950s. Only recently have the unique benefits of ECT, which include a rapid response, low side effect profile, and relatively low morbidity, been used to advantage in the treatment of depression in the elderly. In comparison, the side effect profile of most antidepressant medications may preclude their use in NH patients.

For some NH residents, ECT is clearly indicated as the first choice of treatment. Patients most likely to require ECT are the severely depressed who suffer marked changes in their vegetative functions (10). Those refusing to eat, drink, or move or who are not sleeping have little reserve and are subject to dehydration, malnutrition, exhaustion, and the effects of psychomotor retardation (skin breakdown, etc.). These patients must be treated on an emergency basis, and standard antidepressant medications may take 3 to 6 weeks to be effective. Patients who have attempted or are threatening suicide and others who are at high suicide risk also must be given treatment that is fast acting and effective. Other patients who are candidates for ECT include those whose depression has been refractory to antidepressant medications.

ECT has been reported to be the most effective treatment in episodes of severe major depression (84). Several recent studies focus on the effects of ECT in the elderly. Burke et al. (1985) reported that in a group of patients 60 years and older, with both major affective and schizoaffective disorders, 83% of all patients who underwent ECT improved. This study also demonstrated that the oldest patients were at increased risk to experience medical complications following ECT. In a larger sample of older patients, Burke et al. (1987) found similar rates of improvement. Cattan et al. (1990) compared the effectiveness of ECT in two groups of geriatric patients. Young-old patients (65-80 years) had significantly more improvement than old-old patients (over 80 years). Additionally, the latter group was more likely to experience cardiovascular complications and falls.

However, these patients had a greater need for an ECT trial because of their increased frequency of depression-associated life-threatening symptoms (refusal to eat, amotivation, dehydration). Babigian and Guttmacher (1984) as well as Robinson (1989) reported lower mortality in depressed elderly patients who receive ECT when compared those not receiving ECT. Robinson also reports a lower rate of recurrence of major depression in patients treated with ECT in a 15-year longitudinal study.

As noted above, elderly patients treated with ECT can have a variety of medical complications. In addition to falls, which can be avoided, and cardiovascular complications, which can be treated, a major complication of ECT is its well-documented cognitive effects (30). The use of ECT is associated with confusion and memory loss during the course of the treatment (95). Memory problems usually resolve after 7 months, although there is a small number of individuals in whom the amnesia persists (89). Patients with preexisting cognitive impairment may be susceptible to prolonged confusion and memory effects and should be given ECT only when absolutely necessary (23). The effects of the procedure on memory can be lessened by using unilateral electrode placement. Some controversy exists regarding the difference in efficacy of bilateral versus unilateral electrode placement in treating depression. Additionally, differences in antidepressant effects between dominant and nondominant hemisphere unilateral electrode placement have been documented (2). It also should be noted that these cognitive effects are a function both of the number of treatments given and the age of the patient, with older patients and patients having more treatments experiencing more memory deficits for a longer time period. Several studies indicate that elderly patients receiving ECT do not develop permanent cognitive changes (at least changes that can be readily measured) (32,82). The question of whether brain damage can be secondary to ECT has been controversial. Recent studies using computed tomography (9) and magnetic resonance imaging (66) revealed no structural changes. Yet a study by Figiel et al. (1990) reported structural changes, notably in the basal ganglia and subcortical white matter in elderly patients who had prolonged interictal delirium induced by ECT.

Additionally, it should be noted that many case reports (1) and one recent study (25) have reported the palliative effects of ECT on motor dysfunction in patients with Parkinson's disease. It should be noted that all of these reports involve patients who are being treated with ECT for depression and not primarily for their movement disorder. However, significant improvement in motor dysfunction has been documented. Douyon et al. (1989) showed improvement in seven patients in both their movement disorder and their mood after an average of seven treatments. There are several possible mechanisms of action for these noted improvements. Because ECT effects the blood-brain barrier by making it more permeable, neurotransmitters including dopamine and norepinephrine are more available to the synapses (11). Additionally, ECT may directly effect the neuroreceptors by making them more sensitive to the dopamine (Fochtman, 1988).

Unlike other psychiatric treatments, the use of ECT is often governed by institutional and governmental restrictions. Despite the minimal risk and the known benefits, ECT continues to be controversial. Additionally, patients and their families are often reticent to use ECT due to misrepresentations of the procedure and its results in the lay media. All of this contributes to the difficulty of conducting research using ECT in the NH. Most states require that patients sign complicated consent forms before receiving ECT. This can be especially difficult for those elderly patients most likely to need ECT. These patients are often so depressed that they are unwilling or unable to give consent. In such cases consent must be obtained from a conservator. It should be noted that many NH patients have no conservator and that lengthy court proceedings may be needed to appoint one. Many NH patients who would benefit from ECT are not treated because of these obstacles. Understandably, from the above information, it is difficult to conduct research using ECT as a treatment modality in the NH. There are no studies using the NH as a specific source of subjects for ECT. Yet many areas need to be further explored. Issues concerning severity and time span of cognitive deficits, courses of maintenance ECT as a way of preventing relapses, efficacy of ECT in patients with disorders other than depression, and many other pertinent questions about ECT can be studied in the NH, but often with great difficulty.

Somatic treatment of depression is a difficult task in the NH. It was estimated that 10% to 30% of depressive episodes are resistant to treatment (63). Along with somatic therapeutic interventions, there are other treatment modalities that may be not only beneficial but essential in treating depression in the NH.

PSYCHOSOCIAL INTERVENTIONS

There are few studies evaluating the effectiveness of the various forms of psychotherapy in the elderly NH patient. These therapies may play an important role in the treatment of depression in the NH when used with the appropriate patient. The psychotherapeutic modalities include psychodynamic psychotherapy (8), cognitive and behavioral therapies (93), group psychotherapy (18), and family therapy (68). Individual psychodynamic psychotherapy is rarely used because of concerns with reduced personnel, time, and cost-effectiveness. However, this treatment of depression has been found to be effective (92). Psychotherapy has also been described as being beneficial for demented patients and caregiving family members (61). Teri and Gallagher-Thompson (1991) describe effective cognitive-behavioral interventions in depressed Alzheimer's patients. These interventions have been measured clinically before and after administration of the treatments using the Beck Depression Inventory (7) and the Hamilton Depression Rating Scale (42) with appreciable declines in depression scores.

Cognitive and behavioral therapies are more focused and time limited than insight-oriented psychotherapy and therefore may be more appropriate for treatment in the NH. Morris and Morris (1991) reviewed six studies using cognitive and behavioral approaches with elderly depressed patients. They concluded that these psychological treatments generally resulted in improvement, especially when compared to placebo groups. Research that seeks to evaluate cognitive-behavioral interventions is somewhat less limited than the research on the other therapeutic approaches. However, many of the studies are limited in their research design, especially with regard to subject selection and the ability to randomly assign subjects to groups. Jarvik et al. (1982) compared the efficacy of either imipramine or doxepin to cognitive-behavioral group therapy. Their study was limited by the severity of the physical and emotional distress of their patients, which made it impossible to assign them to random groups. However, they were able to conclude that 45% of the drug treatment group showed a complete remission of depression compared to 12% of the psychotherapy group. There are no research studies that report the efficacy of cognitive-behavioral treatment with NH patients specifically. Inasmuch as many of the depressed patients in NHs are similar to other depressed older patients, it would be safe to conclude that similar positive outcomes would be likely. Clearly more studies are indicated comparing the outcomes for depressed NH patients of medications alone, of psychotherapy, or a combination of the two.

There are many other psychosocial interventions that have not been or are only beginning to be explored in the research being done in the NH. These include pet therapy and recreational and occupational therapies (including all creative learning opportunities, art, music, and literature, etc.) (26). Reminiscence and genealogy review exercises also have been beneficial. Haight (1988) studied the effects of a structured life review process with 60 homebound elderly patients, concluding that this was indeed a therapeutic intervention. The NH environment itself also provides many opportunities to examine its effect on the depressed patient. Structured therapeutic gardens have also been found to improve morale and mood in the NH (44,14).

In conclusion, the NH has many residents that are suffering from depression, an often treatable disease that can be devastating if left untreated. Research in the NH could ultimately help identify these patients and delineate the most appropriate interventions needed for this difficult treatment population.

REFERENCES

1. Abrams, R. (1989). ECT for Parkinson's disease. *American Journal of Psychiatry, 146,* 1391-1393.
2. Abrams, R., Swartz, C. M., & Vedak, C. (1989). Antidepressant effects of right versus left unilateral ECT and the lateralization theory of ECT action. *American Journal of Psychiatry, 146,* 1190-1192.
3. Alexopoulos, G. S. (1992). Treatment of depression. In C. Salzman (Ed.), *Clinical geriatric psychopharmacology* (pp. 137-169). Baltimore, MD: Williams & Wilkins.
4. Ames, D. (1991). Epidemiological studies of depression among the elderly in residential and nursing homes. *International Journal of Geriatric Psychiatry, 6,* 347-354.
5. Askinazi, C., Weintraub, M. D., & Karamouz, N. (1986). Elderly depressed females as possible subgroup of patients responsive to methylphenidate. *Journal of Clinical Psychiatry, 47*(9), 467-469.
6. Babigian, H. M., & Guttmacher, L. B. (1984). Epidemiologic considerations in electroconvulsive therapy. *Archives of General Psychiatry, 41,* 246-253.
7. Beck, A. T, Ward, C., Mendelson, M., Mock, J., et al. (1961). An inventory for measuring depression. *Archives of General Psychiatry, 4,* 561-571.
8. Berezin, M. A. (1972). Psychodynamic considerations of aging and the aged: An overview. *American Journal of Psychiatry, 128,* 33-41.
9. Bergsholm, P., Larsen, J. L., Rosendahl, K., et al. (1989). Electroconvulsive therapy and cerebral computed tomography. *Acta Psychiatrica Scandinavica, 80,* 566-572.
10. Bidder, T. G. (1981). Electroconvulsive therapy in the medically ill patient. *Psychiatric Clinics of North America 4,* 391-405.
11. Bolwig, T., Hertz, M., & Paulson, O. B. (1977). The permeability of the blood brain barrier during electrically induced seizures in man. *European Journal of Clinical Investigation, 7,* 87-93.
12. Borson, S., & Raskind, M. (1986). Antidepressant-resistant depression in the elderly. *Journal of the American Geriatrics Society, 34,* 245-249.

13. Branconnier, R. J., & Cole, J. O. (1980). The therapeutic role of methylphenidate on senile organic brain syndrome. In J. O. Cole & J. Barrett (Eds.), *Psychopathology of the aged* (pp. 183-195). New York: Raven.
14. Bryant, W. (1991). Creative group work with confused elderly people: A development of sensory integration therapy. *British Journal of Occupational Therapy, 54,* 187-192.
15. Burke, W. J., Rubin, E. H., Zorumski, C. F., et al. (1987). The safety of ECT in geriatric psychiatry. *Journal of the American Geriatrics Society 35,* 516-521.
16. Burke, W. J., Rutherford, J. L., Zorumski, C. F., et al. (1985). Electroconvulsive therapy and the elderly. *Comprehensive Psychiatry, 35,* 480-486.
17. Burns, B. J., Larson, D. B., Goldstrom, I. G., et al. (1988). Mental disorder among nursing home patients: Preliminary findings from the National Nursing Home Survey pretest. *International Journal of Geriatric Psychiatry, 3,* 27-35.
18. Burnside, I. (1984). *Working with the elderly: Group process and techniques.* Monterey, CA: Brooks/Cole.
19. Cattan, R. A., Barry P. P., Mead, G., et al. (1990). Electroconvulsive therapy in octogenarians. *Journal of the American Geriatrics Society, 38,* 753-758.
20. Chandler, J. D., & Chandler, J. E. (1988). The prevalence of neuropsychiatric disorders in a nursing home population. *Journal of Geriatric Psychiatry and Neurology, 1,* 71-76.
21. Chiarello, R. J., & Cole, J. O. (1987). Psychostimulants: A reconsideration. *Archives of General Psychiatry, 44,* 286-295.
22. Clark, A. N., & Mankikar, G. (1979). d-Amphetamine in elderly patients refractory to rehabilitation procedures. *Journal of the American Geriatric Society, 27,* 174-177.
23. Daniel, W. F., Weiner, R. D., Crovitz, H. F., et al. (1983). ECT-induced delirium and further ECT. *American Journal of Psychiatry, 140,* 922-924.
24. deMontigny, C., Grunberg, F., Mayer, A., et al. (1981). Lithium induces rapid relief of depression in tricyclic antidepressant drug non-responders. *British Journal of Psychiatry, 138,* 252-256.
25. Douyon, R., Serby, M., Klutchko, B., et al. (1989). ECT and Parkinson's disease revisited: A "naturalistic" study. *American Journal of Psychiatry, 146,* 1451-1455.
26. Erikson, E. H., Erikson, J. M., & Kivinick, H. Q. (1986). *Vital involvement in old age.* New York: Morton.
27. Feighner, J. P., Boyer, W. F., Meredith, C. H., et al. (1988). An overview of fluoxetine in geriatric depression. *British Journal of Psychiatry, 153*(Suppl. 3), 105-108.
28. Feighner, J. P., & Cohen, J. B. (1985). Double-blind comparative trials of fluoxetine and doxepin in geriatric patients with major depressive disorder. *Journal of Clinical Psychiatry, 46,* 20-25.
29. Figiel, G. S., Coffey, C. E., Djang, W. T., et al. (1990). Brain magnetic resonance imaging findings in ECT-induced delirium. *Journal of Neuropsychiatry, 2,* 53-58.
30. Fink, M. (1979). *Convulsive therapy: Theory and practice.* New York: Raven.
31. Fochtman, L. (1988). A mechanism of efficiency of ECT and Parkinson's disease. *Convulsive Therapy, 4,* 321-327.
32. Fraser, R. M., & Glass, I. B. (1978). Recovery from ECT in elderly patients. *British Journal of Psychiatry, 133,* 524-528.
33. Georgotas, A., McCue, R. E., Hapworth, W., et al. (1986). Comparative efficacy and safety of MAOIs versus TCAs in treating depression in the elderly. *Biological Psychiatry, 21,* 1155-1166.
34. Gitlin, M. J., Weiner, H., Fairbanks, L., et al. (1987). Failure of T3 to potentiate tricyclic antidepressant response. *Journal of Affective Disorders, 13,* 267-272.

35. Glassman, A. H., Walsh, T., & Roose, P. (1982). Factors related to orthostatic hypotension associated with tricyclic antidepressants. *Journal of Clinical Psychiatry, 43,* 35-38.
36. Goff, D. C., & Jenike, M. A. (1986). Treatment-resistant depression in the elderly. *Journal of the American Geriatrics Society, 34,* 63-70.
37. Goodwin, F. K., Prange A. J., Jr., Post, R. M., et al. (1982). Potentiation of antidepressants effects of L-triiodothyronine in tricyclic antidepressants. *American Journal of Psychiatry, 139,* 34-38.
38. Gurian, B., & Rosowsky, E. (1990). Low dose methylphenidate in the very old. *Journal of Geriatric Psychiatry and Neurology, 3,* 152-154.
39. Gurland, B. J. (1976). The comparative frequency of depression in various adult age groups. *Journal of Gerontology, 31,* 283-292.
40. Gurland, B. J., Kuriansky, J., & Sharpe, L. (1977). The Comprehensive Assessment and Referral Evaluation (CARE)—rationale, development and reliability. *International Journal of Aging and Human Development, 8,* 9-42.
41. Haight, B. K. (1988). The therapeutic role of a structured life review process in homebound elderly subjects. *Journal of Gerontology, 43,* 40-44.
42. Hamilton, M. (1967). Development of a rating scale for primary depressive illness. *British Journal of Social and Clinical Psychology, 6,* 278-296.
43. Heninger, G. R., Charney, D. S., & Sternberg, D. E. (1983). Lithium carbonate augmentation of antidepressant treatment. *Archives of General Psychiatry, 40,* 1335-1339.
44. Hill, C. O., & Relf, P. O. (1982). Gardening as an outdoor activity in geriatric institutions. *Activities, Adaptation and Aging, 3,* 47-54.
45. Horiguchi, J., & Inami, Y. (1991). A survey of the living conditions and psychological states of elderly people admitted to nursing homes in Japan. *Acta Psychiatrica Scandinavica, 83,* 338-341.
46. Hyer, L., & Blazer, D. G. (1982). Depressive symptoms: Impact and problems in long term care facilities. *International Journal of Behavioral Geriatrics, 1,* 33-44.
47. Jacobsen, F. M. (1991). Possible augmentation of antidepressant response by buspirone. *Journal of Clinical Psychiatry, 52,* 217-220.
48. Jarvik, L. F., Mintz, J., Steuer, J., et al. (1982). Treating geriatric depression: A 26-week interim analysis. *Journal of the American Geriatrics Society, 30,* 713-717.
49. Jenike, M. A. (1984). The use of monoamine oxidase inhibitors in the treatment of elderly, depressed patients. *Journal of the American Geriatrics Society, 32,* 571-575.
50. Kafonek, S., Ettinger, W. H., Roca, R., et al. (1989). Instruments for screening for depression and dementia in the long-term care facility. *Journal of the American Geriatrics Society, 37,* 29-34.
51. Kaplitz, S. E. (1975). Withdrawn, apathetic geriatric patients responsive to methylphenidate. *Journal of the American Geriatrics Society, 23,* 271-276.
52. Katon, W., & Raskind, M. (1980). Treatment of depression in the medically ill elderly with methylphenidate. *American Journal of Psychiatry, 137,* 963-965.
53. Katz, I. R., Lesher, E., Kleban, M., et al. (1989). Clinical features of depression in the nursing home. *International Psychogeriatrics, 1,* 5-15.
54. Katz, I. R., Simpson, G. M., & Curlick, S. M. (1990). Pharmacologic treatment of major depression for elderly patients in residential care settings. *Journal of Clinical Psychiatry* (Suppl.), *51*(7), 41-47.
55. Kaufmann, M. W., Tesar, G. E., Murray, G. B., et al. (1982). Use of psychostimulants in medically ill depressed patients. *Psychosomatics, 23,* 817-819.

56. Kay, D. W., Beamish, P., & Roth, M. (1964). Old age mental disorders in New Castle upon Tyne: 1. A study prevalence. *British Journal of Psychiatry, 110,* 146-158.

57. Lantz, M., Louis, A., Lowenstein, G., et al. (1990). A longitudinal study of psychotropic prescriptions in a teaching nursing home. *American Journal of Psychiatry, 147,* 1637-1639.

58. Lesher, E. (1986). Validation of the geriatric depression scale among nursing home residents. *Clinical Gerontology, 4,* 21-28.

59. Louie, A. K., & Meltzer, H. Y. (1984). Lithium potentiation of antidepressant treatment. *Journal of Clinical Psychopharmacology, 4,* 316-321.

60. Lowther, C. P. & McLeod, H. M. (1974). Admissions to a welfare home. *Health Bulletin, 32,* 14-18.

61. Miller, M. D. (1989). Opportunities for psychotherapy in the management of dementia. *Journal of Geriatric Psychiatry and Neurology, 2,* 11-17.

62. Morris, R. G., & Morris, L. W. (1991). Cognitive and behavioral approaches with the depressed elderly. *International Journal of Geriatric Psychiatry, 6,* 407-413.

63. Nierenberg, A. A., & Amsterdam, J. D. (1990). Treatment-resistant depression: Definition and treatment approaches. *Journal of Clinical Psychiatry, 51*(Suppl.), 39-50.

64. Norris, J. T., Gallagher, D., Wilson, A., et al. (1987). Assessment of depression in geriatric medical outpatients: The validity of two screening measures. *Journal of the American Geriatrics Society, 35,* 989-995.

65. Parmelee, P. A., Katz, I. R., & Lawton, M. P. (1989). Depression among institutionalized aged: Assessment and prevalence estimation. *Journal of Gerontology, 44,* M22-29.

66. Pande, A. C., Grunhaus, L. J., Aisen, A. M., et al. (1990). A preliminary magnetic resonance study of ECT-treated depressed patients. *Biological Psychiatry, 27,* 102-104.

67. Phillips, C. J., & Henderson, A. S. (1991). The prevalence of depression among Australian nursing home residents: Results using draft ICD-10 and DSM-III-R criteria. *Psychological Medicine, 21,* 739-748.

68. Pinsof, W. M. (1989). A conceptual framework and methological criteria for family therapy process research. *Journal of Consulting and Clinical Psychology, 57,* 53-64.

69. Plotkin, D. A., Gerson, S. C., & Jarvik, L. F. (1987). Antidepressant drug treatment in the elderly. In H. Y. Meltzer (Ed.), *Psychopharmacology: The third generation of progress* (pp. 1149-1158). New York: Raven.

70. Quitkin, F. M., Rabkin, J. G., Ross, D., et al. (1984). Duration of antidepressant drug treatment. *Archives of General Psychiatry, 41,* 238-245.

71. Rabkin, J., Quitkin, F. M., Harrison, W., et al. (1984). Adverse reactions to monoamine oxidase inhibitors: 1. A comparative study. *Journal of Clinical Psychopharmacology, 4,* 279-288.

72. Ranzi, J., White, K. L., White, J., et al. (1983). The safety and efficacy of combined amitriptyine and tranylcypromine antidepressant treatment. *Archives of General Psychiatry, 40,* 657-660.

73. Risch, S. C., Groom, G., & Janowsky, D. S. (1989). Cardiovascular effects of tricyclic antidepressants in depressed patients. *Journal of Clinical Psychiatry, 50,* 1-18.

74. Robinson, J. R. (1989). The natural history of mental disorder in old age: A long term study. *British Journal of Psychiatry, 154,* 783-789.

75. Robinson, R. G., Kubos, K. L., Starr, L. B., et al. (1983). Mood changes in stroke patients: Relationship to lesion location. *Comprehensive Psychiatry, 24,* 555-566.

76. Rockwell, E., Lam, R. W., & Zisook, S. (1988). Antidepressant drug studies in the elderly. *Psychiatric Clinics of North America, 11*(1), 215-233.
77. Rosenberg, P. M., Ahmed, I., & Hurwitz, S. (1991). Methylphenidate in depressed medically ill patients. *Journal of Clinical Psychiatry, 52,* 263-266.
78. Rosenthal, N. E., Sack D. A., Carpenter, C. J., et al. (1985). Antidepressant effects of light in seasonal affective disorder. *American Journal of Psychiatry, 142,* 163-170.
79. Rovner, B. W., German, P. S., Brant, L. J., et al. (1991). Depression and mortality in nursing homes. *Journal of the American Medical Association, 265,* 993-996.
80. Rovner, B. W., German, P. S., Broathead, J., et al. (1990). The prevalence and management of dementia and other psychiatric disorders in nursing homes. *International Psychogeriatrics, 2,* 13-24.
81. Rovner, B. W., Kafonek, S., Filipp, L., et al. (1986). Prevalence of mental illness in a community nursing home. *American Journal of Psychiatry, 143,* 1446-1449.
82. Russ, M. J., Ackerman, S. H., Burton, L., et al. (1990). Cognitive effects of ECT in the elderly: Preliminary findings. *International Journal of Geriatric Psychiatry, 5,* 115-118.
83. Salzman, C. (1985). Clinical guidelines for the use of antidepressant drugs in geriatric patients. *Journal of Clinical Psychology, 46*(Suppl.), 38-44.
84. Scovern, A. W., & Kilmann, P. R. (1980). Status of electroconvulsive therapy: Review of the outcome literature. *Psychological Bulletin, 87,* 260-303.
85. Snowdon, J., & Donnelly, N. (1986). A study of depression in nursing homes. *Journal of Psychiatric Research, 20,* 327-333.
86. Sorensen, B., Kragh-Sorensen, P., & Larsen, N. E. (1978). The practical significance of nortriptyline plasma control. *Psychopharmacology, 59,* 35-37.
87. Spagnoli, A., Foresti, G., MacDonald, A., et al. (1986). Dementia and depression in Italian geriatric institutions. *International Journal of Geriatric Psychiatry, 1,* 15-23.
88. Spitzer, R. L., Endicott, J., & Robins, E. (1978). Research Diagnostic criteria rationale and reliability. *Archives of General Psychiatry, 35,* 773-782.
89. Squire, L. R. (1982). Neuropsychological effects of ECT. In R. Abrams & W. B. Essman (Eds.), *Electroconvulsive therapy: Biological foundations and clinical applications.* New York: Spectrum.
90. Teeter, R. R., Garetz, F. K., Miller, W. R., et al. (1976). Psychiatric disturbances of aged patients in skilled nursing homes. *American Journal of Psychiatry, 133,* 1430-1434.
91. Teri, L., & Gallagher-Thompson, D. (1991). Cognitive-behavioral interventions for treatment of depression in Alzheimer's patients. *Gerontologist, 31,* 413-416.
92. Thompson, L. E., Gallagher, D., & Breckenridge, S. (1987). Comparative effectiveness of psychotherapies for depressed elders. *Journal of Consulting and Clinical Psychology, 55,* 385-390.
93. Thompson, L. E., Gantz, F., Florsheim, Del Maestro, S., et al. (1991). Cognitive-behavioral therapy for affective disorders in the elderly. In W. A. Myers (Ed.), *New techniques in the psychotherapy of older patients* (pp. 3-19). Washington, DC: American Psychiatric Press.
94. Veith, R. C. (1982). Depression in the elderly: Pharmacologic considerations in treatment. *Journal of the American Geriatrics Society, 30,* 581-586.
95. Weiner, R. D. (1984). Does electroconvulsive therapy cause brain damage? *Behavioral and Brain Sciences, 7,* 1-53.
96. Woods, S. W., Tesar, G. E., Murray, G. B., et al. (1986). Psychostimulant treatment of depressive disorders secondary to medical illness. *Journal of Clinical Psychiatry, 47,* 12-15.

Table 10.2 Psychostimulant Studies

Study	Population	Intervention	Study Design	Outcome Measures	Adverse Effects	Outcome
1. Kaplitz, 1975	N=44 26 male, 18 female 25 drug, 19 placebo Psychiatric diagnosis: withdrawn, apathetic institutionalized patients	Methylphenidate 20 mg daily for 6 wks	Double-blind randomized	1. Clinical evaluation 2. Mental status check list (MSCL) 3. Nurse's Observation Scale for Inpatient Evaluation (NOSIE)	No side effects observed; no weight changes reported in either treatment or placebo group.	Statistically significant improvement in interest, competence, and psychomotor retardation was noted in 24 of 25 patients (pts).
2. Clark & Mankikar, 1979	N=88 15 males, 73 females Age range= 66-94 Psychiatric diagnosis: poor motivation syndrome	Dextroamphetamine given for 3 wks in increasing doses from 2.5 mg-10 mg BID	Open trial, prospective	Clinical evaluation of three measures: mobility, motivation, and self-care	23 pts terminated treatment (22 females, 1 male) due to aggressive and uncooperative behavior (10 pts), confusion or delusions (7 pts), hypomania (1 pt), vomiting (1 pt). Appetite stimulation also noted. All side effects disappeared when medication was discontinued.	48 pts responded to the treatment, becoming more alert, communicative, and self-caring; 28 were discharged in an independent state; 17 showed age-related resistance to the drug; the response to the drug in PMS was noted to be prompt when it occurred.

Study	Sample	Medication/Dose	Design	Outcome Measure	Side Effects	Results
3. Woods et al., 1986	N=66 32 males, 32 females X age=72 Age range= 37-87 Pt character-istics: seriously medically ill Psychiatric diagnosis included: major depression, adjustment disorder, organic affective disorder	Dextroampheta-mine: given to 35 pts, average maximal dose: 12 mg/day, range: 2.5-30 mg/day Methylpheni-date: given to 36 pts, average maximal dose: 13.5 mg/day, range: 5-30 mg/day	Retrospective review	Clinical Global Impression Scale (CGIS)	7% of pts terminated treatment because of side effects rated as possibly related to medication; these included confusion, sinus tachycardia, nausea, diaphoresis, maculopapular rash. None of the side effects was severe; all were reversible.	In 34 (48%) of 71 retrospectively reviewed clinical psychostimulant trials, an overall result of marked or moderate improvement was obtained; relapse was observed in only 5 pts.
4. Askinazi et al., 1986	N=13 5 males, 8 females Age range= 58-89 Psychiatric diagnosis: major depression (medically ill)	Methylphenidate 2.5 mg-20 mg/day	Retrospective chart review	Clinical evaluation scale similar to the CGI scale above	Few side effects were noted. One case of drug-related rash and one case of ventricular ectopic activity (9 of 13 pts initially had significant cardiovascular disease).	Of 29 pts, 16 (55%) had moderate to marked improvement within 2 days of initial treatment. Therapeutic response was significantly correlated with maximum methylphenidate dose.

continued

Table 10.2 Continued

Study	Population	Intervention	Study Design	Outcome Measures	Adverse Effects	Outcome
5. Rosenberg et al., 1991	N=29 12 males, 17 females X age=64.5 Age range= 23-85 Psychiatric diagnosis: major depression (medically ill)	Methylphenidate mean maximal dose=14.6 mg/day (range= 5-30 mg/day)	Retrospective chart review	Clinical Global Impression Scale (CGIS)	28% of pts reported side effects, rated as mild; these included cardiac side effects (3 pts), agitation (4 pts), visual hallucinations (1 pt). All side effects were reversible.	16 (55%) of pts had moderate or marked improvement within 2 days of initiation of treatment. Improvement seen in pts with a diagnosis of both major depression and adjustment disorder.
Case Reports of Psychostimulant Use						
1. Katon & Raskind, 1980	2 females; 1 male X age: 80 Diagnosis: major depression	Methylphenidate 10 mg BID			None reported	Improvement noted after 2-3 days. Drug treatment continued for 2-4 months. No relapse reported.
2. Kaufmann et al., 1982	3 females; 1 male X age: 62.5 Diagnosis: major depression; S/P cardiac surgery (thus use of tricyclics contraindicated)	Methylphenidate 10 mg BID			None reported	Clinical improvement noted after 1-2 days. Drug treatment continued for 8-14 days. No relapse noted at 6-month follow-up.
3. Gurian & Rosowsky, 1990	2 females X age: 97.5	Methylphenidate 1.2 mg QD and 2.5 mg BID			None reported	Improvement noted after 5-14 days. No relapse noted at 8 months.

11

Assessment and Management of Behavior Problems in the Nursing Home

JISKA COHEN-MANSFIELD, PH.D.
PERLA WERNER, M.A.
MARCIA S. MARX, PH.D.
STEVEN LIPSON, M.D., M.P.H.

INTRODUCTION

Behavior problems pose a major challenge to the provision of quality care in the nursing home (NH). Behavior problems seem to indicate distress in at least some NH residents. In turn, these behaviors are a source of distress to both family caregivers and staff caregivers. Further, they frequently interfere with the actual provision of services to NH residents. A few examples will illustrate this: a resident who is so restless that she does not stay in one place, gets out of her chair immediately after being seated in the dining room and cannot be adequately fed; another NH resident resists assistance at showering; a third screams every evening, thereby disturbing other residents' rest. An understanding of behavior problems and their management is therefore essential for the functioning of a NH, yet current research has only started to explore this area. In this chapter, we will review and analyze the current literature as it pertains to the following:

The definition and description of behavior problems in the frail elderly

Assessment of behavior problems

Prevalence of behavior problems

The authors acknowledge support from the National Institute on Aging grant AG-08675.

Characteristics of NH residents manifesting behavior problems
Management of behavior problems
Future directions in the management of behavior problems in the NH

DEFINITION AND DESCRIPTION OF
BEHAVIOR PROBLEMS IN THE FRAIL ELDERLY

Behavior problems in the frail elderly have been referred to as behavior disturbances, behavioral problems, disruptive behaviors, and agitation. The range of behaviors varied widely among different investigators. In 1986, Cohen-Mansfield and Billig defined agitation as inappropriate behavior, where the origin of the behavior is not apparent to an observer. It included behaviors that are abusive or aggressive; behaviors that would otherwise be appropriate, but are manifested at an inappropriate frequency, such as constant requests for attention; and behaviors that are under inappropriate stimulus control, such as disrobing in a public area. Several investigators (e.g., Reisberg et al., 1987b) also included psychiatric symptoms such as delusions and hallucinations.

There are several systems of classifying behavior problems. Based on a factor analysis, Cohen-Mansfield et al. (1989a) classified behavior problems into four syndromes: (a) aggressive behaviors, such as hitting or kicking, (b) physically nonaggressive behaviors such as aimless wandering or inappropriate disrobing, (c) verbally agitated behaviors such as repetitious phrases, and (d) hiding and hoarding. Zimmer et al. (1984) classified behaviors as disturbing behaviors, behaviors endangering self, and behaviors endangering others (used also by Winger et al., 1987). Other investigators classified subgroups of these behaviors. For example, Hussian and Brown (1987) identified four types of institutionalized wanderers: (a) akathisiacs, that is, neuroleptic-induced pacing and restlessness; (b) exit seekers, that is, newly admitted residents who try to open locked exit doors; (c) self-stimulators, that is, persons who perform other self-stimulating activities, such as turning doorknobs, in addition to pacing; and (d) modelers, or persons who tag onto other persons. Ryan et al. (1988) identified six categories of noise making among elderly residents of long-term care facilities: noise making that appears purposeless and perseverative, noise making that is a response to the environment, noise making that elicits a response from the environment, "chatterbox" noise making, noise making due to deafness, and other noise making.

ASSESSMENT OF BEHAVIOR PROBLEMS

Assessment of behavior problems is generally performed either through caregivers' ratings (including family caregivers or formal caregivers, i.e., institution staff members) or through direct observations. In comparison to observations, caregiver ratings usually assess the behavior over a longer time period and are easier to perform and therefore less costly. Their disadvantage lies in their subjective nature, that is, they capture caregivers' perceptions, which may be tainted by their relationship to the elderly person or by the burden they are experiencing. Direct observations are very costly, and if a behavior is infrequent, great amounts of observation time are needed to detect occurrences of the target behavior. Some observational studies have utilized videotapes (48,66). The advantage is that long periods of time can be taped, and the tapes can be scanned more quickly with a fast-forward mechanism. This system also has its disadvantages, however. If the videotaping is automatic, then no person may be in view for significant proportions of the videotape. If the videotaping is manual, a person carrying the camera and following residents has to be present throughout the videotaping sessions, rendering the procedure at least as costly and time consuming as direct observation.

Assessments that have a major focus on behavior problems are summarized in Table 11.1. Only instruments that were used more than once or for which reliability values were given were included in the table. There are many other instruments in which agitation is either an item or is represented in several items. For example, the Alzheimer's Disease Assessment Scale (ADAS) (56,73) has items concerning pacing, increased motor activity, delusions, and hallucinations.

As seen in Table 11.1, the most frequently utilized assessments are caregiver ratings using frequency rating scales. The assessment instruments vary on a number of dimensions: (a) *detail and degree to which the instrument is comprehensive:* the amount of detail provided by examining many different behaviors and the detail provided by the rating scale used; (b) *focus:* the extent to which instruments focus on behavior problems or on general decline in dementia; (c) *subscales:* the examination of the component subscales of the instrument; and (d) *validation:* the degree to which reliability and validity have been examined. These dimensions are discussed below.

Detail and Degree of Comprehensiveness

The different assessment instruments presented in Table 11.1 vary in the degree of detail and comprehensiveness provided. For example, the CMAI (19) includes 29 detailed disruptive behaviors as its items. The BEHAVE-AD (69) includes delusions and hallucinations, but is less detailed in examining other disruptive behaviors. Several instruments were not included in Table 11.1 because they only include a few items related to behavior problems. Some of these have nevertheless been frequently used in medication studies (79). For example, the Brief Psychiatric Rating Scale (BPRS) (6,62) and the Sandoz Clinical Assessment-Geriatric Scale (SCAG; 78,81) do not cover as many behavior problems as other instruments presented in Table 11.1. (Related items on the BPRS are: tension, mannerisms and posturing, hostility, suspiciousness, hallucinatory behavior, and uncooperativeness, out of 16 items, all rated on a severity rating scale. Related items on SCAG are: irritability, emotional lability, hostility, bothersome, and uncooperativeness, out of 19 items, rated on a severity scale.)

Most instruments use frequency rating scales, but these vary in their sensitivity, ranging from 3-point to 7-point scales. Several instruments measure other dimensions, including: severity, distress to staff, duration, and reaction (Table 11.1). In our experience, caregivers are more comfortable with very specific and detailed frequency rating scales (e.g., several times a day, several times an hour) than with the more general ones (e.g., never, sometimes, frequently). Additionally, because raters tend not to use the extreme categories, a larger number of categories allows a more detailed presentation of the variability in the sample. Obviously, such detail also has a cost, as raters need to become familiar with all categories of the rating scale and longer instruments require more time to complete. It is very important that each assessment instrument specify not only the scope of each behavior and the categories for rating it, but also the time frame the rater needs to consider when rating a person (e.g., Teri et al., 1989, considered behavior problems within the month prior to rating with a community-based sample; Cohen-Mansfield et al., 1989a, considered the 2 weeks prior to rating with a NH sample). This last consideration is not specified in some of the published instruments.

Focus

Several instruments examine decline in general and include items assessing cognitive decline in addition to those assessing behavior problems (e.g., Teri et al.'s, 1989, Behavioral Problems Checklist, which includes items relating to loss of memory and confusion; or Zarit & Zarit's, 1983, Memory and Behavior Problem Checklist, MBPC); some instruments have items pertaining to mood (e.g., Greene et al., 1982, Behavior and Mood Disturbance Scale, BMD; or Reisberg et al., 1987a, BEHAVE-AD), whereas others such as the Cohen-Mansfield Agitation Inventory (CMAI) concentrate specifically on behavior problems.

Subscales

In several instruments, subscales have been identified, most frequently through factor analytic techniques (19,24,30). The identification of subscales is of special importance, because although many behavior problems tend to co-occur, it seems that different types of behaviors represent different constructs and tend to be manifested in different subgroups of the NH population and occur under different environmental conditions. Therefore the summation of all behaviors into one score may be misleading for certain purposes, particularly for clinical practice.

Validation

Reliability measures vary greatly: Some use interrater, others utilize test-retest measures, and still others examine internal consistency within the instrument as in Cronbach alpha. Further, the actual values given represent either agreement rates, Pearson correlations, Kendall coefficients, or Kappa values. Whereas all the behavioral assessment instruments have face validity, other validation has usually not been investigated because of a lack of an adequate external measure. Baumgarten et al. (1990) established the validity of the Dementia Behavior Disturbance (DBD) scale by correlating scores with the active/disturbed subscale of Greene et al.'s (1982) BMD scale. The examination of behavior problems in relation to other constructs, such as cognitive impairment, and the convergence of these findings across studies suggest that several instruments have construct validity (e.g., CMAI) (20).

PREVALENCE OF BEHAVIOR PROBLEMS

Several studies examined the prevalence of behavior problems in institutional settings. Studies with a subject population of over 40 persons are summarized in Table 11.2. These studies ranged in their scope from the examination of 50 residents in one facility (75) to surveying 103 intermediate and skilled nursing facilities in Rhode Island and rating over 3,000 residents (41). Aside from the differences in the populations studied, there are major differences in the criteria used to ascertain a problem. For example, Zimmer et al. (1984) considered patients as having significant behavior problems if their care plan indicated that they required constant or active consideration in patient care for a behavior problem. Cohen-Mansfield et al. (1989a) considered the frequency at which 29 behavior problems were manifested during the 2 weeks prior to rating by nursing staff. Because of these vast differences in methodologies, different estimates of the prevalence of behavior problems are to be expected.

Despite the fluctuations in the prevalence rates reported in different studies, some generalizations can still be made. First, behavior problems are very frequent in the NH, with several studies citing rates of over 50% of the residents (75,96,99,102), and one definition (of one behavior manifested at a frequency of at least once a week) corresponding to a rate of about 90% (21). Second, although different studies examined different subtypes of behavior problems, there are general trends: General restlessness and verbal behaviors were the most common problems. Wandering was also quite frequent. Aggressive behaviors occurred in a significant proportion of residents, in a higher proportion than wandering (see Table 11.2). (Note, however, that Winger et al.'s [1987] estimates of aggressive behaviors are probably inflated, as the aggression scale included behaviors not considered aggressive in others' assessments, such as saying sarcastic things or refusing to eat.) This finding (of higher prevalence of aggression than wandering in Table 11.2) should, however, be interpreted cautiously because, although a larger number of persons may manifest aggressive behaviors, the frequency at which these behaviors are manifested is much lower (e.g., Cohen-Mansfield et al., 1989a; Cohen-Mansfield et al., 1991; Marx et al., 1990; U.S. Congress, 1987). Prevalence rates should generally be studied together with the frequency distribution of the behaviors under study. This approach is, however, quite rare. Samples from community-dwelling elderly persons reflect a slightly younger population, but do not seem to indicate lower rates of behavior problems (although the variation in methodology precludes a direct comparison). The high rates of behavior problems in studies of community-dwelling persons is due to the selection of only persons diagnosed as suffering from dementia in most of the community samples. Receiving a diagnosis of dementia may in itself reflect a selection process in which those who manifest behavior problems are most likely to be referred for evaluation.

CHARACTERISTICS OF RESIDENTS MANIFESTING BEHAVIOR PROBLEMS

The most commonly noted characteristic of NH residents manifesting behavior problems is that of dementia. For example, Zimmer et al. (1984) noted that 67% of those with serious behavior problems had a diagnosis of organic brain syndrome. Wandering was associated with cognitive deficits in NH (26,23) and community samples (24,89). One should note, however, (a) a large proportion of residents suffer from dementia, so that findings of a high percentage of demented persons among residents manifesting behavior problems could theoretically only reflect the populations studied rather than the specific phenomenon under investigation; and (b) not all demented individuals manifest behavior problems. Nevertheless, there appears to be a significant relationship between declining cognitive function and some behavior problems, such as aggression, screaming, wandering, and other physical (rather than verbal) forms of inappropriate behaviors (20,99). Similar findings have been reported in the community (10,11,37,64,71).

The characterization of the relationship between behavior problems and cognitive decline in terms of specific brain function or specific stage of dementia is yet to be clarified. Cohen-Mansfield et al. (1990b) found that the frequency of both aggressive behaviors and physically nonaggressive behavior problems correlated with the level of cognitive decline in a sample of NH residents. Similarly, Swearer et al. (1988), in a study of an Alzheimer's Disease and Related Disorders clinic of a hospital, reported that severity of behavior disturbances was related to the severity of dementia. Reisberg et al. (1989), in a study of patients from mixed settings, concluded that activity disturbances and aggression were seen most often in persons with moderately severe to severe levels of cognitive impairment, with secondary peaks in persons with very severe cognitive impairment. Burns et al. (1990b), in a study of Alzheimer's disease, found that aggression was associated with more severe temporal lobe atrophy and wandering was linked with increased size of the Sylvian fissure.

Different types of behavior problems have been associated with different characteristics of NH residents. Specifically, *aggressive behaviors* were associated with males, cognitive impairment, poor quality of social interactions, and manifestations of aggressive behaviors prior to NH entry (50). These findings are strengthened by Hamel et al.'s (1990) survey of community-dwelling persons in which aggression was related to memory problems, premorbid aggression, and a troubled premorbid social relationship between patient and caregiver. *Pacing and wandering* were associated with fewer medical diagnoses, better appetites, shorter length of stay in the NH, cognitive impairment, and past exposure to life-threatening experiences during the resident's lifetime (23). Snyder et al. (1978) found that wanderers had significantly greater involvement in nonsocial behaviors (i.e., behaviors that occur when alone and are not oriented to others) than nonwanderers. Monsour and Robb (1982) found that prior to the onset of incapacitating illness, wanderers (as compared to nonwanderers) were more likely to have expended physical energy in the pursuit of social/leisure activities, to have experienced more stressful events, and to have responded to stress with considerable psychomotor activity (rather than more emotional reactions). *Screaming* was associated with cognitive impairment, depressed affect, social networks of poor quality, sleep problems, physical pain, and severe impairment in the performance of activities of daily living (22). Similarly, Cariaga et al. (1991) reported that disruptive vocalizers in the NH were more functionally impaired, more likely to receive a diagnosis of dementia, and experienced more sleep disturbances than a comparison group of NH residents. Hallberg et al. (1990a) also reported that vocally disruptive behavior related significantly to physical dependence and to confusion. Based on a case study, Greenwald et al. (1986) suggested that screaming may be related to depression in elderly persons with dementia.

MANAGEMENT OF BEHAVIOR PROBLEMS

Several approaches have been utilized in an attempt to manage behavior problems: pharmacological, behavioral, environmental, stimulation, and others. These are described below.

Pharmacological Approaches

Although for 15 years or more, psychotropic drug use in the NH has been labeled as "chemical restraint," "drug misuse," "doping," or other pejorative terms, it has become the "standard of care" for residents with behavior problems. Jenike (1985, 1989) and others have argued that the use of psychotropic agents in the elderly must be undertaken with the same clinical care that is used in treating other medical conditions. Specific diagnosis based on careful evaluation should precede treatment. The physician should select a drug and the dosage to be used, based on the diagnosis and the characteristics of the patient. Drug effectiveness and the need for continued use must be monitored on a regular basis, with careful attention to side effects. Use of a single agent at a time is preferable to minimize side effects, particularly those due to drug-drug interactions.

Despite this widely repeated advice, recent descriptive studies listed in Table 11.3 show that about half of NH residents are prescribed psychotropic agents. These are conservative estimates of annual or lifetime risk of receiving these drugs, as exemplified by Lantz et al.'s (1990) finding that over a 5-year period, a total of 70% of NH residents received psychotropics at some point. Garrard et al. (1991) found that for half of those residents receiving antipsychotic agents there was no documentation of a condition justifying their use according to recently established federal criteria (38).

Including psychotropic agents, the average resident takes 4.7 different medications a day (83). In addition to antipsychotics, anxiolytics, antidepressants, and sedative-hypnotics, NH residents receive a wide variety of other drugs that may affect behavior. These include antihistamines, analgesics, antihypertensives, corticosteroids, anticonvulsants, and many others (4). For the purposes of this review, discussion is limited to those psychotropic drugs or substances administered specifically for the purpose of limiting or reducing problematic behavior.

Even where the patient record documents that the choice of a psychotropic agent and dose were appropriate for the diagnosis and condition of the patient, Johnson and DiBona (1990) were unable to find evidence of monitoring of the therapeutic effects or side effects of treatment. Changes in this situation are mandated by the interpretive guidelines implementing the 1989 Health Care Financing Administration regulations, which require documentation of diagnosis related to the problem behavior, monitoring of side effects, and attempts to reduce dose or discontinue use of psychotropic agents. At this time, NH facilities have just begun implementation of these efforts, and no reports of their effectiveness are yet available.

Despite the widespread use in the NH population, it is difficult to identify studies that demonstrate the effectiveness of psychotropic agents in terms of controlling behavior problems as opposed to changes in patient symptoms or sedation (61). A recent metaanalysis (79) of controlled trials of neuroleptic treatment in dementia suggests that neuroleptics had a small significant benefit over placebo accounting for 3.2% of the variance; there was no clear advantage of any specific medication. In the metaanalysis, only seven studies were found that used a double-blind, placebo-controlled, parallel-group design to assess subjects who probably had dementia. Group sizes ranged from 5 to 22, and study location varied across studies. According to Schneider et al. (1990), no significant difference between neuroleptic and placebo was obtained in any single study when analyzed by chi-squared tests, although the direction of effect was in favor of the neuroleptic in six of the seven reports. There was a high placebo response and medication nonresponse in many of the studies. Several studies reported clinical worsening or disabling side effects with neuroleptic treatment. An editorial accompanying this article points to the problems in conducting such a metaanalysis, including the varying definitions of behavior problems, and urges more research in this area (32). Indeed, the different studies utilized a variety of ratings, including clinical impressions, anxiety scales, and scales that assess psychopathology in general. All these studies taken together provide limited guidance for the practitioner confronted with an "unmanageable" patient.

We know little of the natural history of behavior problems. Rather, we have some limited data describing characteristics of those patients who are more likely to be treated with psychotropics (82), but we have no answers to questions like, "How long does a demented patient who screams manifest this behavior and need antipsychotic treatment?" If the monitoring required under the HCFA regulations is effective, we should have better information in future years.

Behavioral Approaches

Behavioral approaches apply behavioral principles such as contingent reinforcement, extinction, shaping, and discrimination to appropriate and inappropriate behaviors, in order to decrease the frequency of behavior problems or redirect the manifestations of these behaviors to appropriate circumstances. Several studies have demonstrated the use of these principles with behavior problems in older persons (see Table 11.4). Only one single-subject study utilized this approach in the NH (2). The only large study was by Mishara and Kastenbaum (1973); although innovative, this study did not specify cognitive level of the patients. The token economy utilized in this study would require substantial cognitive skills. However, many of those who manifest behavior problems in the NH are severely cognitively impaired. This brings up the broader question of the effect of dementia on learning and the implications for using behavioral approaches for demented persons. Although behavioral interventions have been used with NH residents to increase social behaviors and activities of daily living (1,72), finding reinforcers for this population may pose a problem (90). For the more cognitively intact residents, cognitive and self-control procedures have also been suggested (33). The understanding of the applicability of behavioral principles for this population and of their specific utilization in managing behavior problems awaits further study.

Environmental Approaches

Environmental interventions involve a change in the elderly person's environment that will (a) directly cause a change in the manifestation of the behavior problem or (b) change the impact of the behavior. An example of the first category is physical restraints, which have been shown to be associated with increased levels of behavior problems (97). In this case, the physical environment may be exacerbating the behavior problems, and the removal of physical restraints should decrease the manifestation of these behaviors. Another environmental attribute that may be contributing to behavior problems is the dreary institutional environment of NHs, which is frequently unaesthetic and uncomfortable (e.g., inappropriate chairs) for frail persons. A different example is the use of semilocked doors on units (using a lock that requires cognitive skills), so as to control the area in which wanderers can actually move. A fourth example is the use of a two-dimensional grid on the floor in front of the exit door that prevents exits through the door. This is the only environmental approach for which published intervention studies were found (13,40), and unfortunately, these were inconclusive in terms of the efficacy of this intervention (see Table 11.4).

The second category of environmental approaches to management of behavior problems involves changing the environment to accommodate the behaviors with minimal interference. Most of these interventions are provided for wanderers and include indoor or outdoor special areas for wandering (e.g., enclosed outdoor park), electronic monitors that alert caregivers to the person's passage through exit doors, and identity bracelets that help in relocating wanderers who get lost (68).

Stimulation, Activities, Exercise, and Music

Many approaches pertain to the delivery of care to older individuals. Some programs (7,52,100) provide stimulations such as music, touch, exercise, and activities to persons who may be bored or even suffering from stimulus deprivation because of the sterile and static environment in the NH. Cleary et al. (1988) combined reduction of stimulation (by eliminating telephones, radios, and televisions) with provision of structured times for activities and rest. Both of these approaches were successful with a small number of persons (see Table 11.4).

Other Approaches

Other approaches included individualization of care (65), enhanced instructions (39), a social skills training program (94), and a combination of approaches (25,54).

It should be noted that many of the "pure" approaches are actually combined approaches; for example, a behavioral management program that includes social reinforcement or even a token economy, by their very nature, increase the social activity and stimulation of participants. Carefully controlled studies need to be conducted to discern which component (or which combination of elements) is necessary to produce change in behavior problems in this population. Additional discussion of approaches to management of behavior problems can be found in Cohen-Mansfield (1989), Mace (1990), and Maletta (1988).

FUTURE DIRECTIONS IN THE MANAGEMENT OF BEHAVIOR PROBLEMS IN THE NH

As is evident from the above review, the understanding of behavior problems in elderly persons is still in its infancy. This stems from several reasons: (a) interest in this field is relatively recent; (b) NH residents suffer from multiple physical and emotional problems; (c) residents are frequently unable to communicate; and (d) research staff has to interact not only with the elderly person, but also with formal and/or informal caregivers and with the facility in which the person resides. All these factors make the investigation of behavior problems in this population very complex.

The understanding of behavior problems in residents is crucial for deciding which behaviors are to be considered problem behaviors. For example, several researchers (23,49) have suggested that wandering may be an adaptive behavior in the face of cognitive decline, as it provides exercise and stimulation to people who would otherwise suffer from inactivity and boredom. If wandering is adaptive for the elderly person, then caregivers need to learn to accommodate it through both environmental changes and changes in their own attitudes.

A second crucial component of the study of behavior problems is the differentiation between actual behavior problems and those that are directly related to a medical condition, such as physical pain (18), which should be treated. Similarly, the role of medication in causing or exacerbating behavior problems needs to be assessed. Third, the impact of environmental attributes, such as furnishings or room temperature levels, needs to be investigated. Finally, as is all too clear from Table 11.4, larger and better designed intervention studies are needed to ascertain the utility of available interventions for managing specific behavior problems within the heterogeneous population of the NH.

REFERENCES

1. Baltes, M. M., & Barton, E. M. (1977). New approaches toward aging: A case for the operant model. *Educational Gerontology, 2,* 383-405.
2. Baltes, M. M., & Lascomb, S. L. (1975). Creating a healthy institutional environment for the elderly via behavior management: The nurse as a change agent. *International Journal of Nursing Studies, 12,* 5-12.
3. Baumgarten, M., Becker, R., & Gauthier, S. (1990). Validity and reliability of the Dementia Behavior Disturbance scale. *Journal of the American Geriatrics Society 38(3),* 221-226.
4. Beardsley, R., Larson, D., Burns, B., et al. (1989). Prescribing of psychotropics in elderly nursing home patients. *Journal of the American Geriatrics Society, 37,* 327-330.
5. Beers, M., Avorn, J., Soumerai, S. B., et al. (1988). Psychoactive medication use in intermediate-care facility residents. *Journal of the American Medical Association, 260(20),* 3016-3020.
6. Beller, S. A., & Overall, J. E. (1984). The Brief Psychiatric Rating Scale in geropsychiatric research: 2. Representative profile patterns. *Journal of Gerontology, 39(2),* 194-200.
7. Birchmore, T., & Clague, S. (1983). A behavioural approach to reduce shouting. *Nursing Times, 79,* 37-39.
8. Buck, J. (1988). Psychotropic drug practice in nursing homes. *Journal of the American Geriatrics Society, 36,* 409-418.
9. Burgio, L. D., Jones, L. T., Butler, F., et al. (1988). Behavior problems in an urban nursing home. *Journal of Gerontological Nursing, 14(1),* 31-34.
10. Burns, A., Jacoby, R., & Levy, R. (1990a). Behavioral abnormalities and psychiatric symptoms in Alzheimer's disease: Preliminary findings. *International Psychogeriatrics, 2,* 25-36.

11. Burns, A., Jacoby, R., & Levy, R. (1990b). Psychiatric phenomena in Alzheimer's disease: 4. Disorder of behaviour. *British Journal of Psychiatry, 157*, 86-94.

12. Cariaga, J., Burgio, L., Flynn, W., et al. (1991). A controlled study of disruptive vocalizations among geriatric residents in nursing homes. *Journal of the American Geriatrics Society, 39*, 501-507.

13. Chafetz, P. K. (1990). Two-dimensional grid is ineffective against demented patients' exiting through glass doors. *Psychology and Aging, 5*(1), 146-147.

14. Chafetz, P. K., & West, H. L. (1987). *Longitudinal control group evaluation of a special care unit for dementia patients: Initial findings.* Paper presented at the 40th Annual Scientific Meeting of the Gerontological Society of America, Washington, DC.

15. Cleary, T. A., Clamon, C., Price, M., et al. (1988). A reduced stimulation unit: Effects on patients with Alzheimer's disease and related disorders. *Gerontologist, 28*(4), 511-514.

16. Cohen-Mansfield, J. (1989). Agitation in the elderly. In N. Billig & P. Rabins (Eds.), *Advances in psychosomatic medicine: Geriatric psychiatry* (pp. 101-113). Basel, Switzerland: S. Karger.

17. Cohen-Mansfield, J., & Billig, N. (1986). Agitated behaviors in the elderly: 1. A conceptual review. *Journal of the American Geriatrics Society, 34*(10), 711-721.

18. Cohen-Mansfield, J., Billig, N., Lipson, S., et al. (1990a). Medical correlates of agitation in nursing home residents. *Gerontology, 36*(3), 150-158.

19. Cohen-Mansfield, J., Marx, M. S., & Rosenthal, A. S. (1989a). A description of agitation in a nursing home. *Journals of Gerontology: Medical Sciences, 44*(3), M77-M84.

20. Cohen-Mansfield, J., Marx, M. S., & Rosenthal, A. S. (1990b). Dementia and agitation in nursing home residents: How are they related? *Psychology and Aging, 5*(1), 3-8.

21. Cohen-Mansfield, J., Werner, P., & Marx, M. S. (1989b). An observational study of agitation in agitated nursing home residents. *International Psychogeriatrics, 1*(2), 153-165.

22. Cohen-Mansfield, J., Werner, P., & Marx, M. S. (1990c). Screaming in nursing home residents. *Journal of the American Geriatrics Society, 38*, 785-792.

23. Cohen-Mansfield, J., Werner, P., Marx, M. S., et al. (1991). Two studies of pacing in the nursing home. *Journals of Gerontology: Medical Sciences, 46*(3), M77-M83.

24. Cooper, J. K., Mungas, D., & Weiler, P. G. (1990). Relation of cognitive status and abnormal behaviors in Alzheimer's disease. *Journal of the American Geriatrics Society, 38*, 867-870.

25. Davis, A. (1983). Behavioural techniques for elderly patients: 2. *Nursing Times, 43*, 26-27.

26. Dawson, P., & Reid, D. W. (1987). Behavioral dimensions of patients at risk of wandering. *Gerontologist, 27*(1), 104-107.

27. Donat, D. C. (1986). Modifying wandering behavior: A case study. *Clinical Gerontologist, 6*, 41-43.

28. Evans, L. K. (1987). Sundown syndrome in institutionalized elderly. *Journal of the American Geriatrics Society, 35*, 101-108.

29. Garrard, J., Makris, L., Dunham, T., et al. (1991). Evaluation of neuroleptic drug use by nursing home elderly under proposed Medicare and Medicaid regulations. *Journal of the American Medical Association, 265*, 463-467.

30. Greene, J. G., Smith, R., Gardiner, M., et al. (1982). Measuring behavioural disturbance of elderly demented patients in the community and its effects on relatives: A factor analytic study. *Age and Ageing, 11*, 121-126.

31. Greenwald, B. S., Marin D. B., & Silverman, S. M. (1986, December). Serotoninergic treatment of screaming and banging in dementia. *Lancet, 20*(27), 1464-1465.

32. Grossberg, G. T. (1990). The pitfalls of meta-analysis. *Journal of the American Geriatrics Society, 38,* 607.
33. Haley, W. E. (1983). Behavioral self-management: Application to a case of agitation in an elderly chronic psychiatric patient. *Clinical Gerontologist, 1*(3), 45-52.
34. Haley, W. E., Brown, S. L., & Levine, E. G. (1987). Family caregiver appraisals of patient behavioral disturbance in senile dementia. *Clinical Gerontologist, 6*(4), 25-34.
35. Hallberg, I. R., Norberg, A., & Eriksson, S. (1990a). A comparison between the care of vocally disruptive patients and that of other residents in psychogeriatric wards. *Journal of Advanced Nursing, 15,* 410-416.
36. Hallberg, I. R., Norberg, A., & Eriksson, S. (1990b). Functional impairment and behavioural disturbances in vocally disruptive patients in psychogeriatric wards compared with controls. *International Journal of Geriatric Psychiatry, 5,* 53-61.
37. Hamel, M., Gold, D. P., Andres, D., et al. (1990). Predictors and consequences of aggressive behavior by community-based dementia patients. *Gerontologist, 30*(2), 206-211.
38. Health Care Financing Administration. (1989). Medicare and Medicaid: Requirements for long term care facilities. *Federal Register, 54,* 5316-5336.
39. Hussian, R. A. (1988). Modification of behaviors in dementia via stimulus manipulation. *Clinical Gerontologist, 8*(1), 37-43.
40. Hussian, R. A., & Brown, D. C. (1987). Use of two-dimensional grid patterns to limit hazardous ambulation in demented patients. *Journal of Gerontology, 42*(5), 558-560.
41. Jackson, M. E., Drugovich, M. L., Fretwell, M. D., et al. (1989). Prevalence and correlates of disruptive behavior in the nursing home. *Journal of Aging and Health, 1*(3), 349-369.
42. Jenike, M. A. (1985). *Handbook of geriatric psychopharmacology.* Littleton, MA: PSG.
43. Jenike, M. A. (1989). *Geriatric psychiatry and psychopharmacology: A clinical approach.* Chicago: Year Book Publishers.
44. Johnson, J. F., & DiBona, J. R. (1990). A concurrent quality assurance review of psychotropic prescribing in elderly patients: Process and outcome measures. *Journal of Geriatric Drug Therapy, 4*(4), 43-80.
45. Lantz, M., Louis, A., Lowenstein, G., et al. (1990). A longitudinal study of psychotropic prescriptions in a teaching nursing home. *American Journal of Psychiatry, 147*(12), 1637-1639.
46. Mace, N. L. (1990). The management of problem behaviors. In N. L. Mace (Ed.), *Dementia care: Patient, family, and community* (pp. 74-112). Baltimore, MD: Johns Hopkins University Press.
47. Maletta, G. J. (1988). Management of behavior problems in elderly patients with Alzheimer's disease and other dementias. *Clinics in Geriatric Medicine, 8*(4), 719-747.
48. Martino-Saltzman, D. (1989). Systematic observation of wandering behavior. *Gerontologist, 29*(128) Special Issue, 141A-142A.
49. Martino-Saltzman, D. (1990). When managed, wandering can help residents. *Brown University Long Term Care Letter, 2*(6), 5-6.
50. Marx, M. S., Cohen-Mansfield, J., & Werner, P. (1990). A profile of the aggressive nursing home resident. *Behavior Health and Aging, 1*(1), 65-73.
51. Mayers, K., & Griffin, M. (1990). The play project: Use of stimulus objects with demented patients. *Journal of Gerontological Nursing, 16*(1), 32-37.
52. McGrowder-Lin, R., & Bhatt, A. (1988). A wanderer's lounge program for nursing home residents with Alzheimer's disease. *Gerontologist, 28*(5), 607-609.

53. Meer, B., & Baker, J. A. (1966). The Stockton Geriatric Rating Scale. *Journal of Gerontology, 21*, 392-403.

54. Mentes, J. C., & Ferrario, J. (1989). Calming aggressive reactions: A preventive program. *Journal of Gerontological Nursing, 15*(2), 22-27.

55. Mishara, B. L., & Kastenbaum, R. (1973). Self-injurious behavior and environmental change in the institutionalized elderly. *International Journal of Aging and Human Development, 4*(2), 133-145.

56. Mohs, R. C., & Cohen, J. (1988). Alzheimer's Disease Assessment Scale (ADAS). *Psychopharmacology Bulletin, 24*(4), 627-628.

57. Monsour, N., & Robb, S. S. (1982, September). Wandering behavior in old age: A psychosocial study. *Social Work, 27*(5), 411-416.

58. Moore, J. T., Bobula, J. A., Short, T. B., et al. (1983). A functional dementia scale. *Journal of Family Practice, 16*(3), 499-503.

59. Mungas, D., Weiler, P., Franzi, C., et al. (1989). Assessment of disruptive behavior associated with dementia: The disruptive behavior rating scales. *Journal of Geriatric Psychiatry and Neurology, 2*(4), 196-202.

60. Niederehe, G. (1988). TRIMS behavioral checklist (BPC). *Psychopharmacology Bulletin, 24*(4), 771-778.

61. Olsen, R. B., Gydesen, S. U., Kristensen, M., et al. (1990). Psychotropic medication in the elderly: A survey of prescribing and clinical outcome. *Danish Medical Bulletin, 37*(5), 455-459.

62. Overall, J. E., & Gorham, D. R. (1962). The Brief Psychiatric Rating Scale. *Psychological Reports, 10*, 799-812.

63. Palmstierna, T., & Wistedt, B. (1987). Staff Observation Aggression Scale, SOAS: Presentation and evaluation. *Acta Psychiatrica Scandinavica, 76*, 657-663.

64. Patterson, M. B., Schnell, A. H., Martin, R. J., et al. (1990). Assessment of behavioral and affective symptoms in Alzheimer's disease. *Journal of Geriatric Psychiatry and Neurology, 3*, 21-30.

65. Raber, W. C., Lamboo, F., & Mitchell-Pederson, L. (1987). From duckling to swan. *Clinical Gerontologist (Special Issue: The elderly uncooperative patient), 6*(2), 179-188.

66. Rabinovich, B., Cohen-Mansfield, J., & Stein, B. (1990). The relationship between structured activities and agitated behavior: An observational study. *Gerontologist, 30*(85) Special Issue, 94A-95A.

67. Rabins, P. V., Mace, N. L., & Lucas, M. J. (1982). The impact of dementia on the family. *Journal of the American Medical Association, 248*(3), 333-335.

68. Rader, J. (1987). A comprehensive staff approach to problem wandering. *Gerontologist, 27*(6), 756-760.

69. Reisberg, B., Borenstein, J., Franssen, E., et al. (1987a). BEHAVE-AD: A clinical rating scale for the assessment of pharmacologically remediable behavioral symptomatology in Alzheimer's disease. In J. J. Altman (Ed.), *Alzheimer's disease: Problems, prospects, and perspectives* (pp.1-16). New York: Plenum.

70. Reisberg, B., Borenstein, J., Salob, S. P., et al. (1987b). Behavioral symptoms in Alzheimer's disease: Phenomenology and treatment. *Journal of Clinical Psychiatry, 45*(5), 9-15.

71. Reisberg, B., Franssen, E., Sclan, S. G., et al. (1989). Stage specific incidence of potentially remediable behavioral symptoms in aging and Alzheimer disease: A study of 120 patients using the BEHAVE-AD. *Bulletin of Clinical Neurosciences, 54*, 95-112.

72. Rosberger, Z., & MacLean, J. (1983). Behavioral assessment and treatment of "organic" behaviors in an institutionalized geriatric patient. *International Journal of Behavioral Geriatrics, 1*(4), 33-46.

73. Rosen, W. G., Mohs, R. C., & Davis, K. L. (1984). A new rating scale for Alzheimer's disease. *American Journal of Psychiatry, 141*(11), 1356-1364.
74. Rovner, B., German, P., Broadhead, J., et al. (1990). The prevalence and management of dementia and other psychiatric disorders in nursing homes. *International Psychogeriatrics, 2*(1), 13-24.
75. Rovner, B. W., Kafonek, S., Filipp, L., et al. (1986). Prevalence of mental illness in a community nursing home. *American Journal of Psychiatry, 143*(11), 1446-1449.
76. Ryan, D. P., Tainsh, S. M. M., Kolodny, V., et al. (1988). Noise-making among the elderly in long-term care. *Gerontologist, 28*(3), 369-371.
77. Ryden, M. (1988). Aggressive behavior in persons with dementia who live in the community. *Alzheimer's Disease and Associated Disorders, 2,* 342-355.
78. Salzman, C. (1983). The Sandoz Clinical Assessment Geriatric scale. In T. Crook, S. Ferris, & R. Bartus (Eds.), *Assessment in geriatric psychopharmacology* (pp. 53-58). New Canaan, CT: Mark Powley.
79. Schneider, L. S., Pollock, V. E., & Lyness, S. A. (1990). A meta-analysis of controlled trials of neuroleptic treatment in dementia. *Journal of the American Geriatrics Society, 38,* 553-563.
80. Sclan, S. G. (1993). *Reliability and score analysis of behavioral symptoms of Alzheimer's disease.* Paper presented at the 140th Meeting of the American Psychological Association, San Francisco, CA.
81. Shader, R. I., Harmatz, J. S., & Salzman, C. (1974). A new scale for clinical assessment in geriatric populations: Sandoz Clinical Assessment-Geriatric (SCAG). *Journal of the American Geriatrics Society, 22,* 107-113.
82. Sloane, P. D., & Mathew, L. J. (1991). An assessment and care planning strategy for nursing home residents with dementia. *Gerontologist, 31*(1), 128-131.
83. Sloane, P. D., Mathew, L. J., Scarborough, M., et al. (1991). Physical and pharmacologic restraint of nursing home patients with dementia. *Journal of the American Medical Association, 265*(10), 1278-1282.
84. Snyder, L. H., Rupprecht, P., Pyrek, J., et al. (1978). Wandering. *Gerontologist, 18*(3), 272-280.
85. Spector, W. D. (1991). Cognitive impairment and disruptive behaviors among community-based elderly persons: Implications for targeting long-term care. *Gerontologist, 31*(1), 51-59.
86. Sternberg, J., Spector, W. D., Drugovich, M. L., et al. (1990). Use of psychoactive drugs in nursing homes: Prevalence and residents' characteristics. *Journal of Geriatric Drug Therapy, 4*(4), 47-60.
87. Swearer, J. M., Drachman, D. A., O'Donnell, B. F., et al. (1988). Troublesome and disruptive behaviors in dementia: Relationships to diagnosis and disease severity. *Journal of the American Geriatrics Society, 36*(9), 784-789.
88. Teri, L., Borson, S., Kiyak, H. A., et al. (1989). Behavioral disturbance, cognitive dysfunction, and functional skill: Prevalence and relationship in Alzheimer's disease. *Journal of the American Geriatrics Society, 37, 109-116.*
89. Teri, L., Larson, E. B., & Reifler, B. V. (1988). Behavioral disturbance in dementia of the Alzheimer's type. *Journal of the American Geriatrics Society, 36*(1), 1-6.
90. Teri, L., & Logsdon, R. G. (1991). Identifying pleasant activities for Alzheimer's disease patients: The Pleasant Events Schedule-AD. *Gerontologist, 31*(1), 124-127.
91. U.S. Congress. Office of Technology Assessment. (1987, April). *Losing a million minds: Confronting the tragedy of Alzheimer's disease and other dementias* (OTA-BA-323). Washington, DC: U.S. Government Printing Office.

92. Vaccaro, F. J. (1988a). Application of operant procedures in a group of institution-alized aggressive geriatric patients. *Psychology and Aging, 3*(1), 22-28.
93. Vaccaro, F. J. (1988b). Successful operant conditioning procedures with an insti-tutionalized aggressivegeriatric patient. *International Journal of Aging and Human Development, 26*(1), 71-79.
94. Vaccaro, F. J. (1990). Application of social skills training in a group of institution-alized aggressive elderly subjects. *Psychology and Aging, 5*(3), 369-378.
95. Verstraten, F. J. (1988). The GIP: An observational ward behavior scale. *Psycho-pharmacology Bulletin, 24*(4), 717-719.
96. Wayne, S. J., Rhyne, R. L., Thompson, R. E., et al. (1991). Sampling issues in nursing home research. *Journal of the American Geriatrics Society, 39*, 308-311.
97. Werner, P., Cohen-Mansfield, J., Braun, J., et al. (1989). Physical restraints and agitation in nursing home residents. *Journal of the American Geriatrics Society, 37*(12), 1122-1126. Also published in *Restraints and the frail elderly patient: Practical considerations for hospitals and nursing homes*. Hospital Association of New York State, June 1990, pp. 155-159.
98. Wilkinson, I. M., & Graham-White, J. (1980). Psychogeriatric dependency rating scales (PGDRS): A method of assessment for use by nurses. *British Journal of Psychiatry, 137*, 558-565.
99. Winger, J., Schirm, V., & Stewart, D. (1987). Aggressive behavior in long-term care. *Journal of Psychosocial Nursing, 25*(4), 28-33.
100. Zachow, K. M. (1984). Helen, can you hear me? *Journal of Gerontological Nursing, 10*(8), 18-22.
101. Zarit, S. H., & Zarit, J. M. (1983). Cognitive impairment. In P. M. Lewinsohn & L. Teri (Eds.), *Clinical geropsychology* (pp. 38-81). New York: Pergamon.
102. Zimmer, J. G., Watson, N., & Treat, A. (1984). Behavioral problems among patients in skilled nursing facilities. *American Journal of Public Health, 74*(10), 1118-1119.

Table 11.1A Assessment Instruments—Caregiver Ratings

Assessment	Facility	# Items	Measure	Scales and Items (pertaining to behavior problems)	Reliability
In Institutional Settings					
Chafetz & West, 1987	LTC	29: 21 tap behavior problems	7-pt frequency	*Excesses:* physical aggression, self-injurious behavior, climbing, fecal smearing or digging, excessive movement, distressed facial expression, excessive speech, loud speech, complaining about self *Stimulus control:* inappropriate voiding, inappropriate masturbation, trespassing within unit, unauthorized exit from unit, exposure, spitting, inappropriate sexual advances, awake at night and disturbing others, complaining about external things or other people, unkind speech, multiple dressing *Deficits:* difficulty cooperating with staff	Interrater: Kendall's coefficient ranged from .35 to .80 for Excesses, .38 to .79 for Control, .27 to .64 for Deficits
Cohen-Mansfield Agitation Inventory (CMAI) (Cohen-Mansfield et al., 1989a)	SNF	29	7-pt frequency	*Aggressive behaviors:* hitting, kicking, pushing, scratching, grabbing, tearing things, biting, spitting, cursing, hurting self or others *Physically nonaggressive behaviors:* inappropriate robing/disrobing, repetitious mannerisms, trying to get to a different place, pacing, handling things inappropriately, general restlessness, throwing things	Interrater agreement rate=.92

continued

293

Table 11.1A Continued

Assessment	Facility	# Items	Measure	Scales and Items (pertaining to behavior problems)	Reliability
				Verbally agitated behaviors: complaining, constant requests for attention, negativism, repetitious sentences or questions, screaming, strange noises *Other behaviors:* hiding, hoarding, intentional falling, eating/drinking inappropriate substances, verbal sexual advances, physical sexual advances	
Stockton Geriatric Rating Scale (SGRS) (Meer & Baker, 1966)	Hospital	33: 8 tap behavior problems	3-pt frequency	*Socially Irritating Behavior (SIB):* objectionable during the day, makes repetitive vocal sounds, threatens verbally to harm others, objectionable during the night, accuses others of harm, destructive of surrounding materials, engages in useless repetitive motor activity, hoards meaningless items	Interrater reliability for SIB: $r = .75$
Functional Dementia Scale (FDS) (Moore et al., 1983)	LTC	20: 8 tap behavior problems	4-pt frequency	*Orientation:* wanders at night, wanders during day *Affect:* hears things, threatens others, destructive, shouts or yells, accuses others, moans	Interrater agreement for the 8 items from 76% to 90%, test-retest over 2 weeks for the 8 items: $.31 < r < .75$
Disruptive Behavior Rating Scale (DBRS) (Mungas et al., 1989)	SNF	21	5-pt severity; 3-pt distress to staff	*Physical aggression:* hitting, kicking, biting, spitting, throwing things, using weapons, other physical aggression	Interrater: $.71 < r < .93$

				Verbal aggression: yelling and screaming, swearing, threatening physical harm, criticizing, scolding, other verbal aggression *Agitation:* pacing, hand wringing, inability to sit or lie still, rapid speech, increased psychomotor activity, repeated expressions of distress, other signs of agitation *Wandering* (includes walking aimlessly in areas that are not authorized)	
GIP (Verstraten, 1988)	Psychogeriatric units	82: half tap behavior problems	4-pt frequency	Scales (a mean of 6 items per scale) pertain to: loss of decorum, rebellious behavior, senseless repetitive behavior, restless behavior, suspicious behavior, anxious behavior, nonsocial behavior	Interrater: $.53 < r < .90$ Cronbach alpha from .61 to .90
Psychogeriatric Dependency Rating Scales (PGDRS) (Wilkinson & Graham-White, 1980)	Psychogeriatric & LTC units; community dwelling	26: 15 of these tap behavior problems	3-pt frequency	*Behavior section:* disruptive, manipulating, wandering, demanding interaction, communication difficulties, noisy, active aggression, passive aggression, verbal aggression, restless, destructive (property), destructive (self), delusions/hallucinations, socially objectionable, speech content	Interrater: Kappa from .40 to .63 (for Behavior section)
In the Community					
Dementia Behavior Disturbance Scale (DBD) (Baumgarten et al., 1990)	Community residing seen at geriatric assessment unit	28: 22 of these tap behavior problems	5-pt frequency	Items: Asks same question repeatedly; loses, misplaces, or hides things; makes unwarranted accusations; paces up and down; repeats same action over and over; verbally abusive, curses; dresses inappropriately; cries or	Test-retest over 2 weeks for entire DBD: $r = .71$

continued

Table 11.1A Continued

Assessment	Facility	# Items	Measure	Scales and Items (pertaining to behavior problems)	Reliability
				laughs inappropriately; refuses to be helped with personal care; hoards things for no obvious reason; moves arms/legs in restless or agitated way; empties drawers/closets; wanders in the house at night; gets lost outside; refuses to eat; wanders aimlessly outside or in house during day; makes physical attacks; screams for no reason; makes inappropriate sexual advances; exposes private body parts; destroys property or clothing; throws food	
Behavior and Mood Disturbance (BMD) Scale (Greene et al., 1982)	Psychiatric day hospital	34: 10 of these tap behavior problems	5-pt frequency or severity	*Active-Disturbed Behavior:* has to be prevented from wandering outside the house, hoards useless things, talks nonsense, appears restless and agitated, gets lost in the house, wanders outside the house at night, wanders outside house and gets lost, endangers self, paces and wrings hands, talks aloud to self	Test-retest over 3 weeks for entire Active-Disturbed subscale (15 items): $r = .87$
Behavior Problem Checklist (BPC) (Niederehe, 1988)	Private home	52: 16 of these tap behavior problems	5-pt frequency 5-pt duration 5-pt reaction	Items: Asks same questions over and over again, auditory hallucinations, visual hallucinations, suspicious/accusative, verbal threats to another person, threats to harm self, restless/agitated, shout/yell, take/hide/hoard, wander, destroy property, uncooperative, temper outbursts, physical threats to others, physically aggressive, inappropriate sexual behavior	Cronbach's alpha for the 52 items = .93

Measure	Population	Number of items	Response format	Items/categories	Reliability
Behavioral Pathology in Alzheimer's Disease Rating Scale (BEHAVE-AD) (Reisberg et al., 1987b)	Out-patients at an aging and dementia research center	25: 18 of these tap behavior problems	4-pt severity	Symptomatic categories are: paranoid and delusional ideation (7 items), hallucinations (5 items), activity disturbances (3 items), and aggressivity (3 items)	Rater agreement coefficient for BEHAVE-AD total score=.96 (Sclan et al., 1993)
Ryden Aggression Scale (RAS) (Ryden, 1988)	Community dwelling	25	6-pt frequency	*Physical aggression:* threatening gestures, pushing/shoving, throwing an object, damaging property, pinching/squeezing, hitting/punching, elbowing, slapping, kicking, brandishing a weapon, striking a person with an object, spitting, biting, scratching, tackling, using a weapon *Verbal aggression:* hostile/accusatory language, cursing directed at a person, verbal threats, name calling *Sexual aggression:* hugging, kissing, touching body parts, intercourse, making obscene gestures	Test-retest (interval of 8-12 weeks)=.86
Behavioral Problems Checklist (BPC) (Teri et al., 1989)	Community-residing patients with Alzheimer's disease	48: 21 of these tap behavior problems	5-pt frequency	Items: Overactive, pacing; tendency to wander off and get lost; verbally aggressive to others; tense, jittery; follows strict rituals in behavior; unpredictable behavior; unusual mannerisms or facial expressions; refusal to eat; unpredictable crying; grandiose, unreal thoughts about himself/herself; belief there was a conspiracy against him/her; hearing imaginary voices; destruction of	Test-retest over 1 week=.90

continued

Table 11.1A Continued

Assessment	Facility	# Items	Measure	Scales and Items (pertaining to behavior problems)	Reliability
				property; seeing imaginary things or people; feeling of being watched or talked about by others; threats to hurt oneself; attempts to hurt others; threats to hurt others; attempts to hurt himself/herself; unpredictable giggling; inappropriate dress	
Memory and Behavior Problems Checklist (MBPC) (Zarit & Zarit, 1983)	Community residing	29: 11 of these tap behavior problems	6-pt frequency 5-pt caregiver distress	Items: Wandering or getting lost; asking repetitive questions; hiding things; being suspicious or accusative; losing or misplacing things; not completing tasks; destroying property; being constantly restless; constantly talkative; engaging in behavior that is potentially dangerous to others/self; seeing/hearing things that are not there	Test-retest: Frequency=.80 Distress=.56

298

Table 11.1B Assessment Instruments—Direct Observations

Assessment	Facility	Behaviors Assessed	Aspects Assessed	Reliability
Agitation Behavior Mapping Instrument (ABMI) (Cohen-Mansfield et al., 1989b)	SNF	Requests for attention; strange noises, constant talk, babble, screaming, crying or weeping; negative, complains; walks aimlessly, paces; strange movements, makes faces; walks, stands, or sits when inappropriate; hides things; repetitious mannerisms; robes inappropriately; disrobes inappropriately; peeps; tries to get to a different place; moves toward someone, touches or rubs against; throws things, picks at things, grabs onto things; total rigidity; tries to get out of restraints; refusals or uncooperative; aggressive: hurts self or others, tears things, pushes or pulls people, bites or scratches, etc.; other inappropriate behavior	Direction, Social environment, Reaction, Activity and initiation, Body position, Location, Physical environment	Interobserver agreement rates for the behaviors on the ABMI averaged .93
Confusion Inventory (Evans, 1987)	SNF and ICF	Wandering, tapping, picking at bedclothes, scratching, rubbing self or object, banging, attempting to remove restraints, screaming, crying, calling for help, etc.	Psychomotor and psychosocial behavioral indicators of mental confusion	Interrater reliability in a pretest from .86 to .93
Staff Observation Aggression Scale (SOAS) (Palmstierna & Wistedt, 1987)	Psychogeriatric long-stay wards	Aggressive behaviors	Provocation, means used by patient, aim of aggression, consequence(s) for victim(s), measure to stop aggression	Intraclass correlation, r=.96

Table 11.2A Prevalence of Behavior Problems—Institutional Setting

Reference	Facility/Population	Demographics	Overall Agitation	Aggression	Wandering	Verbal Behaviors	Other[1]
Burgio et al., 1988	LTC N=160	60 years and older		26% tantrum-like behaviors 20% physical aggression 9% self-injurious 4% property destruction 3% spilling	10% wandering	22% verbal abuse	DIS 14% SEX 7%
Cariaga et al., 1991	2 LTC facilities N=700					11% disruptive vocalizations	
Cohen-Mansfield et al., 1989a, 1990c, 1991; Marx et al., 1990a	SNF N=408	Mean age=85 23% M, 77% F 100% Jewish	93% manifested one or more agitated behaviors at least once a week	49% were categorized as aggressive	39% of the residents paced (out of 402)	25% of the residents screamed at least once a week	
Hallberg et al., 1990a, 1990b	Psychogeriatric hospital wards N=264					15% exhibited vocally disruptive behavior	
Jackson et al., 1989	ICFs and SNFs in Rhode Island N=3,351	94% over 65 23% M, 77% F 98% white	26% engaged in at least one disruptive behavior over a 2-week period	12% abusiveness	6% wandering	10% noisiness	

Rovner et al., 1986	ICF N=50 94% had a major psychiatric disorder, most often dementia	Mean age=83 16% M, 84% F 98% white	76% manifested at least one behavioral problem	26% active aggression 14% self-destructive	24% wandering	26% verbal aggression 24% noisy behaviors 36% demands interaction 20% incoherent speech	DEL/HAL 38% DIS 34% REST 38%
Ryan et al., 1988	2 LTC facilities N=400 (pilot study) N=636 (replication study)					10% noise making that is purposeless and perseverative 5% noise making that elicits a response from the environment 2% "chatterbox" noise making	
Sloane & Matthew, 1991	32 nonspecialized nursing home units N=318, all with a diagnosis of dementia	Mean age=83.2 15% M, 82% F 87% white	30% major disruptive behaviors				

continued

Table 11.2A Continued

Reference	Facility/ Population	Demographics	Overall Agitation	Aggression	Wandering	Verbal Behaviors	Other[1]
Wayne et al., 1991	3 university-affiliated community nursing homes N=112	Mean age=76 39% M, 61% F 67% diagnosis of dementia		61% exhibited inappropriate (aggressive/violent) behavior			
Winger et al., 1987	LTC units of a VA medical center N=43 (NH) N=58 (intermediate care)	Mean age=69 (nursing home) 64 (intermediate care) 97% M, 3% F		91% of the nursing home patients and 66% of the intermediate care manifested a form of aggressive behavior[2]			
Zimmer et al., 1984	42 skilled nursing facilities N=1,139	Median age=84	64% moderate and serious behavior problems	8.3% physically aggressive behaviors 4.3% physical self-abuse 0.4% indirectly endangering others	5.4% dangerous ambulation 3.8% inappropriate ambulation	12.6% verbal behaviors such as noisy	DIS 2% HOR 0.6% NEG 11% SEX 0.4%

Table 11.2B Prevalence of Behavior Problems—In the Community

References	Facility/ Population	Demographics	Overall Agitation	Aggression	Wandering	Verbal/Vocal	Other[1]
Baumgarten et al., 1990	96 community-residing patients, all diagnosed as having dementia or Alzheimer's disease (AD)	Mean age=73 45% M, 55% F		7% makes physical attacks 3% destroys property	27% paces up and down 15% wanders at night 10% wanders during day 13% gets lost outside	72% repetitious questions 33% unwarranted accusations 25% verbally abusive 20% cries or laughs inappropriately 6% screams	DRES 24% HAND 15%, 1%, HID 65% HOR 19% NEG 20%, 12% REST 26%, 18% SEX 5%
Burns et al., 1990a, 1990b	178 community-dwelling, residential homes, and long-stay care; all had AD			20% aggressive 35% going into rages	18% wanderers		DEL 16% HAL visual 13%, auditory 9%, SEX 7%
Haley et al., 1987	44 community-dwelling patients, all cognitively impaired	Mean age=79		32% dangerous to self 11% dangers to others 9% destroy property	41% wandering	77% repetitive questions 34% constantly talking	HAL 36% HID 30% REST 61%

continued

Table 11.2B Continued

References	Facility/Population	Demographics	Overall Agitation	Aggression	Wandering	Verbal/Vocal	Other[1]
Hamel et al., 1990	213 community-dwelling patients, all with a diagnosis of progressive dementia disorder	Mean age=75 40% M, 60% F		34% physical aggression 7% sexual aggression		51% verbal aggression	
Rabins et al., 1982	55 patients with diagnosis of dementia (3 in nursing homes)	29% M, 71% F		47% physical violence 32% hitting	59% daytime wandering	60% making accusations	DEL 47% HAL 49% HID 69% SEX 2%
Reisberg et al., 1987a, 1987b	Outpatients N=57 All had a diagnosis of AD & GDS ≥4	Mean age=75 42% M, 58% F	58% had significant behavioral symptomatology 48% agitation of a non-specific nature	30% violence	3% wandering	24% verbal outbursts	DEL 21%, 12% HAL 12%, 12% REST 36%

Study	Setting	Demographics					
Reisberg et al., 1989	Outpatients of aging and dementia research center N=120	Mean age=73 32% M, 68% F	9%-27% physical threats and/or violence 7%-64% nonverbal anger[3]		9%-50% wandering[3]	7%-45% verbal outbursts[3]	HAL visual 6-23%, auditory 4-17% HID 12-59%, 18-68% fidgeting, pacing[3]
Ryden, 1988	Community-dwelling patients with dementia N=183	Mean age=71 46% M, 54% F		47% physically aggressive		50% verbally aggressive	17% sexually aggressive
Spector, 1991	Community dwelling N=over 4 million	Over 65 years	6.5% experienced disruptive behaviors	1% frequent temper tantrums	5% wanders and loses way		
Swearer et al., 1988	126 patients with dementia	Mean age=69 45% M, 55% F	83% exhibited 1 or more of 9 disruptive behaviors	21% assaultive/ violent		51% angry outbursts	DEL/HAL 22%
Teri et al., 1988	Outpatient geriatric and family services clinic at a hospital N=127	Mean age=77 30% M, 70% F			26% wandering		DIS 24% HAL 21% REST 45%
	All met DSM-III criteria for Primary Degenerative Dementia						

continued

Table 11.2B Continued

References	Facility/ Population	Demographics	Overall Agitation	Aggression	Wandering	Verbal/Vocal	Other[1]
Teri et al., 1989	Outpatient geriatric and family services clinic at a hospital N=56 All had a diagnosis of Alzheimer's disease	Mean age=71 57% M, 43% F		11% verbally aggressive to others 4% destruction of property	16% pacing 5% tendency to wander off and get lost	2% threats to hurt self	DEL 4%, 4%, 2%, DRES 14% HAL 4%, 2% NEG 7% REST 20%, 7%

NOTES: 1. DEL=Delusions; DIS=disruptive; DRES=dressing inappropriately; HAND=handling things inappropriately, throwing things; HAL=hallucinations; HID=hiding things; HOR=hoarding things; NEG=negativism; NOISE=crying, laughing, making strange noises; REST=general restlessness, repetitious actions; SEX=sexual advances.
2. Includes several behaviors not defined by other researchers as aggressive, such as: says sarcastic things, refuses treatment.
3. Prevalence varies with the stage of dementia according to the Global Deterioration Scale (GDS). Maximum and minimum values are shown.

Table 11.3 Frequency of Psychotropic Drug Use in Elderly Nursing Home Residents

Reference	Site	Criteria	Drug	Percent Receiving Drug	
Beers et al., 1988	All residents in 12 ICFs in eastern Massachusetts N=850	Exclude ICFs with >20% mental hospital patients or with nurse practitioner prescribing	All Psychoactives	OBS (n=150)	63%
				AD (n=228)	72%
				Psychosis (n=51)	82%
				Depression (n=116)	83%
			Antipsychotics	OBS	39%
				AD	43%
				Psychosis	71%
				Depression	40%
			Antidepressants	OBS	5%
				AD	14%
				Psychosis	14%
				Depression	40%
			Sedative/Hypnotics	OBS	38%
				AD	41%
				Psychosis	29%
				Depression	48%
Buck, 1988	Yearlong Medicaid recipients in Illinois NHs in 1984 N=33,351 Matched pharmacy billing records to NH listings.	Excludes those in ICFs for the mentally retarded and those <18 years of age	All psychotropics reimbursed by Medicaid	60.1% Data provided by diagnosis and drug for those <65 and 65+	

continued

Table 11.3 Continued

Reference	Site	Criteria	Drug	Percent Receiving Drug	
Lantz et al., 1990	Teaching NH in Queens, NY N=91	Continually resident in NH during 5-year study	Any Psychotropic	42-51% in a year	
			Antipsychotic	17-21%	
			Antidepressant	12-21%	
			Antianxiety	10-22%	
			Antihistamine	11-22%	
			Episodic Psychotropic	46% sometime in 5 yrs	
			Continuous Psychotropic	24% for 5 years	
Rovner et al., 1990	454 consecutive admissions to 8 Baltimore, MD, area NHs of one proprietary chain N=454	Exclude patients who had resided in NH within prior 6 months	Neuroleptics	DO n=183	34%
				DC n=123	44%
				OPD n=58	24%
				NPD n=90	7%
Sloane et al., 1991	31 dementia units, 32 traditional units in 5 states N=304 and N=314 respectively	Units matched for state, ownership type, size, certification level, % Medicaid	Pharmacological restraints	Dementia units	45%
				Traditional units	43%
Sternberg et al., 1990	Sample of residents in all Medicare/Medicaid certified facilities in RI N=3352	Residents evaluated between Dec 1984 and Dec 1985	Psychoactive drugs	<65 years old	61%
				65-74	61%
				75-84	56%
				85+	50%
				All ages	54%
				>1 drug	15%

NOTE: OBS=Organic brain syndrome; AD=Alzheimer's disease; DO=Dementia only; DC=Dementia complicated; OPD=Other psychiatric disorder; NPD=No psychiatric disorder.

Table 11.4 Intervention Studies

Reference	Behavior	Design	Facility	Subject Characteristics	Intervention	Findings
Behavioral Approaches						
Baltes & Lascomb, 1975	Screaming	ABA N=1	Nursing home	80-year-old F, confused and paranoid	Contingent positive reinforcement and modified timeout	Reduced screaming during treatment phase.
Mishara & Kastenbaum, 1973	Self-injurious behaviors	Experimental (N=80) vs. control group (N=55)	State mental hospital	Mean age 69—experimental, 70—control 50% M, all communicative	Enrichment (social stimulation, improved environment, empowering residents) vs. token rewards	Both interventions were found to be successful.
Rosberger & MacLean, 1983	Fecal smearing, kicking or tripping others, throwing dishes, pushing, banging, and exposing self	Case study N=1	Chronic care unit for interim care within an acute care facility	79-year-old F, post-CVA, hemiparesis	Social reinforcement of appropriate behaviors by staff and ignoring the person when target behaviors are manifested	The intervention resulted in a marked decline in the frequency of the inappropriate behaviors.
Vaccaro, 1988a, 1988b	Aggressive behaviors	ABA and phaseout N=6	Adult ward in a state-operated developmental center	Functionally psychotic Mean age=70 100% M	Positive reinforcements of nonaggressive behavior, verbal reprimand, and timeout	Aggressive behaviors were significantly reduced in the reinforcement condition and during phaseout.

continued

Table 11.4 Continued

Reference	Behavior	Design	Facility	Subject Characteristics	Intervention	Findings
Environmental Approaches						
Chafetz, 1990	Exit seeking (wandering)	ABA N=30	Special care unit of a retirement and LTC facility	Mean age=81 7% M, 93% F, all demented	Placement of 2-dimensional grid in front of glass exit doors	No intervention effect, i.e., installing the tape grid did not reduce exiting behavior.
Hussian & Brown, 1987	Exit-seeking ambulation	ABA N=8	A ward of a public mental hospital	Mean age=78 100% M 7—severe dementia 1—moderate dementia	2-dimensional grid (made from masking tape) placed on floor in front of exit door	2-dimensional grid reduced exit door contact.
Stimulation, Activities, and Music						
Birchmore & Clague, 1983	Vocalizations	AB single-subject study	Hospital	70-year-old F, blind and with a diagnosis of senile dementia	Increased sensory stimulation (e.g., music and touch)	Music did not decrease the manifestation of vocalizations, but touch did.
Cleary et al., 1988	Agitation	Pretest-posttest N=11	SNF and ICF	Mean age=87 27% M, 73% F All suffered from Alzheimer's disease or related disorders	Special care unit designed to reduce stimulation (e.g., neutral colors, no radios, telephones, or televisions) Scheduled rest and small-group activity periods	Agitation levels decreased.

Study	Behavior	Design	Setting	Sample	Intervention	Outcome
Mayers & Griffin, 1990	Extreme agitation, assaultiveness	Case studies N=9	Geropsychiatric medical unit in a state psychiatric hospital	Mean age=76; 100% M 5—Alzheimer's disease 4—dementia secondary to alcohol abuse	Sensory stimulation provided by different stimulus objects	Patients seemed more calm and less agitated after exploring stimulus objects.
McGrowder-Lin & Bhatt, 1988	Aggressive behaviors, shouting, wandering, hallucinations and others	Evaluation over time	SNF	Dementia was the most prevalent diagnosis; residents exhibited a strong propensity to wander	The wanderers' lounge provided structured activities (e.g., music, exercise, poetry)	Wandering behavior decreased; participants seek each other out when not in the wanderers' lounge.
Zachow, 1984	Screaming, shrillness, perseveration, restlessness	Case study N=1	Nursing home	F, presenting multiple sclerosis and heavily medicated with tranquilizers	Music; relaxation/guided imagery; validation/fantasy therapy; sensory stimulation	The subject was quieter after 8 weeks of intervention.
Other Approaches						
Davis, 1983	Talking, grabbing people, screaming, actual falling to the ground	Case study N=1	Long-term geriatric ward	78-year-old F	Positive social contact, an activities program, and an agitation management routine, including instructions to staff to look for precursors of agitation and to keep silent when she is screaming	Screaming and grabbing were much reduced.

continued

Table 11.4   Continued

Reference	Behavior	Design	Facility	Subject Characteristics	Intervention	Findings
Donat, 1986	Wandering	Case study N=1	Geriatric treatment center	79-year-old F, white	Relocation of subject into a room into which she had often wandered (with a window and a mirror)	Intrusions into other patients' rooms decreased from 16/hour to less than 2/hour after the room change.
Hussian, 1988	Inappropriate toileting, bed misidentification, inappropriate entry, exit seeking	AB$_1$AB$_2$ N=5	Long-term care institution	Mean age=71 100% M Psychogeriatric patients with diagnosis of dementia	Two interventions: 1. Stimulus enhancement with verbal and/or physical prompts 2. Stimulus enhancement only	All patients showed at least an 86% change in the desired direction.
Mentes & Ferrario, 1989	Physical abuse of staff (including hitting, scratching)	AB N=8	Teaching nursing home	25% M, 75% F Subjects had physically abused staff within the 3 months prior to study	Calming Aggressive Reactions in the Elderly (C.A.R.E): education program for nurse aides, focusing on early identification of risk factors and preventive approaches to aggression, e.g., use of verbal/nonverbal communication, touch, and building therapeutic relationship	There was a decline in the number of incidents of staff abuse following the implementation of the intervention.

| Raber et al., 1987 | Aggressive behaviors (e.g., banging, swearing, hitting) | Case studies N=5 | Geriatric unit of hospital | 40% M, 60% F | "One-to-one approach," i.e., developing a therapeutic relationship of one nurse to one patient | Positive changes in patients' behaviors, as well as in staff perceptions and staff behaviors |
| Vaccaro, 1990 | Verbally aggressive behaviors | ABAB N=6 | Adult ward in a state-operated developmental center | Mean age=66 50% M, 50% F Schizophrenic with no recorded organic impairment; all received psychotropic medication for aggressive behavior | A social skills training program consisting of instructions, modeling, role playing, and feedback | Verbally aggressive behavior was significantly decreased. |

12

Managing Nurse Aides to Promote Quality of Care in the Nursing Home

JOHN F. SCHNELLE, PH.D.
M. PATRICK MCNEES, PH.D.
SANDRA F. SIMMONS, M.A.
MARK E. N. AGNEW, M.D.
VALERIE C. CROOKS, D.S.W.

Nurse aides (NAs) comprise 66% of the work force in nursing homes (NHs) and provide most of the basic care for NH residents who require substantial assistance (63). Seventy-seven percent of residents exhibit severe functioning problems and 68% severe dementia (29). Many of these residents are not capable of simple life activities such as toileting, independent ambulation, or even self-feeding. NAs are responsible for providing such assistance. "Neglect" occurs when such daily assistance is not consistently delivered (26).

Unfortunately, neglect has often been documented in NHs. Reports issued by the Institute of Medicine (1986), Special Committee on Aging (1986), and the General Accounting Office (1987) suggest that a large number of NHs continue to deliver inadequate care, and direct regulation of care, even if it were possible, may not provide adequate quality of care in NHs (41). Moreover, consistently assisting residents with daily life functioning has to be regarded as only the foundation of good resident care. In addition to providing such basic assistance, NAs also have frequent opportunity to talk and interact with residents. How well this interaction occurs can determine the resident's quality of life. Interviews with NH residents have revealed that three of the most desired staff attributes were courtesy, cheerfulness, and helpfulness (60). These human qualities were rated as more important than higher staff credentials, training, or even adequate staffing. Yet, there is no way to evaluate these characteristics or provide the NH resident with viable means of feedback regarding how an aide performs. Currently, measures of quality of care often focus on the availability and training level of the caretakers who are primarily NAs (41).

In short, residents need to be consistently and competently assisted with their physical needs and treated well interpersonally. If such care is not delivered, the overall quality of care and quality of life in a NH cannot be good even if the home is otherwise staffed by competent physicians and professional nurses. Because NAs are the *primary* caregivers in NHs, in this chapter we examine how NAs provide resident care and how deficits in the provision of this care originate and can be identified. In the first part of the chapter, the literature review will point to serious problems with how NAs are retained, trained, and managed. In the final part of the chapter, a management model to improve training and quality of care will be briefly described.

NURSE AIDES

The importance of the NA job position is widely acknowledged by health care providers (61). This public acknowledgment quickly rings hollow, however, when the reality of how NAs are trained, paid, and managed is considered. NAs are among the lowest paid of all occupational groups in the NH (30). They are often paid minimum wages (18). Reflecting this low pay and the high physical and emotional effort required to do the job well, the turnover rate of NAs is extraordinarily high. It is not unusual to see reports of 100% turnover rates in the course of a year (23). Demographic statistics indicate that NAs are typically women with education below the high school level and members of a minority group (66). Foreign-born aides often predominate in urban NHs, and NAs often work more than one job. One descriptive study reported that the single most common denominator across all groups of NAs was their low socioeconomic class (60). In most cases, they were barely above the poverty level. It is clear that NAs do not bring to the job the skills produced by formal education or the motivation produced by high salary. The question thus arises: How are NAs retained, trained, and managed?

Nurse Aide Training and Management

Review of the literature concerning the effectiveness of training and management programs for NAs revealed no controlled evaluations or even comprehensive descriptive evaluations of training/management systems. The virtually complete lack of evidence and effort in this area belies the frequent claims that the NA job is viewed as important. This alleged importance is not supported by either salary considerations or attention to training and management details. There is minimal evidence to answer even the most basic training and management questions. First, given existing resident to aide staffing ratios, do NAs have time to complete all assigned responsibilities? Also, how well and efficiently do NAs sequence their work activities? One study (see Table 12.1) provides anecdotal evidence that suggests that aides are not able to complete all responsibilities and often cut corners and organize patient needs according to their own task priorities (5). Another equally important question is: Do training programs have an effect on job performance? To date, published studies are sparse and the findings often inconclusive. Finally, what types of management approaches could be used to improve nurse aides' job performance? The absence of effective systematic training and management approaches are well documented (8). Except for the total quality control approach described in the latter section of this chapter, no specific training and management system for NAs has been fully implemented or studied.

Although there is a dearth of research on these questions, a number of descriptive reports and studies have examined NA characteristics and their effects on the NH organization and performance. These studies, many with relatively small samples of NAs, have examined turnover, attitudes, stress, training, and management. Several of the larger sample studies are highlighted in Table 12.1.

Descriptive studies that have been conducted to examine turnover among NAs in NHs have found that management practices may be a factor that contributes to job turnover and the level of care provided by aides (32). In one study, staff turnover statistics were significantly reduced in homes with the implementation of new management practices including orientation of new employees, training, ongoing supervision, and systematic recruitment efforts (66). Turnover was reduced by 50% in another 120-bed NH after the implementation of a formal orientation and ongoing in-service program (62). Another study showed that turnover rates were related more to administrative control and supervision procedures than to low wages and benefits (22). Other studies identify a variety of characteristics related to turnover. Aide characteristics that contribute to high turnover are younger age (less than 30), overqualification, previous short-term employment (64); inexperience, low pay, lack of RN role model (7); concern about extrinsic rewards (pay and benefits) (19); and routinization of work (42). Factors that were often associated with low turnover are lower staffing ratios, improved orientation, perceived need of patients, ability to criticize, and higher pay (12,13); attachment to others, recognition, decision-making power, and teamwork (37); interpersonal relationships and supervision (27); and accurate information regarding nature of job and mistakes (42). Many of these same factors are described in the larger studies cited in Table 12.1.

Attitudes and stress may also impact on the NA work performance and resident care. One study of NAs found that an experiential education program may positively affect attitudes toward NH residents (14). Another analysis found that the sociocultural environment within the individual NH is a prime determiner of attitudes and could be used to predict quality of care (69). Another study of NAs and LPNs examined the effects of a 6-week training program on knowledge and attitudes about aging. Pre- and posttest results showed an overall favorable change in knowledge and attitudes in both groups (1). In an ethnographic study of 132 nurse aides in Illinois, attitudes toward elderly residents were negatively affected by both the institutional culture of the NH and the burdens of personal life (60). In large part, these findings were repeated in another study on nursing personnel burnout (25). Positive aspects of resident care have also been found to reduce stress and to increase NH staff satisfaction (16). Specific training for work with cognitively impaired residents, workload reductions, and job rewards have also been cited as stress reducers (15).

Most studies relevant to NA training have evaluated effects of in-service lectures on knowledge but rarely effects on patient outcomes. For the most part, these studies do not use control groups, have limited if any pretraining data, and use relatively small samples or report anecdotal results. A study that evaluated knowledge of NAs regarding common mental health problems of residents recommended an interactive learning format to sustain knowledge (58). In one study the efficacy of an in-service on the topic of behavior therapy was tested and trained observers described positive effects of NAs applying interventions with difficult residents (4). Yet, in a quasi-experimental behavior study of 166 NAs in four NHs, the

Table 12.1 Nurse Aides: Studies of Turnover, Performance, and Training in Nursing Homes

Source	Study Description	Findings
Waxman et al., 1984	Descriptive study of factors related to turnover and job satisfaction in 7 randomly selected Philadelphia NHs. Several group interviews were conducted using a sample of 234 aides.	Low turnover was related to more loosely organized administration, where aides have high control in daily decisions and care planning. Highest turnover and satisfaction occurred in highest quality homes.
Halbur & Fears, 1986	Descriptive study of 122 North Carolina NHs analyzed effects of nursing personnel turnover on resident discharge and death rates.	Turnover rates of RNs and LPNs (not aides) were positively related to discharge rates and not with death rates. Suggests that turnover can have positive effects on patient outcomes.
Wagnild, 1988	A descriptive study of 11 randomly selected NHs in rural and urban Texas involved interviews of 119 day- and night-shift aides and examined effects of aide characteristics and management factors on aide turnover.	In order of importance, factors affecting aide turnover included understaffing, low pay and poor benefits, and interpersonal problems with staff. Management factors affecting aides included no opportunity for advancement, no expectation of wage raise, and inadequate orientation.
Caudill, 1989	Descriptive study of factors related to turnover rates in 77 skilled NHs in Washington state. A 36-item questionnaire was completed by 996 aides of varying ages, shifts, and types of NHs.	Aides with longer employment were more likely to experience: 1. Charge nurse who listened, 2. Freedom to criticize, 3. Effect on policy or care plan changes, and 4. Attendance at case conferences.
Gottesman & Bourestom, 1974	A descriptive study, using a probability sample of 40 Michigan NHs, 1,144 residents and 200 NAs, measured through observation in a predetermined sequence the level of basic care and activities of residents.	Level of value placed on aides' training by management had a strong relationship to quantity of care observed. Prior experience as NA was strongly correlated to higher level of basic care.

Bowers & Becker, 1992	A descriptive study using participant observation and in-depth interviews of 30 NAs in 3 NHs in a midwestern city to determine factors that contribute to quality of care	Strategies to better organize work by individual aides is positively related to quality of care (as defined by supervisors) and is negatively associated to turnover.
Smyer et al., 1992	A multiple-treatment nonequivalent control group design was used with a cluster sampling of 120 NAs in 3 NHs to determine the effects of skills training or job redesign or both on job performance. Forty NAs in a 4th NH served as a control. Measures were taken pre-/postintervention and 3 to 6 months later.	Pre-/postknowledge over time was improved in experimental sites only. Job redesign sites did not significantly increase job motivation potential. Performance on caregiver rating scales showed no significant changes in single or combined intervention groups.
Cohn et al., 1990	An evaluation study of behavior management training for approx. 77 NAs in 2 NHs in Pennsylvania. The training included five 1½-hr. sessions at 1-month intervals re: depression, disorientation, and agitation.	Significant improvement in overall knowledge of problems was reported. A positive relationship was found between test performance and self-reported caregiving performance, suggesting training may alter behavioral performance of NAs.

experimental group ($N = 96$ aides) was pretested for baseline attitude and knowledge regarding urinary incontinence, then trained in a resident toileting program. Although there was a slight increase in knowledge, the training resulted in minimal to no effect on attitudes and compliance with the toileting protocol (10). Poor performance on written tests corresponded with unsatisfactory performance of basic nursing procedures in another study of NA training (68). A competency-based approach, which included resources, feedback, and reinforcement, resulted in mastery of some required skills for beginning NAs (59). Another study found that a short course in rehabilitation care resulted in improved learning and retention (39). In a study by Gottesman and Bourestom (1974), a relationship was found between aide training and the level of basic care delivered by NAs. The researchers found that the level of value management placed on aide training was one of the four characteristics most strongly related to the amount of nursing care observed. Additionally, in NHs where new aides were expected by management to have prior experience, a higher level of basic care was observed by the research staff. In this study, an observation-based measure of actual behavior in NHs was utilized. The procedures used for recording behavior employed two trained assistants who observed residents during 24 one-hour segments between 6:30 a.m. and 7:30 p.m. on 2 days. In each hour the resident was observed for 1 full minute in a predetermined sequence. Each time, a record was made of the services given or the activity of the patient and of his or her location, position, and involvement with other people. This latter report is suggestive, but there remains no strong evidence concerning how NA management and training programs affect resident care. There does not even appear to be a standardized approach to training and management in NHs. For example, a survey revealed that even aides within the same NH received dramatically different training and orientation procedures. Some aides could not even remember being oriented or trained (63). Even when training effects are found, permanent changes in aide performance is not the result.

Studies that examine management attributes and approaches specific to improving NA jobs and skills are minimal. Poor human resource management policies and practices were found to contribute to inadequate resident care in a study of 25 NHs and 530 nursing staff (53). Another descriptive study analyzed management use of job redesign as a means to enhance worker motivation and effectiveness (6). In a study reviewing the impact of organizational structure and supervision on staff satisfaction, results indicated that staff satisfaction was positively associated with an organization in which individual efforts are rewarded and negatively associated with coercive approaches (38). Management styles and negative stereotypes of aides may also contribute to turnover rates and poor care, according to a NH study conducted in Florida (11). In another study of 296 Iowa NHs, homes with a higher percentage of nurse supervisory hours were found to be more efficient. Higher general staffing levels also were associated with quality of life measures (defined as 13 tasks related to adequate custodial care) (40). In a study of 80 Rhode Island NHs and 2,500 residents, higher staff levels and low RN turnover also were found to be related to functional improvements in residents (57). In a study of NA training conducted by Burgio et al. (1990), a management system of regular self- and supervisory monitoring was used along with group performance feedback to improve resident incontinence care. This resident toileting training resulted in a 87% rate of compliance by aides, which in turn showed improvement in resident dryness at 2-week and 3-month follow-ups. However, without persistent feedback in the 4th and 5th months, compliance declined; and reinitiation of individual feedback was necessary to restore previous compliance levels (9).

Despite the number and variety of these studies related to management of NAs, there are limited reports to link management approaches to job performance or job performance to resident outcomes, the Burgio et al. study being one exception to this generalized conclusion. More important, few studies examine interventions that may mitigate these conditions. To summarize the NA work situation, minimally paid workers are asked to perform critically important resident care tasks that require high physical and emotional effort, and there is no evidence regarding the best approach to training and supervising these workers in this difficult effort. There is not even evidence to suggest that aides have time to complete all of the required job tasks, assuming that they are working at a maximally productive level. Given these salary, labor pool, training, and management considerations, what is known about how well NAs perform their job?

Nurse Aides—Quality of Care

Problems with the quality of care in NHs have been discussed in many places (28,55). Many of these documented problems, such as overuse of medication and overuse of restraints, are clearly the responsibilities of physicians and nurses who work in long-term care. There can be no argument that responsibility for deficiencies in resident care lies across all occupational groups. However, because NAs provide the majority of hands-on care, this group warrants particular attention. The failure to provide basic care consistently and the tendency to reinforce dependency during the times that they do provide care are perhaps the major quality of care problems attributed to NAs.

A series of descriptive studies with the institutionalized elderly documented that aides are more likely to be supportive of dependent behaviors shown by elders than independence-related behaviors (2,3). For example, observations indicated that residents were able to perform many required behaviors, for example, dressing themselves, but they were prevented from doing so by the NAs, who intervene simply to get the "job" completed more quickly, thereby reinforcing dependency. There are a number of potential explanations for the failure of NAs to provide consistent care and for supporting dependency in the care they do provide. Lack of time, excessive paperwork, and pessimistic stereotypical attitudes about the capabilities of residents have all been discussed (3). One study related quality of care to staff encouragement of independence among NH residents. It was recommended that NH staff should adopt the role of "staging opportunities for resident independence" as opposed to constantly doing tasks for the resident (22).

A specific reason for quality of care problems related to the dynamics of the work situation has been identified and discussed in a series of articles describing urinary incontinence care in NHs (43,45-48). The point of these articles is that excessive resident dependency, in this case incontinence, may be supported by staff because it is more time efficient for staff to do so. The urinary incontinence research has made the following major points: (a) 25% to 33% of NH residents are incontinent primarily because of the failure of NAs to deliver consistent toileting assistance, and (b) identifying the residents who can be responsive to toileting and training staff how to implement toileting procedures will not motivate aides to render consistent toileting assistance.

This failure of aides to maintain toileting programs could perhaps be expected if they were asked to toilet residents who could not be responsive. However, the failure of aides to maintain programs with only responsive residents was surprising. This maintenance failure was explored in several follow-up investigations that came to the following conclusions: (a) It took staff significantly more time to render toileting assistance than it did to simply change residents when wet. A single toileting episode averaged 7.5 minutes, whereas a changing episode averaged 4.3 minutes. (b) Staff minimized the work involved in caring for incontinent residents by not changing residents after each incontinent episode. Resident incontinence frequency averaged 3.2 per day and staff changed the residents only 1.3 times per day. (c) Staff spent approximately 8 minutes per resident in changing and rendering occasional toileting assistance to residents. To maintain continence, it was necessary to contact these same residents consistently on a 2- or 3-hour schedule and to offer toileting assistance. The staff time involved in maintaining dryness with this schedule was approximately 18 minutes per patient per shift.

In conclusion, these incontinence studies make several important points about the quality of care and the work dynamics that exist in NHs. One is that ignoring incontinence episodes by not systematically changing residents saves a great deal of time. The major cost of such neglect is borne only by the residents. Maintaining resident continence and a higher degree of independence by being responsive to the residents' requests for toileting assistance will require more work from NAs. This same work dynamic applies to other areas of resident care. The rule across many care areas is that it is more time efficient to ignore problems or to maintain dependence than to promote higher levels of resident independence. The question must now be posed: What type of management system is required to promote more consistent care and a higher quality of care?

QUALITY ASSURANCE AND QUALITY CONTROL

Attempts to promote higher levels of care in NHs are often labeled *quality assurance* (QA). Most of these efforts involve setting specific standards for care and then evaluating whether such standards are met. The feedback from the evaluations is designed to motivate NH caregivers to provide higher levels of resident care. Controlled evaluations of the results of these QA studies have not been promising (see Table 12.2). In one major study, over 100 NHs in Rhode Island were randomly divided into experimental and control groups (56). Experimental homes received a new regulatory survey process in which state surveyors reduced the amount of time spent in reviewing policies and increased the amount of time spent in evaluating direct patient care. For example, there was an increased emphasis on interviewing residents about the quality of their care. The new survey process resulted in more deficiencies being cited in the experimental

Table 12.2 Studies of Quality Assurance in Nursing Homes

Source	Study Description	Findings
Weissert et al., 1983	A controlled field experiment of 36 skilled NHs in California used an incentive-based reimbursement system to alter access, use of beds, and quality of care in NHs.	No resident quality of care outcome effects were found by setting standards and offering financial incentives.
Mohide et al., 1988	Randomized trial of quality assurance program pre/post intervention in 30 experimental and 30 control NHs in Canada used a sample of 1525 NH residents. The intervention included predeveloped quality assurance packages re. hazardous mobility and constipation.	There were statistically significant differences yet small improvement in management of constipation and mobility in experimental NHs.
Spector & Drugovich, 1989	Randomized control design study of 51 experimental and 52 control NHs with a sample of 3,271 NH residents in Rhode Island evaluated the impact of a new federal review process on documentation, environmental deficiencies, and resident outcomes.	Although the experimental survey identified more deficiencies, no significant differences in resident outcomes (functional status) were noted.
Geron, 1991	Descriptive study of 809 Illinois NHs that participated in a Quality Incentive Program (QUIP) of bonus payments to improve quality of care in terms of structure and environment, resident participation and choice, community and family participation, resident satisfaction, care plans, and specialized services.	High participation rates and qualification for bonus payments for multiple standards increased over time. However, the questionable validity and insensitivity of the measures precluded any correlation between the QUIP and resident quality of life.

homes, and more important, an increase in citations for patient care deficiencies. However, despite the fact that the NHs were very motivated by the implications of the state survey reports, there were no differences between the experimental and control homes in terms of resident outcome.

In a second controlled QA intervention study, the approach of setting standards and evaluating whether standards were met was supplemented by intense educational efforts and the targeting of specific patient conditions (36). In this study, 60 NHs were randomized to experimental and control groups. Experimental groups received a QA package directed toward either constipation or hazardous mobility conditions. The quality assurance package involved a plan of assessing for the targeted condition and a listing of potential management actions that direct care staff could initiate. Experimental homes did show small but statistically significant changes in regard to chart notations of how the targeted conditions were treated. For example, there was an increase in the number of assessments ordered for hazardous mobility conditions and a change of medications ordered for constipation. There was no evidence, however, of improvements or changes in resident outcomes (36).

In other excellent efforts, financial incentives or public recognition was offered for achieving improved standards of care. For example, a recent report evaluated a quality incentive program for NHs in Illinois. Eight hundred and nine participating NHs received a separate bonus payment for achievement of six quality control standards. There was evidence that NHs were highly motivated to obtain both the financial incentives and the recognition received for participating in the program. However, there was no evidence that resident care quality improved (21). This study replicates the "no resident outcome" conclusions of a previous field experiment designed to effect quality of care by setting standards and offering financial incentives (67).

Numerous plausible reasons for the failure of QA efforts to improve resident care have been discussed; however, one potential reason has received very little attention. There have been no systematic efforts in any of the studies to involve NAs in the QA efforts. The projects set care standards for NH management to achieve but did not plan management techniques to change how NAs deliver resident care. Thus, NHs were encouraged to meet care standards but were not given a technology to change how NH care was delivered. In addition, even though financial incentives were provided for NHs for improvement in care, there were no provisions to deliver these incentives to NAs.

Efforts to improve care by giving administrators money for attainment of standards but no technology to improve NA performance ignore the realities of the resident care situation. Until recently, there have been no published studies of QA programs that target the resident care performance of NAs.

Schnelle et al. have described the implementation of a quality control management system in maintaining continence in NH residents (44,49-52). This important research demonstrates the effectiveness of a prompted voiding toileting training and management program with indigenous NAs. Seventy-six of 190 incontinent residents in seven NHs were targeted and placed on a prompted voiding maintenance program. The system included the establishment of performance standards, a toileting chart procedure, quality control monitoring, prompted voiding training and maintenance evaluation. Residents were assessed at prebaseline, baseline, prompted voiding, and 6-month management periods. Results showed a reduction in wetness from 43% to 21% ($p < .0001$), which was sustained over the full 6-month period. The characteristics of the quality control management system are briefly summarized below.

A QUALITY CONTROL MODEL

It has been suggested that there are several key elements inherent in successful quality improvement systems. The management model is based on the quality control technology successfully used in business and industry to improve quality and consistency of work behaviors (31,65). Job processes must be identified and clearly related to objective outcomes. There must be a system allowing ongoing monitoring of work processes. Continuous improvement is achieved by judging actual outcomes with expected outcomes. These expected outcomes are based on the past level and variability of previous outcomes and not on arbitrary standards. There have been attempts to incorporate these premises into a working system to address urinary incontinence in NHs. However, early attempts necessitated considerable ongoing involvement and support from research staff to maintain anticipated wetness levels. One reason for this difficulty in maintaining the system was thought to involve data-analytical requirements of NH staff.

In an attempt to provide NH staff with the analytical tools needed for maintaining the incontinence management system, the assessment and quality control features of the system were automated. The basic computer system characteristics have been described in an article by

McNees and Schnelle (1992). The results of an evaluation in one NH are described in another article by McNees et al. (1992). Wetness rates were reduced from preintervention levels of approximately 25% to about 12% during the implementation of the system. Follow-up checks reflected wetness rates of approximately 8%, indicating that staff were able to utilize the computer system to maintain the overall continence management system. Anecdotal reports reflect the facilities continued utilization of the system after over 18 months. User feedback suggests that staff was able to detect when wetness rates indicated the system was out of control and also identify controllable sources of variability.

For example, although overall wetness levels were within ranges that were assumed acceptable, the automated system detected unusual elevations in wetness levels on the weekends. Further staff analysis resulted in the determination that most of the staff on the weekends had not been trained in the prompted voiding system. Subsequent training resulted in wetness dropping to levels comparable with other days. This example provides a basis for illustrating how continuous improvement might occur, even in cases where the overall system appears to be in control.

The quality control model described in this chapter extends traditional quality assurance efforts in many important ways. Most important, the quality control model addresses the critical issue of the job performance of NAs and the critical role that NAs play in changing resident outcomes. Unlike the relatively simplistic quality assurance approach, arbitrary quality standards for resident outcomes are not set. Instead, the exact job processes that produce changes in resident outcomes are specifically defined and validated in the actual work environments. Resident care standards are set based on how these job processes actually impact the outcomes for the unique set of residents. Follow-up monitoring systems and computerized information technology permit the ongoing analysis of the factors that limit the effective implementation of this work process. The net result is an empirically guided, continuous improvement approach that changes how the work environment supports the work process. This quality control model is applicable to other areas of resident care. For example, a recent paper illustrates the application of this model to managing physical restraints (52).

There is strong evidence that the quality control model described in this chapter can improve the quality and consistency of supervisory and clinical employee performance across a diverse range of health care settings and nursing homes. We argue that the unique set of problems that characterize long-term care and NA performance can be particularly well approached with this validated quality control management technology. The net result of the application of the quality control technology to long-term care should be to improve employee performance and the quality of life for NH residents. Future clinical research should be directed at using such technologies and other training and management approaches that can be directly linked to patient outcomes.

REFERENCES

1. Almquist, E., Stein, S., Weiner, A., et al. (1981). Evaluation of continuing education for long-term care personnel: Impact upon attitudes and knowledge. *Journal of the American Geriatrics Society, 29*(3), 117-122.
2. Baltes, M. M., Burgess, R. L., & Stewart, R. B. (1980). Independence and dependence in self-care behaviors in nursing home residents: An operant-observational study. *International Journal of Behavioral Development, 3,* 489-500.
3. Baltes, M. M., & Hans-Werner, W. (1988). The behavioral and social world of the institutionalized elderly: Implications for health and optimal development. In M. Ory & R. P. Abeles (Eds.), *Aging, health, and behavior.* Baltimore, MD: Johns Hopkins University Press.
4. Block, C. B., Boczkowski, J. A., Hansen, N., et al. (1987). Nursing home consultation: Difficult residents and frustrated staff. *Gerontologist, 27*(4), 443-446.
5. Bowers, B. L., & Becker, M. (1992). Nurse's aides in nursing homes: The relationship between organization and quality. *Gerontologist, 32,* 360-366.
6. Brannon, D., Smyer, M., Cohen, M. et al. (1988). A job diagnostic survey of nursing home caregivers: Implications for job redesign. *Gerontologist, 28*(2), 246-252.
7. Brown, M. (1988). Nursing assistants' behavior toward institutionalized elderly. *Quality Review Bulletin, 14*(1), 15-17.
8. Burgio, L. D., & Burgio, K. L. (1990). Institutional staff training and management: A review of the literature and a model for geriatric, long-term care facilities. *International Journal of Aging and Human Development, 30*(4), 287-302.
9. Burgio, L. D., Engel, B. T., Hawkins, A., et al. (1990). A staff management system for maintaining improvements in continence with elderly nursing home residents. *Journal of Applied Behavior Analysis, 23*(1), 111-118.
10. Campbell, E. B., Knight, M., Benson, M., et al. (1991). Effect of an incontinence training program on nursing home staff's knowledge, attitudes, and behavior. *Gerontologist, 31*(6), 788-794.
11. Carter, R. Y., Kooperman, L., & Clare, D. A. (1988, Summer). Importance of perceived personal values in nursing home management. *Journal of Long-Term Care Administration,* pp. 10-13.
12. Caudill, M. (1989). Nursing assistant involvement in patient care planning pays off. *Nursing Management, 20,* 111Z-112DD.
13. Caudill, M., & Patrick, M. (1989). Nursing assistant turnover in nursing homes and need satisfaction. *Journal of Gerontological Nursing, 15*(6), 24-30.

14. Chandler, J. T., Rachal, J. R., & Kazelskis, R. (1986). Attitudes of long-term care nursing personnel toward the elderly. *Gerontologist, 26*(5), 551-555.
15. Chappell, N. L., & Novak, M. (1992). The role of support in alleviating stress among nursing assistants. *Gerontologist, 32*, 351-359.
16. Cohen-Mansfield, J. (1989). Sources of satisfaction and stress in nursing home caregivers: Preliminary results. *Journal of Advanced Nursing, 14*, 383-388.
17. Cohn, M. D., Horgas, A. L., & Marsiske, M. A. (1990). Behavior management training for nurse aides: Is it effective? *Journal of Gerontological Nursing, 16*(11), 21-25.
18. Diamond, T. (1986). Social policy and everyday life in nursing homes: A critical ethnography. *Social Science Medicine, 23*(12), 1287-1295.
19. Garland, T. N., Oyabu, N., & Gipson, G. A. (1988, Winter). Stayers and leavers: A comparison of nurse assistants employed in nursing homes. *Journal of Long-Term Care Administration*, pp. 23-29.
20. General Accounting Office. (1987). *Medicare and Medicaid: Stronger enforcement of nursing home requirements needed.* Washington, DC: Author.
21. Geron, S. M. (1991). Regulating the behavior of nursing homes through positive incentives: Analysis of Illinois' Quality Incentive Program (QUIP). *Gerontologist, 31*, 292-301.
22. Gottesman, L. E., & Bourestom, N. C. (1974). Why nursing homes do what they do. *Gerontologist, 14*, 501-506.
23. Grau, L., Burton, B., & Kolditz, D. (1991). Institutional loyalty and job satisfaction among nurse aides in nursing homes. *Journal of Aging and Health, 3*, 47-65.
24. Halbur, B. T., & Fears, N. (1986). Nursing personnel turnover rates turned over: Potential positive effects on resident outcomes in nursing homes. *Gerontologist, 26*, 70-76.
25. Hare, J., Pratt, C. C., & Andrews, D. (1987). Predictors of burnout in professional and paraprofessional nurses working in hospitals and nursing homes. *International Journal of Nursing Studies, 25*(2), 105-115.
26. Haviland, S., & O'Brien, J. (1989). Physical abuse and neglect of the elderly: Assessment and intervention. *Orthopaedic Nursing, 8*, 11-18.
27. Holtz, G. A. (1982). Nurses' aides in nursing homes: Why are they satisfied? *Journal of Gerontological Nursing, 8*(5), 265-271.
28. Institute of Medicine. Committee on Nursing Home Regulation. (1986). *Improving the quality of nursing homes.* Washington, DC: National Academy Press.
29. Kaeser, L., Musser L. A., & Andreoli, K. (1989). Developing an effective teaching nursing home: The planning process. *Nurse Educator, 13*, 37-41.
30. Kane, R. A., & Kane, R. L. (1987). *Effective long term care.* New York: Springer.
31. Laffel, G., & Blumenthal, D. (1989). The case for using industrial quality management science in health care organizations. *Journal of the American Medical Association, 262*, 2869-2873.
32. LeSar, K. W. (1987). Who provides for the nursing assistant? *Provider, 13*, 20-21.
33. Mainstone, L. E., & Lev, A. S. (1987). Fundamentals of statistical process control. *Journal of Organizational Behavior Management, 9*, 4-21.
34. McNees, M. P., & Schnelle, J. F. (1992). Computer aided management of urinary incontinence in nursing homes. *Western Journal of Nursing Research, 14*(4), 516-519.
35. McNees, M. P., Schnelle, J. F. Agnew, M., et al. (1992, Spring). Alaska nursing home takes role in addressing urinary incontinence. *Alaska Medicine*, pp. 101-102.
36. Mohide, E. A., Tugwell, P. X., Caulfied, P. A., et al. (1988). A randomized trial of quality assurance in nursing homes. *Medical Care, 26*, 554-564.

37. Monahan, R. S., & McCarthy, S. (1992). Nursing home employment: The nurse's aide's perspective. *Journal of Gerontological Nursing, 18*(2), 13-16.

38. Mullins, L. C., Nelson, C. E., Busciglio, H., et al. (1988, Spring). Job satisfaction among nursing home personnel: The impact of organizational structure and supervisory power. *Journal of Long-Term Care Administration*, pp. 12-18.

39. Nikjeh, D. A., & Shein, M. M. (1989). Rehabilitative care: Who teaches paraprofessionals? *Nursing Management, 20*(1), 80Q-80S.

40. Nyman, J. A., Bricker, D. L., & Link, D. (1990). Technical efficiency in nursing homes. *Medical Care, 28*(6), 541-551.

41. Nyman, J. A., & Geyer, C. R. (1989). Promoting the quality of life in nursing homes: Can regulation succeed? *Journal of Health Politics, Policy and Law, 14*, 797-815.

42. Rublee, D. A. (1985, Summer). Predictors of employee turnover in nursing homes. *Journal of Long-Term Care Administration*, 5-8.

43. Schnelle, J. F. (1990). Treatment of urinary incontinence in nursing home patients by prompted voiding. *Journal of the American Geriatrics Society, 38*, 356-360.

44. Schnelle, J. F. (1991). *Managing urinary incontinence in the elderly.* New York: Springer.

45. Schnelle, J. F., Sowell, V. A., Hu, T. W., et al. (1988). Reduction of urinary incontinence in nursing homes: Does it reduce or increase costs? *Journal of the American Geriatrics Society, 36*, 34-39.

46. Schnelle, J. F., Traughber, B., Sowell, V. et al. (1989). Prompted voiding treatment of urinary incontinence in nursing home patients. *Journal of the American Geriatrics Society, 37*, 1051-1057.

47. Schnelle, J. F., Newman, D., & Abbey, J. (1990a). Urodynamic and behavioral analysis of incontinence in nursing home patients. *Behavior, Health and Aging, 1*, 41-49.

48. Schnelle, J. F., Newman, D., & Fogarty, T. (1990b). Patient continence in long-term care nursing facilities. *Gerontologist, 30*, 373-376.

49. Schnelle, J. F., Newman, D. R., & Fogarty, T. (1990c). Statistical quality-control in nursing homes: Assessment and management of chronic urinary incontinence. *Health Services Research, 25*(4), 627-637.

50. Schnelle, J. F., Newman, D. R., Fogarty, T. E., et al. (1991). Assessment and quality control of incontinence care in long-term nursing facilities. *Journal of the American Geriatrics Society, 39*, 165-171.

51. Schnelle, J. F., Newman, D., White, M., et al. (1993). Maintaining continence in nursing home residents through the application of industrial quality control. *Gerontologist, 33*(1); 114-121.

52. Schnelle, J. F., Newman, D. R., & Volner, T., et al. (1991). Reducing and managing restraints in long term care. *Journal of the American Geriatrics Society, 40*, 381-385.

53. Sheridan, J. E., White, J., & Fairchild, T. J. (1992). Ineffective staff, ineffective supervision or ineffective administration? Why some nursing homes fail to provide adequate care. *Gerontologist, 32*, 334-341.

54. Smyer, M., Brannon, D., & Cohn, M. (1992). Improving nursing home care through training and job redesign. *Gerontologist, 32*, 327-333.

55. Special Committee on Aging, U. S. Senate. (1986). *Nursing home care: The unfinished agenda.* Washington, DC: Author.

56. Spector, W. D., & Drugovich, M. L. (1989). Reforming nursing home quality regulation: Impact on cited deficiencies and nursing home outcomes. *Medical Care, 27*, 789-801.

57. Spector, W. D., & Takada, H. A. (1991). Characteristics of nursing homes that affect resident outcomes. *Journal of Aging and Health, 3*(4), 427-454.

58. Spore, D. L., Smyer, M. A., & Cohn, M. D. (1991). Assessing nurse assistants' knowledge of behavioral approaches to mental health problems. *Gerontologist, 31,* 309-317.
59. Stein, K. Z. (1986). Nursing assistants learn through the competency-based approach. *Geriatric Nursing, 7/8,* 197-200.
60. Tellis-Nayak, V., & Tellis-Nayak, M. (1989). Quality of care and the burden of two cultures: When the world of the nurse's aide enters the world of the nursing home. *Gerontologist, 29,* 307-313.
61. Tobin, S. S., & Lieberman M. A. (1976). *Last home for the aged: Critical implications for institutionalization.* San Francisco: Jossey-Bass.
62. Tynan, C., & Witerall, J. (1984, May/June). Good orientation cuts turnover. *Geriatric Nursing,* pp. 173-175.
63. Wagnild, G. (1988, Spring). A descriptive study of nurse's aide turnover in long-term care facilities. *Journal of Long Term Care Administration,* pp. 19-23.
64. Wagnild, G., & Manning, R. W. (1986, Summer). The high turnover profile screening and selecting applicants for nurse's aide. *Journal of Long-Term Care Administration,* pp. 2-4.
65. Walton, M. (1986). *The Deming management method.* New York: Dodd, Mead.
66. Waxman, H. M., Carner, S. A., & Berkenstock, G. (1984). Job turnover and job satisfaction among nursing home aides. *Gerontologist, 24,* 503-509.
67. Weissert, W. G., Scanlon, W. J., Wan, T. T. H., et al. (1983). Care for the chronically ill: Nursing home incentive payment experiment. *Health Care Financing Review, 5,* 41-49.
68. Woolfork, C. H. (1989). What you can expect of nurse's aides. *Geriatric Nursing, 7/8,* 179-180.
69. Wright, L. K. (1988). A reconceptualization of the "negative staff attitudes and poor care in nursing homes" assumption. *Gerontologist, 28*(6), 813-820.

Index

About the Contributors

Adil A. Abbasi, M.D., is Assistant Professor in the Department of Medicine at the Medical College of Wisconsin in Milwaukee. He also holds an appointment at the Medical Service of the VA Medical Center in Milwaukee. His research interests include nutritional, metabolic, and endocrine problems associated with aging, and he is currently working on the following research projects: the prevalence, causes, and management of protein calorie undernutrition in the elderly; the effects of endogenous and exogenous growth hormone on renal status in old age; and insulinlike growth factor II and aging.

Mark E. N. Agnew, M.D., is a citizen of Great Britain. He was educated at Bedford School and entered the School of Physic at Trinity College Dublin in 1960, graduating in 1966. After graduation, he joined the house staff at Dudley Road Hospital in Birmingham, England, holding a series of appointments there followed by a residency in general practice with special responsibilities for a hospice. In 1972, he moved to Anchorage, Alaska, where he was instrumental in founding Hospice of Anchorage, a community-based program for the terminally ill. An interest in the problems of the frail elderly led to appointments as Medical Director to three long-term care facilities, one of which was recently given the 1991 Order of Excellence Award by Bill Publication of New York. His current areas of clinical interest include nutritional and pharmacologic strategies to reduce the incidence of aspiration pneumonia, anorexia and feeding refusal in the elderly, new pharmacologic approaches to the management of aggressive and agitated behavior in dementia, and use of graphic systems to display clinical data.

Cathy A. Alessi, M.D., is Assistant Professor in the Department of Medicine and the Multicampus Program in Geriatric Medicine and

Gerontology at the University of California, Los Angeles, and Sepulveda VA Medical Center. She is a geriatrician in the Geriatric Research, Education and Clinical Center, and Chief of the Geriatric Evaluation and Management Unit at Sepulveda VA Medical Center. Her prior training included medical training at the University of Illinois School of Medicine in Chicago from 1980 to 1984, and residency in Internal Medicine at Michael Reese Medical Center, also in Chicago, from 1984 to 1987. She then held a 3-year fellowship in Geriatric Medicine at the University of Chicago from 1987 to 1990. She has been in the UCLA program and Sepulveda VA since 1990. Her current research topics include acute illness in the nursing home, the effects of nighttime sleep and medication on daytime behavior in impaired nursing home residents, and geriatric assessment. The topics of her most recent publications have been delirium, constipation in the nursing home, thyroid-function testing in the elderly, and the behavior problems of dementia. The topics of her most recent scientific abstracts have been methods to monitor mental status in the elderly, acute illness in the nursing home, and measuring mental status in the nursing home.

Luca Alverno, M.D., is Chief of Consultation/Liaison Service at the Clement Zablocki Veteran Affairs Medical Center in Milwaukee Wisconsin. He is Associate Professor of Psychiatry at the Medical College of Wisconsin and a member of the American Psychiatric Association and the American Association for Geriatric Psychiatry. His current research interests are health indicators and aggressive and hallucinatory behavior in chronically institutionalized psychiatric patients.

Ariane An, Pharm. D., was born in Saigon, Vietnam, in 1970. In 1978, her family immigrated to the United States as refugees. She attended the University of the Pacific in northern California and received a Doctor of Pharmacy degree in 1992. She is currently completing a residency in clinical geriatric pharmacy at the West Los Angeles VA Medical Center Geriatric Research, Education and Clinical Center (GRECC), after which she plans to enter a pharmacy fellowship program in infectious diseases. Her research interest is the use of antibiotics in the elderly.

Sailendra N. Basu, M.D., is Medical Director at the North Central Health Care Facilities in Wausau, Wisconsin. He has published a variety of papers in India, Europe, and the United States.

Dan R. Berlowitz, M.D., M.P.H., is currently on the staff of the Edith Nourse Rogers Memorial Veterans Hospital in Bedford, Massachusetts, and is Assistant Professor of Medicine at Boston University. Until recently, he served as Assistant Chief of Medicine for Extended Care. In this capacity, he was involved in all aspects of long-term care and maintained an active research program on the clinical epidemiology of pressure ulcers and the use of advanced directives in this setting. Specific projects included a prospective study to identify risk factors for pressure ulcer development and an analysis of the short-term outcome of pressure ulcer patients. Presently, he is the recipient of a Department of Veteran Affairs Research Associate Career Development Award through the Health Services Research and Development Field Program at Bedford. Active research interests center on quality assessment in ambulatory and long-term care settings, with one specific project using the incidence rate of pressure ulcer development as an outcome monitor of the quality of care.

Kenneth V. Brummel-Smith, M.D., is Associate Professor of Medicine and Family Medicine at Oregon Health Sciences University. He is also Program Director of the Geriatric Evaluation and Management Unit and the Geriatric Assessment Clinic at the Portland Veterans Affairs Medical Center in Portland, Oregon. He is coeditor of two textbooks in geriatrics, *Geriatric Rehabilitation* (published by Pro-Ed) and *Ambulatory Geriatric Medicine* (soon to be released by Mosby Year Book). He has written numerous chapters for other textbooks as well. Past research includes a large-scale community survey of the health care status and needs of Hispanic elderly in Los Angeles, the effect of a support group on caregivers of Alzheimer's patients, and methods for establishing the mobility status of community ambulators. His current research interests are in geriatric rehabilitation, late-life effects of postpolio and spinal chord injury, and ethics. He has served as invited reviewer for research grants and as a panelist for the National Consensus Conference on Geriatric Assessment for the National Institutes of Health. He also served on the committee to develop the first certification examination for geriatric physicians and on the Task Force in Geriatric Education for the Society of Teachers of Family Medicine. Prior to moving to Oregon, he served for 8 years as Co-Chief of the Clinical Gerontology Service at Rancho Los Amigos Medical Center in Downey, California, and as Director of the Section of Geriatrics, Department of Family Medicine at the University of Southern California School of Medicine.

Jiska Cohen-Mansfield, Ph.D., founded the Research Institute of the Hebrew Home of Greater Washington in 1984. In addition to her role as Director of the institute, she is Director of Research at the Center on Aging and Professor of Psychiatry, both at Georgetown University. She received her Ph.D. in clinical psychology from the State University of New York at Stony Brook and completed a postdoctoral fellowship at New York University Institute of Rehabilitation Medicine. She also has a master's degree in statistics from the Hebrew University in Jerusalem. She has published numerous articles on the topic of agitation in the nursing home resident and also addressed important issues for the nursing home resident such as sleep, religious beliefs, elderly persons' decisions regarding life-sustaining treatments, and stress in nursing home caregivers. She is a member of many professional organizations, including the Gerontological Society of America, the Maryland Gerontological Association, the American Society on Aging, and the American Psychological Association. She has received grants from various institutions, including the National Institute of Mental Health, the National Institute on Aging, and the National Center for Health Services Research.

Kenneth D. Cole, Ph.D., received his doctorate in clinical psychology with a specialty in life span development from the University of Southern California in 1981. He has published articles and chapters in the areas of depressive and paranoid states in later life, interdisciplinary team development and maintenance, and health care professional relationships. For 7 years, he was Director of the Interdisciplinary Team Training Program at Sepulveda VA Medical Center, and since February 1991, he has been on staff at Long Beach VA Medical Center as a health psychologist providing consultation and liaison services to rehabilitation medicine and hematology/oncology. Since 1985, he has operated a private practice specializing in adult development, particularly at midlife and late in life. He has also consulted with health care organizations on issues of team development and geropsychology.

Valerie C. Crooks, D.S.W., is Research Associate at the Anna and Harry Borun Center for Gerontological Research and the Multicampus Program of Geriatric Medicine and Gerontology at the University of California at Los Angeles. She is also Associate Clinical Professor in the School of Medicine at UCLA. Her research interests have focused on evaluating the effect of geriatric clinical and educational programs on learning in a number of health care disciplines, as well as the impact of these programs on the elderly in community, acute, and long-term care settings. Her most recent research efforts have been directed at developing and refining geriatric assessment instruments to evaluate subjective quality of life in community-dwelling elderly. Her current research is targeted at determining and developing appropriate methods of care and training in the nursing home to aid in measuring resident outcomes. Along with articles on various geriatric patient assessment measures, she has publications in the areas of geriatric mental health and multidisciplinary training strategies in geriatrics.

Bruce A. Ferrell, M.D., is Associate Director for Clinical Programs for the Geriatric Research, Education and Clinical Center (GRECC) at the Sepulveda VA Medical Center and Assistant Professor of Medicine (Geriatrics) at the UCLA School of Medicine. He is also Medical Director of the Hospital-Based Home Care program and Director of the postdoctoral Geriatric Medicine Fellowship program at the Sepulveda GRECC. After receiving his medical degree (1979) and internal medicine training (1982) from the University of Oklahoma, he pursued geriatric medicine training at the UCLA Multicampus Division of Geriatric Medicine. He is board certified in internal medicine (1983) and geriatric medicine (1988). He is a member of the Gerontological Society of America (GSA), the American Geriatrics Society (AGS), the American College of Physicians (ACP), and the American Pain Society (APS). His research interest is applied clinical research. He has conducted studies and authored a number of research articles and book chapters in the areas of geriatric pain management, pressure sores, and geriatric home care.

Steven Lloyd Ganzell, Ph.D., is a neuropsychologist on the geropsychiatry multidisciplinary treatment team at the Sepulveda Veterans Affairs Medical Center. He received his Ph.D. in clinical psychology from Brigham Young University in Salt Lake City, Utah. He completed a postdoctoral fellowship in neuropsychology at the University of California, Los Angeles, in 1989.

Catherine Gill, M.S., M.H.A., P.T., is currently Director of Education and Research for Therapy Management Innovations, Inc. She was previously Research Associate at the Rehabilitation Research and Training Center on Aging, Rancho Los Amigos Medical Center, and practiced therapy in primarily long-term care and home health settings. She received her master of science in physical therapy from the University of Southern California and a master of health care administration from the University of LaVerne. She is currently a member of the American Physical Therapy Association, American Geriatrics Society, Gerontological Society of America, and American Society on Aging and has presented on several research and clinical topics to these organizations. She has also presented numerous workshops and seminars to both professional and community groups.

Cynthia T. Henderson, M.D., M.P.H., F.A.C.N., is Chair of the Department of Geriatric Medicine and Chronic Diseases at Oak Forest Hospital, a 1,000-bed chronic disease hospital in Illinois. She also serves as Director of Nutrition Support Services and consultant in gastroenterology. She is board certified in internal medicine and gastroenterology and holds a certificate of added qualifications in geriatric medicine. She received her M.D. and a master's degree in public health from the University of Illinois and completed residency in internal medicine at Cook County Hospital. She completed fellowship training in gastroenterology and clinical nutrition at the University of Illinois.

Elizabeth H. Hoffman, O.T.R., is currently Corporate Director of Quality Improvement for Integrated Health Services, Hunt Valley, Maryland. Prior to this position, she was Rehabilitation Clinical Coordinator with Therapy Management Innovations. She has more than 20 years' experience in the area of geriatric occupation therapy. She graduated from the occupational therapy assistance program at Mount Aloysius College in Pennsylvania. She received a B.A. in human services from the College of Notre Dame of Maryland. She became licensed through the American Occupational Therapy Association Career Mobility Program. She is currently a master's degree candidate at Johns Hopkins University in administrative science.

Janet A. Howells, M.S., P.T., is Vice President for Therapy Management Innovations, Inc. In her current position, she provides overall program development and direction for the rehabilitation services of Integrated Health Services, Inc. She earned her bachelor's and master's degrees from The Ohio State University. She is a member of the American Physical Therapy Association, in which she has held many state and district offices. She has participated in several research studies and coauthored an article entitled "The Prospective Payment System: Its Realities and Opportunities," which appeared in *Clinical Management in Physical Therapy*.

Karen R. Josephson, M.P.H., is Senior Health Services Researcher for the Geriatric Research, Education and Clinical Center (GRECC) at the Sepulveda VA Medical Center. After receiving her master's degree in public health from UCLA, she continued her training in health services research and gerontology at the Sepulveda VA GRECC and participated in the first randomized trial of a geriatric assessment unit. She coordinated several large health services research projects, including an evaluation of a preventative health screening clinic, a multisite falls intervention trial, and an analysis of quality of health care for elderly persons in the United States. Her current research interests include causes and prevention of falls, exercise among frail older adults, pain management, and ageism in children's literature. She is currently co-investigator on two randomized trials: an exercise intervention for fall-prone elderly veterans and nonpharmacologic pain management for older adults. She has authored a number of research articles and book chapters, especially on the topic of falls.

Karen M. Linderborn, M.S., R.N.-C., is a research nurse at the Geriatric Research, Education and Clinical Center (GRECC), Department of Veterans Affairs Medical Center, Sepulveda, California. She received her nursing degree and a master of science in administration/gerontology from the University of Maryland School of Nursing. She is certified in gerontology through the American Nurses' Association. She is currently involved in several research projects, including an exercise intervention for frail elderly veterans and a study of nursing indicators of acute illness in the nursing home. She was published in the *Journal of Gerontological Nursing* in 1989 and is currently awaiting the publication of several articles.

Steven Lipson, M.D., M.P.H., has been the Medical Director of the Hebrew Home of Greater Washington since 1984 and a full-time member of the faculty of Georgetown University School of Medicine since 1975. A graduate of Cornell University, New York University School of Medicine, and the Johns Hopkins School of Hygiene and Public Health, Dr. Lipson is a board certified specialist in Internal Medicine and in Public Health and General Preventive Medicine. He has extensive experience in medicine, medical administration, and medical education programs, as well as community educational programs. Research experience in the last decade has focused on long-term care of the elderly, including ethical aspects of long-term care decision making, the use of physical and chemical restraints, and the impact of infections in the aging population. He is a member of many national professional organizations, including the American Geriatrics Society, the Gerontological Society of America, the Society for Epidemiologic Research, and the American Society on Aging. He has participated in research projects funded by the National Institute of Mental Health, the National Institute on Aging, and the Retirement Research Foundation.

Marcia S. Marx, Ph.D., who joined the Research Institute of the Hebrew Home of Greater Washington in June 1987, received her doctorate in experimental psychology from Tulane University in 1982. Dr. Marx has extensive experience in research involving the visual system. She worked with Dr. James May at the LSU Eye School of Medicine in New York City, where she studied visual problems in persons with glaucoma as well as in those suffering from Parkinson's disease and other dementing disorders. Since joining the Research Institute, she has developed a test for visual acuity estimation that is appropriate for all nursing home residents, regardless of their ability to communicate. Dr. Marx is a member of the Gerontological Society of America, the Association for Research in Vision and Ophthalmology, and the American Association for the Advancement of Science. She received support from a grant from the Radcliffe Morris and Marion W. Urquhart Memorial Foundation. In addition to her work in vision, Dr. Marx has participated extensively in research projects concerning the nursing home elderly and, in particular, agitation in nursing home residents. She is the principal investigator of a grant from the Alzheimer's Association to study outcome of cataract surgery in the nursing home.

M. Patrick McNees, Ph.D., serves as President of North Rim Systems. His work is directed toward translations of treatment and management protocols that have been validated in controlled (laboratory) settings into complete working systems for use in nursing homes and hospitals. He has a particular focus on incremental (continuous) quality improvement in health care settings. He was the recipient of the National Behavioral Engineering in Business Award. He has contributed numerous articles and chapters to the professional literature and currently serves on a federal grant panel for nursing research. He collaborated with Dr. John Schnelle on the development of an automated urinary incontinence management system for nursing homes and is Principal Investigator for a National Institute on Aging (SBIR Phase II) grant to test the system in nine nursing homes across the nation. He was a visiting researcher at the Mary Conrad Center (Anchorage, Alaska) during the period that Mary Conrad won the Contemporary Long-Term Care Award for Excellence. He currently is involved in nursing home projects in Alaska, Washington, and California.

James Randy Mervis, M.D., completed his psychiatric training at the State University of New York, Downstate Medical Center, in 1988. He currently is Ward Chief of the Geropsychiatry Assessment and Treatment Unit at the Sepulveda Veterans Affairs Medical Center. He has additional board qualifications in geropsychiatry. He is Assistant Clinical Professor at the UCLA School of Medicine, Department of

Psychiatry and Biobehavioral Sciences. He is currently conducting research evaluating various pharmacologic approaches to controlling agitation in patients who are demented.

Dean C. Norman, M.D., was born in New York City in 1950, but moved in 1952 with his family to California, where his father became a faculty member of the Physics Division of the UCLA School of Medicine. He later attended UCLA and graduated in 1972 with a bachelor of science degree in physics. He then entered the UCLA School of Medicine and completed his medical studies in 1976. After graduation from medical school, he entered postgraduate residency training and completed 3 years of internal medicine residency at Los Angeles County-University of Southern California Medical Center. The residency training was followed by a 2-year fellowship in infectious diseases at Harbor General-UCLA Medical Center and then a 2-year fellowship in geriatric medicine at the VA/UCLA Multicampus Program of Geriatric Medicine and Gerontology. In 1980, he joined the faculty of the West Los Angeles VA Medical Center Geriatric Research, Education and Clinical Center (GRECC) and became Assistant Professor of Medicine at UCLA. Currently, he is Clinical Director of GRECC at the West Los Angeles VA Medical Center and Associate Professor of Medicine at UCLA. He has received his boards in internal medicine and infectious diseases and special certification in geriatric medicine. His research focus has been on the pathogenesis and treatment of infections in the elderly.

Joseph G. Ouslander, M.D., is Medical Director of the Eisenberg Village campus of the Jewish Home for the Aging of Greater Los Angeles and Associate Professor of Medicine in the Multicampus Program of Geriatric Medicine and Gerontology, UCLA School of Medicine. He also serves as Director of Research and Education at the Jewish Home, Associate Director of the Borun Center for Gerontological Research, and Director of the Continence Program and Urodynamic Laboratory at Encino Hospital. His primary area of interest has been urinary incontinence in the elderly. He also has begun research on the quality of medical care in nursing homes, initially focusing on improving physician drug prescribing. He is a coauthor of *Essentials of Clinical Geriatrics* and *Medical Care in the Nursing Home.* Currently, he serves on the board of directors of the American Geriatrics Society and the California Association of Medical Directors, and has served on the Geriatric Medicine Test Committee of the American Board of Internal Medicine/American Board of Family Practice. He has lectured extensively on incontinence and nursing home care at national and international meetings, including visiting professorships in Australia, Japan, and China.

Abbas Parsa, M.D., is a faculty member of the Department of Medicine of the Medical College of Wisconsin and the Medical Service of the VA Medical Center, Milwaukee.

Laurence Z. Rubenstein, M.D., M.P.H., is Director of the Geriatric Research, Education and Clinical Center (GRECC) at the Sepulveda VA Medical Center and Associate Professor of Medicine (Geriatrics) at the UCLA School of Medicine. After receiving his M.D. in 1974 from Albert Einstein College of Medicine, he pursued further training in medicine, public health, health services research, and gerontology at Einstein and UCLA and was a UCLA Robert Wood Johnson Clinical Scholar. He is board certified in geriatric medicine (1988) as well as internal medicine (1978) and preventive medicine (1980). He has been on the UCLA geriatric medicine faculty at the Sepulveda GRECC since 1979. He is a GSA Fellow as well as a Fellow in the American Geriatrics Society and American College of Physicians. He serves on the GSA Public Policy Committee and was on the editorial board of the *Journal of Gerontology* (1983-1986). He is section editor of *JAGS* (Heath Services Research) and serves on several other editorial boards, review panels, and advisory boards. He has authored or coauthored more than 90 research articles, books, and book chapters. His primary area of research is geriatric health services, and he has conducted several major studies in the areas of geriatric assessment, long-term care, falls, and instability.

Daniel Rudman, M.D., is Professor of Medicine at the Medical College of Wisconsin and Associate Chief of Staff for Geriatrics and Extended Care at the VA Medical Center in Milwaukee.

John F. Schnelle, Ph.D., is Associate Director of the Borun Center for Gerontological Research and Professor in Residence, Multicampus Program of Geriatric Medicine and Gerontology, School of Medicine, University of California, Los Angeles. He is known for his role as principal investigator on several major clinical trial intervention grants designed to improve care and management in nursing homes and has received awards for his outstanding contributions to behavior therapy. Among his most notable contributions is his innovative work in incontinence care, comprehensively described in his newest book, *Management of Urinary Incontinence Care in the Frail Elderly* (1991). He has published extensively in the areas of quality control in institutional settings and quality of life issues in the frail elderly, with over 70 publications in professional books and journals. He currently serves on the board of editors of the *Journal of Organizational Behavior Management*.

Sandra F. Simmons, M.A., is Staff Research Associate at the Borun Center for Gerontological Research, Multicampus Program of Geriatric Medicine and Gerontology, School of Medicine, University of California, Los Angeles. Her primary focus is on management issues in long-term care, including staff management and related interventions. her most recent publications appear in the *Gerontologist* and the *International Journal of Urogynecology*, reporting research findings on restraint management and incontinence care, respectively. Recent presentations at professional meetings have concerned the effectiveness of exercise programs for frail and demented elderly. She currently serves as a consultant on a Small Business Innovative Research grant designed to disseminate incontinence management systems to nursing homes. She is a member of the Gerontological Society of America.

Fawn Takemoto, Pharm. D., was born in 1960 in Hilo on the island of Hawaii. She graduated from the University of Hawaii at Manoa with a bachelor of arts degree in biology and subsequently attended the University of Southern California, where she received a doctor of pharmacy in 1992. She is currently completing a residency in clinical geriatric pharmacy at the West Los Angeles VA Medical Center Geriatric Research, Education and Clinical Center (GRECC). After completion of residency training, she plans to continue practicing in an environment that combines research, teaching, and a health care team approach to caring for the elderly.

John F. Thompson, Pharm. D., graduated from the University of Southern California in 1973 with a Pharm. D. and did residency in clinical pharmacy at Wadsworth Veterans Administration Medical Center, Los Angeles, California. He became a USC faculty member in 1975 as Assistant Clinical Professor, teaching clinical therapeutics in geriatrics. He became Associate Professor of clinical pharmacy and clinical gerontology in 1991 and 1992, respectively. Currently, he holds the status of Fellow with the American College of Clinical Pharmacology. His research interests center on physician prescribing habits and the elderly, adverse drug reactions, and health services research.

Santiago Deleon Toledo, M.D., was born in Manila, Philippines, in 1959. After completing medical school at the State University of the Philippines, he completed a 3-year postgraduate internal medicine residency at the university-based Philippine General Hospital. In 1991, he completed 1 year of research training at the West Los Angeles VA Medical Center Geriatric Research, Education and Clinical Center (GRECC). Currently, he is enrolled in a 2-year fellowship in geriatric medicine at the VA/UCLA Multicampus Program of Geriatric Medicine and Gerontology. His research interest continues to be in the early detection and treatment of infections in nursing homes.

Perla Werner, M.A., a native of Argentina, received her bachelor's degree from the Hebrew University of Jerusalem, her master's degree from Bar Ilan University in Tel Aviv (in sociology and anthropology), and is a doctoral candidate at the University of Maryland. For 8 years she worked at the Research Department of the National Insurance Institute in Israel. Her research there focused on the evaluation and follow-up demonstration projects for the elderly, including home health care and support programs for the caregivers of disabled elderly in the community. Before joining the Research Institute of the Hebrew Home of Greater Washington, she was a research statistician at the National Institute on Aging, working on a project concerning sleep disturbances among elderly people. In December 1988, she came to the Research Institute where she has been involved in studies of agitation, sleep disturbances in nursing home residents, and other topics. Because of her expertise in data analysis (with both personal computers and mainframe computers), she is an active participant in studies at the Research Institute. Ms. Werner is a member of the Gerontological Society of America and the Southern Society of Aging. She is the recipient of a contract from the National Institute on Aging to study sleep patterns of elderly persons. She is also coprincipal investigator on grants from the Robert Wood Johnson Foundation and the American Society of Consultant Pharmacists Research and Education Foundation to study the effects of removal of physical restraints on psychotropic medication in the nursing home.

Darryl Wieland, Ph.D., is currently Senior Health Services Researcher for the Geriatric Research, Education and Clinical Center (GRECC) at the Sepulveda (California) VA Medical Center and Assistant Research Anthropologist in the Multicampus Program of Geriatric Medicine and Gerontology at the University of California, Los Angeles. He has served as Research Director of the Beverly Foundation, Pasadena, California, and Principal Investigator or Director on numerous research projects in geriatric health services, ranging from hospital-based geriatric assessment to teaching nursing homes and long-term care work force studies. He is also focusing on the implications of ethnic diversity for geriatric care. He has published in the *Journal of the American Medical Association, Social Science and Medicine,* and the *Journal of Cross-Cultural Gerontology,* among others. He was a coeditor of *Anthropology and Aging: Comprehensive Reviews* (1991).

Spencer Van B. Wilking, M.B., B.S., M.P.H., is currently Assistant Clinical Professor of Medicine in the Geriatrics Section of Boston University and Director of Medical Education at Jewish Memorial Hospital and Rehabilitation Center. He received his medical training in Great Britain with a specialty in geriatric medicine. His research interests include the management of pressure ulcers, developing a model for predictors of nursing home placement, and the epidemiology of isolated systolic hypertension in the elderly. He is Clinical Researcher at the Framingham Heart Study, where he is involved with data collection among elderly members of the original Framingham Heart Study cohort. He is actively involved in research and teaching at University Hospital and Jewish Memorial Hospital and Rehabilitation Center.

Bradley R. Williams, Pharm. D., is Associate Professor of Clinical Pharmacy and Clinical Gerontology at the University of Southern California School of Pharmacy and Andrus Gerontology Center and Clinical Pharmacist with the Geriatric Health, Education and Research Center at Rancho Los Amigos Medical Center in Downey, California. He currently is the preceptor for a clinical pharmacy clerkship in geriatrics at Rancho Los Amigos and also teaches a preclinical geriatrics course at the USC School of Pharmacy. His clinical practice includes drug therapy monitoring and management for elderly patients of the Clinical Gerontology Service at Rancho Los Amigos. His research interests focus on drug use evaluation and the appropriate use of medications by elderly patients. Topics of his recent publications include risks of NSAID-induced renal toxicity in institutionalized elderly and conducting drug use evaluation studies in long-term care facilities. He is also coeditor of *Clinical Pharmacology and Nursing.* He is completing a 3-year project investigating interventions of a clinical pharmacist to improve medication use and avoid inappropriate prescribing in residential care facilities for the elderly. This project, sponsored by the John A. Hartford Foundation, has used an educational strategy to improve physician prescribing and increase drug knowledge among staff and residents of rest homes.